Dylan and the Wolf

– A true story of a boy, The World and bio-accumulation

Saving Our Children from the World's Biggest Psychopath

Kalubriah Sage

First Published 2022
Revised Edition

Paperback: 978-1-967820-17-7
eBook: 978-1-967820-18-4
Library of Congress Control Number: 2025908300

This is a work of nonfiction.

Ordering Information:

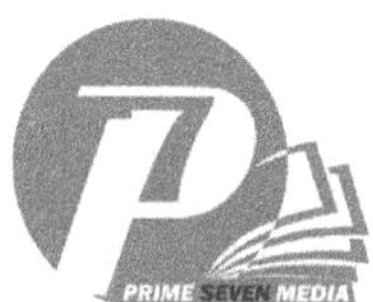

Prime Seven Media
518 Landmann St.
Tomah City, WI 54660

Printed in the United States of America

Table of Contents

Dylan and the Wolf

A story of a real boy and today's world.
Six degrees of separation,
Fractal Geometry...
Bio-Accumulation observably true,
Conscripted Medicine in full view.

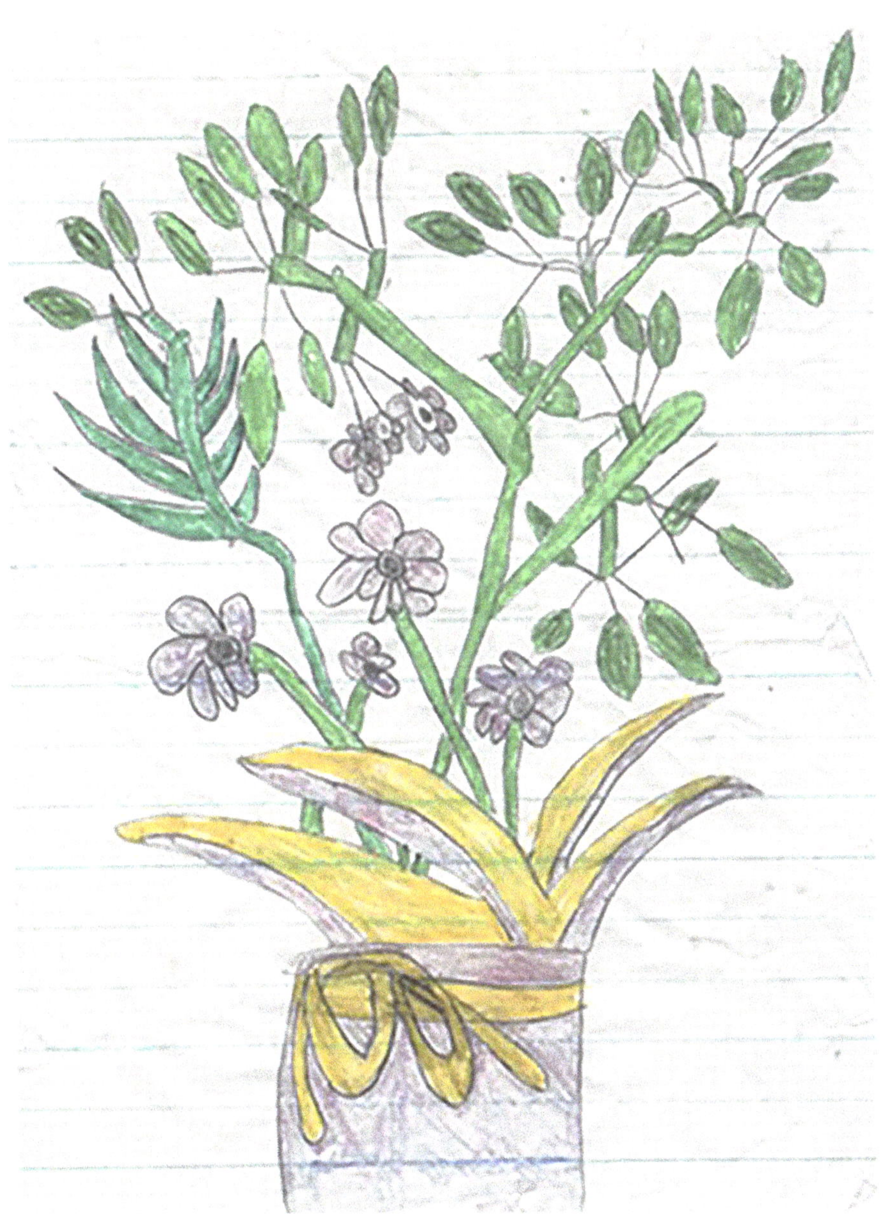

Karma of Life

If souls were racehorses,
Those with good records are weighted accordingly.
It helps alleviate backload, to carry a little extra.
Just as a strong Sherpa does. All karma is combined.
When you carry more, the load is lightened for others,
And everyone reaches the destination.
Teamwork.
As above so below.

Dedication

Thanks to my family and friends for their patience and understanding.

Thanks to my collator for his patience and dedication in collating this material into book form, and to the publishing team that so beautifully present, this ugly duckling of experience, into a beautiful swan of dignified helpfulness.

Thanks to the Heart of Humanity and the dignity of free-will and choice in personal health and living we wish for all our children's children.

What I have written is inspired by a real life experience and conclusions are not intended as exhaustive but a "perspective" for consideration.

Kalubriah S

FWD by David Suzuki

"The way we see the world shapes the way we treat it...
That is the challenge, to look at the world from a different Perspective"
– David Suzuki

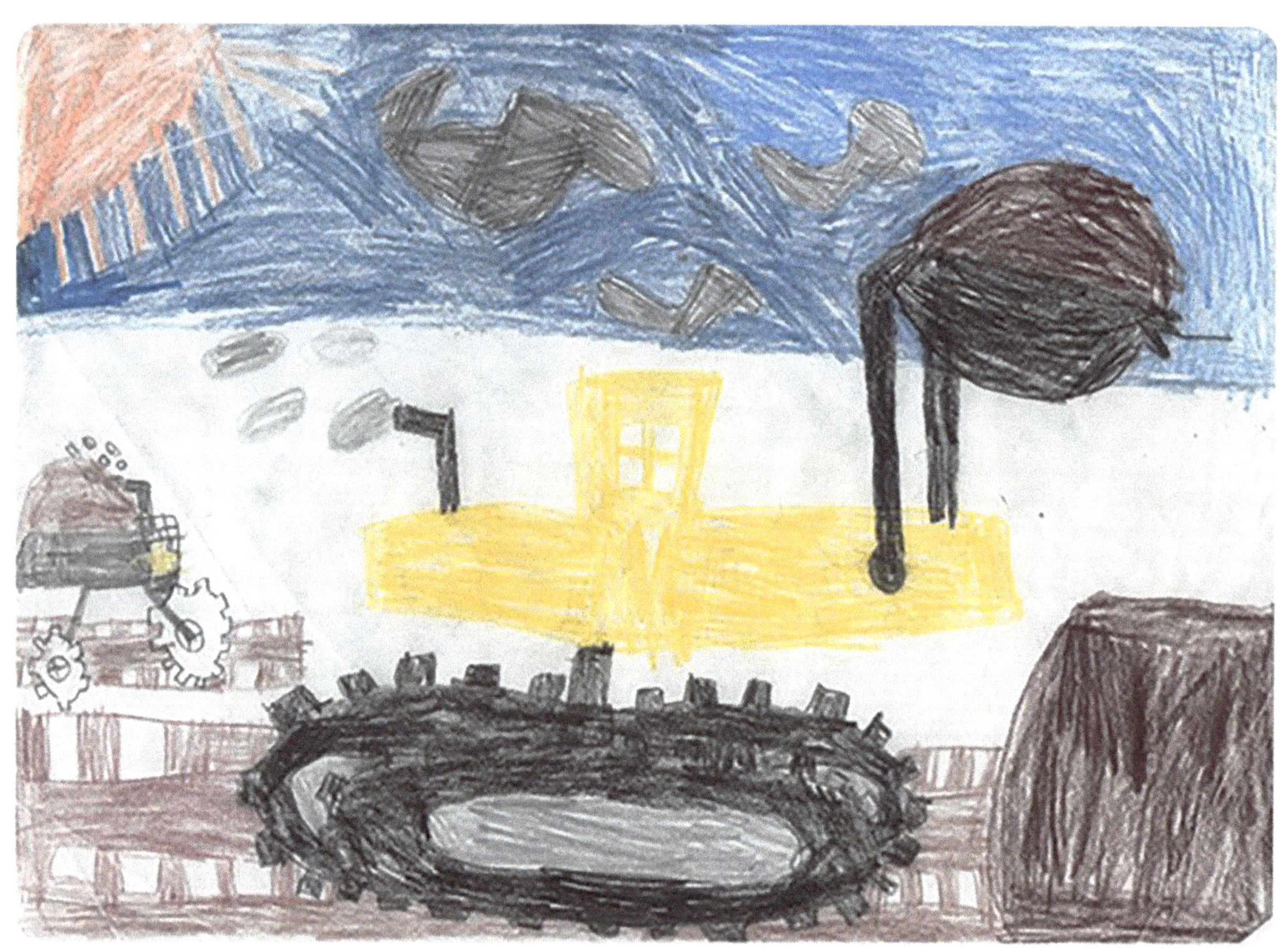

Overview

This work offers a different perspective on the shape of our biology and societal governance. A bio-accumulation story of chemical enslavement, of a boy and the world...
For their own good?

The words here are offered as a different lens through which to look and SEE potential solutions to the toxic bio-accumulation of ignorant modern living, medicine and agriculture. Far from an exhaustive exploration of a multitude of pertinent fields, this perspective aims to educate and promote lateral thinking outside the box we are told we must live within.

Supporting Truth and Choice In Medicine.

Having seen, behind the scenes, I have developed a dislike for most, so called helpful, foundations.
Many have become powerful lobby groups that influence the health of nations.
An old phrase came to mind, "The road to Hell is paved with the best intentions".
Another phrase came to combat, "If you can't beat them Join them" ...
So why not start a new foundation,

For Choice in Medicine

Use anything, 'Just Beat It', any way you can... Yes, I'm sure I could get permission to use the Jacksons' song.
To rally support to provide more choice to suffering children and others.
My son died from chemotherapy induced Leukaemia.
The result of an intensive and prolonged chemotherapy protocol 'Routinely' Forced upon the child and family.
Three years earlier, despite alternative treatments being used and seen to be effective,
Health authorities threatened legal action to force a continuation of the then 36 year old trial,
A cytotoxic protocol – The DNA damage and subsequent cancers admitted and outlined in the Pub Med fine print of each and every substance.

Known to be the most inefficient and damaging methodology of treating the disease through poisoning the whole cell cycle. Only to create more damage than first they sought to fix.

Verdict Guilty!

My child died from the effects of Forced, No-Choice medicines.
Help save our loved ones from this toxic chemical medicine “monopoly” on treatment options.
Effective Harm-Free Alternatives EXIST and are routinely SUPRESSED.
Enough is Enough, give The People the Choice in Medicine.
Stop the “routine” poisoning ‘Monopoly’ from killing our Children.

Chapter 1

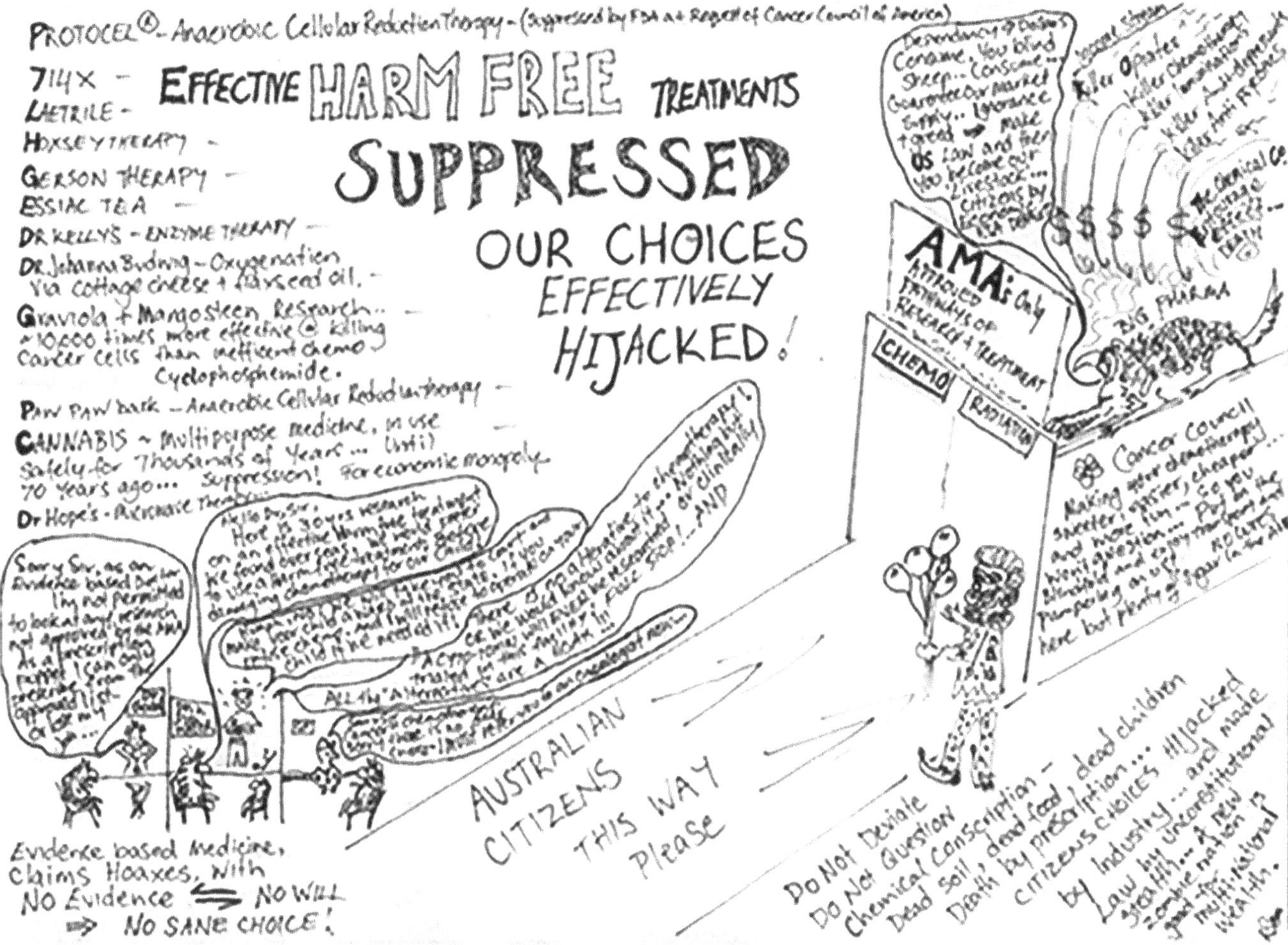

EFFECTIVE HARM FREE TREATMENTS
SUPPRESSED
OUR CHOICES
EFFECTIVELY
HIJACKED!
714X -
LAETRILE -
HOXSEY THERAPY -
GERSON THERAPY -
ESSIAC TEA -
DR KELLY'S - ENZYME THERAPY -
Gravíola + Mangosteen Research.. -
Cyclophosphemide.
Paw Paw bark - Anaerobic Cellular Reduction therapy -
CANNABIS ~ multipurpose medicine. in use
safely for Thousands of Years ... (until)
70 Years ago... Suppression! For economic monopoly.
AMA
CHEMO
RADIATION
BIG PHARMA
Cancer Council
AUSTRALIAN
CITIZENS
THIS WAY
Please
Evidence based Medicine,
Claims Hoaxes, With
No Evidence ⇆ No WILL
⇒ NO SANE CHOICE!
Do Not Deviate
Do Not Question
Chemical Conscription -
Dead soil, dead food, dead children
Death by prescription ...
citizens choices hijacked
by Industry ... and made
Law by unconstitutional
stealth... A new

C HOICE IN MEDICINE – As published in 2015. An article about my story

CHOICE IN MEDICINE –A BASIC HUMAN RIGHT – A CONSTITUTIONAL RIGHT

HIJACKED! "WAKE-UP-AUSTRALIA!"

I am one of those people who has been **forced** to accept a treatment for my child that I knew was deadly harmful.

This is HELL on Earth! UNCONSTITUTIONAL HELL.

Delivered by a Medical Priesthood that deliberately perpetuates harmful "health" modalities to fulfil multinational Trade Agreements and contracts.

Just as the Church Priesthood is being brought to Justice for the Rape of Innocents, so too the Priesthood of Medicine should be brought to account and **Forced** into the new millennium.

So Why hasn't Australia Legalized Medicinal Cannabis, asked Lucy Haslam, headline in the Sydney Morning Herald read a few weeks ago.

Europeans enjoy a wide variety of choices in the treatment of Cancer and other chronic or acute disorders.

Australians are forced into modalities that defy good health, and sensibility.

Who specifically **objected** to legalizing Medicinal Cannabis in Australia? The AMA, Oncologists Australia, and some church groups. Clearly, it is not that there is no evidence but that they want none of it.

When I publish my book, I would like a percentage of sales to go to **Research into HARM FREE ALTERNATIVES to Chemotherapy**, this is the only area of Medicine currently getting NO FUNDING. United in Compassion would be my choice at this time, as it is doing something REAL. Working with Hippocrates oath genuinely.

Many people like Lucy Haslam, lose their children to chemotherapy because of a HOAX, a deliberate ILLUSION of NO CHOICE. Those that question the system get lies and threats. I lost my son to chemotherapy due to a FORCED NO CHOICE!

It is a fact that Big Pharma targets Doctors with Billions of Dollars of incentives to prescribe each year, and that this pathway is the AMA's accepted educational pathway for all graduated Doctors in Australia. It can also be observed over time, that Doctors have been disempowered, the health system costs Australians and we have a growing health deficits of more Millions each year, and we have growing health deficits of "managed" disease that is ballooning out of control. The beneficiary is the Health Arm of our great economic vehicle, which is supporting huge profits overseas and huge health deficits in people here at home. Our current chemicalised medical system, manages disease by inundating people with products of dubious efficiency but denying choice outside the prescription zone. This represents a HOAX on wellness and our constitutional rights.

Do people of Australia put their money into the Cancer Council, or the Leukaemia Foundation or Breast Cancer Research organisations to keep chemotherapy going as our only option? NO!

If Australians knew that these organisations where 'window dressing' for industry, the **wolf in sheep's clothing**, and that their money was only ever going to be used to **prop up** chemotherapy options, or fluff out care assistance while you suffer the protocol, do you think anyone would give their money to this kind of health hoax? NO!

What if the people find out that these organisations advocate to stop, or stall, all alternative pathways other than the chemical trail their funding comes from? NO CURES EVER. If a **cure for cancer** was well known, how long would the CANCER COUNCIL be around? Hmm, and is the Cancer Council actively perpetuating its own existence by thwarting potential cures? Well, this did happen in America, and that is the model of our current path: the "American Dream" Health System. One that props up private health insurance companies and denigrates the concept of a universal health system.

Australia would be better off having a National Office of Wellness to kill off all the cancer in our health system, naturally.

It is a FACT that all Cytotoxins/Chemotherapy is **harmful to all cells**, even healthy tissue. This modality is **inefficient** by its nature as it is **non-discriminatory**, and it harms the DNA, which gives a cell the blueprint to replicate successfully. Damage the blueprint and mutations occur. These mutations are called CANCER. **Many chemotherapy drugs attest in the fine print that they will give rise to further cancers**, particularly relating to blood and bones. This is a poor health outcome for people, yes, but it creates a lot of profit from product use for multi-national pharmaceutical companies.

The AMA in Australia, USA, and NZ lobby government in order to prevent new harm-free choices in cancer medicine, in favour of the WWII Chemotherapy and Radiation technology. The Oncology Australia and AMA submission to the NSW government, considering allowing medicinal cannabis to be publicly available, was objecting on the basis of not having sufficient evidence? These are the same people that ignored the 10-year study by Linus Pauling, Nobel Prize winner, proving that 5g of intravenous vitamin C per day can cure any disease, cancer, auto immune disorder. The Church groups' submissions about Medical Cannabis appear to have forgone the Bible and are siding with the puppet-science of the AMA and Oncology Australia? What intelligent population are these doomsayers hoping to influence? Perhaps they are trusting that the "unthinking livestock mentality" will kick-in to Authority's Rule without question? NO!

Question, Question that is our only safety, our only path to discernment! People are not livestock nor should they be treated as such.

Trade Agreements that our Governments have been making for agricultural progress and medicinal progress since the 1950's and are now preventing progress, away from harmful modalities in both fields. American investment choices made in the 1950's, are still destroying our soils, food, our children's lives and immune systems. Not unlike religious controls, it is the unquestioning arrogance and a passive aggressive approach that has allowed this damaging progress to rule the masses falsely, using fear and guilt across the ages. Doctors also use a passive-aggressive technique to ensure you take their prescriptions and don't ask too many questions. The approach described is used by people, governments and industry that are threatened by change.

When faced with childhood cancer in my own family, I had already gained knowledge about chemotherapy from my mother's experience with her own sister in the 1950's, and in the 1980's working with a Cancer support group that assisted with the Mind/Body connection. I was shocked to see that the same diabolical treatment had barely progressed since the 1950's, and now cancer affected one of my children. I asked a lot of questions; I did a lot of research.

I found a treatment that had been successful in the USA since the 1970's, it even dissolved brain tumours, and was easy to deliver to a child, most importantly Protocel is HARM FREE, completely NON-TOXIC to healthy tissue. The Oncologists were not supportive of me using anything additional to the cyto-toxic protocol assist my child, even vitamin C. It is all about the ANZECC treaty with New Zealand, a (Hoax) trial, for more than 30 years, that states an 80% remission rate with chemo. Well, not actually true … for 5 years perhaps, then cancer is likely to reoccur. And **these positive statistics that are pitched to all people for all cancers, only apply to Acute Lymphoblastic Leukaemia (ALL) patients, a childhood cancer, specifically for the age group 2yrs – 3 yrs.** Older children, Adults and other cancers have no great results, except early death. Breast cancer statistics show only 1 in 6 women surviving 5 years after aggressive treatment, and yet **selenium introduced into the female diet has been researched and shown to have reduced instances of breast cancer by 90%**. Organisations are not investing in Selenium in female diets to prevent cancer, they are researching cyto-toxic chemotherapies and other invasive/ aggressive methods of treatment for Breast cancer. One pathway ends profit and improves health and wellbeing, the other/current path increases profit and resource consumption, while decreasing health and wellbeing. This is a Health and Economics No Brainer!

The Australian catch cry used to be 'COOEE'. Did you know COOEE is a Peruvian word for **Guinee pig?** Have we become a COOEE Nation for **chemical management of our population's life cycle**, birth to death?

It became clear, the more questions I asked the more upset and conflicted the Oncologists became. I brought swathes of research to groups of oncologists for debate. What it came down to was that they all agreed that the current modality was inefficient and harmful, but they were by law, 'not allowed' to look at anything else until the AMA said they could. These Oncologists conditioned by the Medical Priesthood from university to graduation and beyond, are fearful of looking outside the Doctrine that has been handed down. Some thought they would lose their jobs even to question the status quo, which none of them did. Oncologists have such FINE profession to uphold and yet they are not permitted to think outside the square? Free thinkers may be more effective in treating disease but are a threat to the economic status quo of Pharmaceutical Profits.

This **surreptitious 'control drama'** is affecting people's health and rights. It brings **blind** respect for medicine into **healthy question**.

When Medicine is about protecting product lines and protocols and not people's health and choices, something is wrong! The Australian Doctor, Professor Barry Marshall, Nobel Prize Laureate, admits that it took many years to get the medical establishment to acknowledge his finding of the bacterial cause of ulcers. Why? Existing products and market protection.

The same can be said for Vitamin C, another Australian, Professor Linus Pauling, Nobel Prize Winner, spent 10 years studying the effects of Vitamin C on disease, and concluded that doses of 5g intravenous vitamin C could cure any human cancer or auto-immune disease...Ignored by the Oncology profession and AMA.

Therefore **Supporting Medicinal Cannabis will ensure people of Australia have greater choice in their health care**, because for the first time, a natural curative is getting huge public support and has broken through the barrier. Medical Overlords are unable to shut down our collective voices now.

Australian people may not be aware, there exists a **blacklist** that is adhered to by most Public Media outlets. This Blacklist ensures that no damaging Stories/Articles about "Cancer" (or other control sensitive topics) ever get published or broadcast in "Mainstream Media" without a positive chemo /radiation angle attached. This is the reason **no-one has heard of alternatives to treat cancer**, or the health benefits of Raw Milk versus 'bowel damaging' Pasteurization, or the links with Wheat/Gluten Allergies and 'routine' spraying of systemic herbicides to get even crop harvest. etc. ...until the internet, and/or international travel educates.

In 2006 I communicated with a member of the 4Corners team at the height of my plight for 'choice' to save my son. One day I got a call from the Journalist, saying someone higher up had pulled the story, and the explanation was, the **"Blacklist"**. The gentleman apologised, said it was out of his hands; too hot to handle...

Very frightening, I was faced with no choice, legal avenues are costly and no media opportunity to gain support. Alone in the crowd, I went underground, as any caring motivated parent would.

I watched with interest as Ray Martin attempted to assist Australians with the Dr Hope Microwave treatment, which did not get TGA approval in Australia despite Ray Martins best efforts at bringing to light the thousands of patients that were made well by Dr Hope's treatment. Having had personal contact with this good Doctor in the past, I wanted to know why Dr Hope's treatment had not made it through the TGA approval process. I was informed; A Researcher puts in the application for approval, states what the treatment is, what the treatment works for and what the treatment does not work for. Apparently the TGA's authorized testing body only tested Dr Hope's treatment on the specific cancers that the researcher stated were **not treatable**, and **none** of the cancers that the microwave treatment was supposed to be effective for...**Why is it so?** More cigarette science? Multi-Nationals already run our health system. Their profits equal our health costs, which is an escalating percentage of the average income in Australia.

The Following describes an accepted path of official suppression in America, channels of fake testing in the National Cancer Institute, and the refusal to approve by the FDA as a result of HOAX testing. All to thwart the acceptance of 'Cancell 'now '**Protocel**', a cellular reduction therapy that is effective on auto-immune cells and cancer cells, is harm free and non-toxic.

The National Cancer Institute (NCI) in America took the researchers recommendations and instead of trialling the treatment for a minimum of 21 days on cancers other than Leukaemia, they chose to test the treatment for 8 days on **only** leukemic mice. The researcher queried results when the testing was again thwarted/misrepresented from the **NCI** again two years later. The researcher found that the National Cancer Institute of America, had lied about testing to avoid further studies, and The FDA took out an injunction against the distribution of Cancell/Protocel/Entelev at request of the **A**merican **M**edical **A**ssociation who uses the **FDA** as an enforcement arm. It was found that the National Cancer Institute had broken the law to prevent this treatment ever reaching the public domain. **Tanya Harter Pierce, MA, and MFCC covers the topic of alternative cancer treatments and their suppression in her book 'Outsmart your cancer' Alternative Non-Toxic Treatments That Work.**

Think about it... Where will the Cancer Council get money from, when Plants like Cannabis and others, are proven to rectify the condition of cancer with harm-free ease? Big Pharma cannot patent plants and **understanding the "Entourage" effect**, a natural synergy, **makes void synthetic copies**, and gives scientific understanding to synthetic ineffectiveness.

No one chooses chemotherapy, or radiation, it is "recommended" by trusted health professionals that **know no better**. Doctors today are indoctrinated, not educated **how to think**, but **what to think**, both are required, but not in isolation. Unfortunately, it is the nature of our time that economic forces will manipulate and secure their markets in this ever-changing world. **Some "products" have been made law, without anyone agreeing**. A politician was paid $600,000 to get the bill through, to make sure big pharma has a clear Launchpad of multiple **questionable immune system products** to the **unquestioning public.** It is law now, putting foreign animal proteins and mercury poisoning into our children's blood supply. There is Hijacked health in a jiffy.

No more' relatively easy to manage' childhood diseases, now we have new healthcare industries around **chemically managed** Autism spectrum, auto-immune disorders, and cancers, lots and lots of cancers. Great for business, bad for family health and happiness! This is **the progression witnessed and noted by one of Americas leading Paediatricians. Dr Robert Mendelsohn MD** writes extensively on the flaws and effects of chemicalised and mechanized modern health practices that harm more than heal. His books include 'Confessions of a Medical Heretic', and 'How to keep your child healthy in spite of your Doctor'.

In the world of consumerism, gluttony, sanity out of balance, people have become livestock and are only acceptable if they are enslaved into earning and/or consuming more and more products.

You are the market economy in our current system; Big Pharma spends Billions of dollars on incentives for wooing Doctors, Administrators and Politicians right here in Australia in order to **sidestep your personal discernment**. How well can you influence your doctor? **The AMA approved path of Doctor's research, Post University, is let Big Pharma have "Free Trade" upon our overworked Doctors and Administrators of Health systems.**

How do exhausted Doctors who do back-to-back 14-hour shifts, defend their intellect against big money marketing mastery? They cannot. A mad Health system indeed.

Australia's Health system has been hijacked by funding agreements with Big Pharma, and thus **'Disease' is 'Managed' by the 'Prescription for Profit'**. Promising potential cures or harm free treatment options do not get a voice, as there are no ears to listen. This market is perpetuated by illness and dependency. WELLNESS = less profit.

Here is a comforting quote from one of our most trusted health professionals (whose real name shall not be used) in 2006, to reassure all those who may wish to choose their own family's curative options in the future. These are the words that were spoken to myself and my husband when I requested that **"Protocel "**, given its demonstrated e**ffectiveness and 'Nil Toxicity'**, be clinically trialled in a new "clinical trial facility" at a Major Australian Hospital. **Dr Dishwater said "No". I asked "Why?" Dr Dishwater said "Never!" Feeling stonewalled, I asked, "So what you're telling me, Dr Dishwater, is that the only things you will ever allow to be clinically trialled in this new 'clinical trial facility' is 'cyto-toxins'?" Dr Dishwater said, "Yes, that's right."** So, what I was being told is that no alternative to chemotherapy would **EVER** be trialled, **nor would alternative research be pursued**. THIS IS A TRUE STORY. Dr Dishwater spent quality time informing us that **all treatments other than Cyto-toxic Chemotherapy were HOAXES**, yes all, and his evidence was that there was no Evidence!!! Dr Dishwater was passionate about telling me and my husband lies with no evidence, he verbally discredited Dr Hope as a Dr that was immoral for not "treating everyone", my reply was that Dr Hopes Microwave treatment was only appropriate for specific cancers, and that it was honest and discerning of Dr Hope to advise someone if he did not think the treatment would be effective on their particular disease. Dr Dishwater, with arms folded tightly over his chest, "Humphed" so much he sounded like a camel.

Excuse me for losing faith in a corrupt chemical health system, my child was about to enter the Nazi Chemo Chamber of Death and there was nothing I could do about it, except leave the country, if I had money... That same Doctor stated, that if my husband and I refused to submit our child to the CHEMO PROTOCOL, court action would ensue with our child being made a ward of the state. At the end of our conversation, **Dr Dishwater's last jab was, that he would also refuse to do a bone marrow transplant** on our child should one ever be required, if we refused the chemotherapy protocol. **Psychopaths with funding agreements/ties to big Pharma run our children's hospitals and Cancer Clinics. An ignorant plebiscite** attached to this '**chemical trial protocol**' and 'blood transfusions', has removed our **constitutional rights** to choose our family/children's health options. Choosing to be non-medicated or chemical free, had come to an end, without even a public vote? **Unconstitutional!**

People are humans, regardless of qualifications, 'PROFESSIONS OF POWER' are known to have a higher percentage of psychopaths, due to their nature and the structure of organisations. The Church is a classic example, of the damage done to innocents by hidden power abuse that is managed at the TOP, for the purpose of controlling the lower echelons. The same thing can be observed to have occurred in our health system and is harming our health, and our children's' health.

Expose the threads of influence and remove the health damage and financial cost of supporting this overblown, dependency product, un-health economy.

Hidden Treasure (Dr William Lyman and Dr Steven Kaali leading AIDS researchers of the Albert Einstein School of Medicine in New York 1990, micro amperes of electricity used to clean blood of bacteria and viruses including AIDS, 14 device patents and a few newspaper clippings are the only existing evidence that discovery was ever made). Based on sound basic physics and it works simply and efficiently without harming healthy human cells. Drs Lyman and Kaali discovered that healthy human cells have 100,000 times the ability to withstand electrical charge than any bacteria or virus (*One of these patents: 5188738 Dr Kaali. Feb 23 1993. Invention made to attenuate any virus, bacteria, parasites, fungus or disease. Electrode arrays implanted into arm. See more on page 187*). The discovery was briefly seen on the science show, Beyond 2000, during the Aids scare and was touted as a new way to clean blood in blood banks without harming the healthy cells. All of this was cleverly swept away when Bill Clinton announced a 2-billion-dollar boost to Big Pharma to develop pharmaceutical products to **"manage"** Aids. No money in cures, so much that the word "cure" has be made illegal to use in relation to any health issue or product.

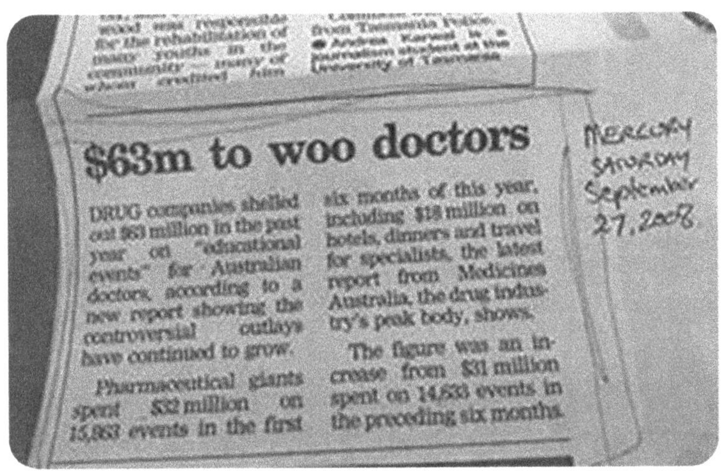

$63m to woo doctors

DRUG companies shelled out $63 million in the past year on "educational events" for Australian doctors, according to a new report showing the controversial outlays have continued to grow.

Pharmaceutical giants spent $32 million on 15,863 events in the first six months of this year, including $18 million on hotels, dinners and travel for specialists, the latest report from Medicines Australia, the drug industry's peak body, shows.

The figure was an increase from $31 million spent on 14,633 events in the preceding six months.

Mercury Saturday September 27, 2008

See full article in Appendix page 308

As reported in an Australian newspaper in September 2008 'Pharmaceutical companies spent $63 million in the 07/08 financial year on "educational events" for Australian Doctors, and these controversial outlays continue to grow. These pharmaceutical giants spent $32 million on 15,863 events in the first six months of 2008, including $18 million on hotels, dinners and travel for specialists, according to the latest report from Medicines Australia, the drug industry's peak body. The figure was an increase from $31 million spent on 14,633 events in the preceding six months. These giant economic players spend millions supporting our universities and controlling curriculum, and once doctors enter the world of service, these same companies ply doctors with their money into junkets to continue a highly controlled ongoing education that focuses exclusively on new pharmaceutical product information.

Doctors of our modern world are no longer allowed to undertake "Real Doctoring", they are no longer allowed to be any more than prescriptive puppets for pharmaceuticals. To this end doctors are actively discouraged from thinking for themselves, all diagnostics are outsourced, and if they question the highly regulated prescriptive bible system, if they prescribe diet for any disease, or mineral therapy they are harassed and threatened with removal of their license. Disempowering Doctors that care and disempowering our health and choices. Our health system empowers greater cost and disease in our nation. A controlling psychopathic Health System for a Zombie Worker Nation? **Sack the AMA** and **elect** fresh representatives that have **no financial ties to Pharmaceutical companies**.

In The Denver Post – 14 April 2014 - Apr 14, 2014 - Pharmaceutical companies wooed academic leaders, ghost-wrote articles. It was just one part of the massive effort by the pharmaceutical industry to drive sales of Pharmaceutical companies in 2008 alone spent nearly $800 million on sales. J&J hired a marketing firm to ghost-write articles attributed to…?

https://www.minnpost.com/.../pharma-companies-spend-millions-wooing...
(See Appendix page 308 for full article)

Jan 9, 2015 - Pharma companies spend millions wooing doctors to prescribe 'me-too' drugs ... As a new investigative article from ProPublica reporters Charles Ornstein ... to doctors typically are not cures or even big medical breakthroughs.

Following the Script: How Drug Reps make friends
By A Fugh-Berman - 2007 - Cited by 147 - Related articles

Apr 24, 2007 - This is an open-access article distributed under the terms of the Creative. In 2000, pharmaceutical companies spent more than 15.7 billion. The average sales force expenditure for pharmaceutical companies is $875 million annually [3]. With reprints from the medical literature and wooed as teachers.

www.wsj.com/articles/as-doctors-lose-clout-drug-firms-redirect-the-sales-...
Sep 24, 2014 - At Big Hospital Systems, Salespeople Woo Administrators to Get on 'Formulary'. Pharmaceutical. companies are refining their sales strategy. Getting a drug on the formulary at a

big hospital system can mean potentially millions of dollars. Today's key-account managers can spend many months trying to...?

The TGA has already shut down of all alternative health/healing clinics in Australia that use to help people overcome cancer, and now the control of labelling of all-natural products to affirm no health benefit. This is Big Pharma's war on Nature, due to industry not being able to profit.

Codex is the name given to a conglomerate of Big Agro Chemical companies and Big Pharma combined. They influence our politicians, trade officials and TGA in relation to trade agreements, and have brought in regulations that affect our food medicine and agriculture, through the side door of trade agreements. Our constitution was written to protect the people from false overlords, and thus, plebiscites are written for the economic benefit of our nation, but the downfall of our soil health, food health, our people's health and our choices. *(See Article, page 233)*

So often you hear Doctors say, "there is no evidence" to some natural remedy or alternative research. So, who decides what gets researched? The same people who pay for the research, pharmaceutical companies; and governments are taking advice from Pharmaceutical companies.

- Crematorium workers are getting cancer from breathing in the chemicals of chemo funeral pyres.
- Hormones cannot be removed from our environment or water ways.
- Medical product runoff is polluting our air and waterways.
- Health is one of the biggest areas of personal and government expenditure, yet little of the consumables or pharmaceutical products are made in Australia.
- The Health industry in Australia is a drain on our financial economy, our people economy and our personal health economy, like flushing money, people and future choices down the toilet.
- It offers no cures, expects you to spend your life on drugs and to give over your trust and personal decision making to a chemical company prescription platform? Not Australian, but a scourge from US multinationals.

Bring forth a tax on products, made for medical or health use, that cause dependence and/or harm to our bodies or the environment/air/water.

- Demand that chemical addictions are treated by the hospital system and that the company related to the product addiction funds the patient care and recovery, particularly if addiction is related to injury where prescription drugs of addiction were prescribed. Thus, taking addiction off our streets and out of our homes, if posing a threat, and making the product originator pay remediation cost to the family.

- Tax Incentives can change the economic platform and commercial will, if people demand products that are quality, tax away obsolescence, making room for quality that lasts and less landfill. The same applies to harmful medical products that create more disease and dependency.
- Demand that our Constitution protect our rights to health choices once again. I do not want to trust my health matters to a prescription puppet.
- That Doctors and Farmers are better educated for discernment acknowledging that pharmaceutical companies, agricultural chemical companies and poisons manufacturers are all owned by the same groups of people. Contaminating our environment, food and medicine is a conflict of interest to our human health, environmental health and our children's future.

Support Harm Free Health, its research and Medicinal Marijuana for our children's health and our health choice freedoms.

Lucy Haslam lost her son to chemotherapy because of an **illusion** of 'NO Choice'. I lost my son to chemotherapy due to law of **force, based on the illusion of, 'No Choice'!**

As with Nazi Fabian Socialism, the wolf in sheep's clothing. The sign above the gate of one famous German death camp reads: "Work your way to freedom" This **LIE** was written by a German chemist, Hitler's friend who discovered Fluoride harmed a part of the hippocampus and intended the substance to invisibly influence the German people. **The Lie on the gate was created to ensure the human livestock moved through facility without resistance**. We live with the same lie in our system, the same substance is used in our water supplies to enhance blind consumerism, and disease, the **drone** media does the rest.

Whole populations medicated without choice or permission? For our good or industry profits? All the evidence about fluoride concludes that there is no benefit to teeth, only harm. Fluoride in soil 'frees up/makes available', calcium for plants. In our bodies fluoride strips calcium making it available to the toilet. Look at the actual studies that can be found on the internet. This waste product of aluminium from phosphate production is routinely put into Australian water supplies, and is damaging to human brains, hearts, immune system and teeth, the scientific studies have been done many years ago, and Europe, Japan, Canada and many other countries refuse to pollute/medicate their water supplies based on this evidence that has been hidden from American and Australian populations.

Most people want to be law abiding citizens and do the right thing, it is easy to be sheep-like, until something occurs that forces one to question the way things are done.

When one does question, one finds that geniuses such as Linus Pauling (Vitamin C), Gaston Nasseans (714X), Jim Sherridan (Protocel), Dr Joanna Budwig (Essential Fatty Acids, Dr Hope (microwave) and many others have produced effective treatments for many of humanities worst health conditions and these treatments are being ignored by mainstream medicine. That is when we see the system is failing our health and wellbeing, in order to support inefficient, dependency driven treatments and economies.

A more intimate view...

Dylan

Chemotherapy products are so toxic that gloves must be worn for a nappy change and

Siblings cannot share a bath...

At age 2, before chemotherapy, Dylan was a vibrant dynamo of a child.

He was doing quite well at the 'reading master' program and was the sort of child who remembered the names of people, children and pets, and who lived where, as we drove around our community.

His wit was as sharp as any adult, and he seemed to laugh, really getting adult jokes and humour in any family style media we watched.

He had to go back into nappies when chemo began, and his short-term memory was never the same again.

At age 7 Dylan was tested by the local university to see why such a bright and intelligent lad, was having trouble with basic reading and writing. The results showed he performed at the level of a 14-year-old, in all areas except short term memory and reading/ writing exercises.

The testing showed that the intensive chemotherapy he had at ages 2,3, 4 and 5 had damaged his brain and central nervous system permanently.

That past treatment also damaged Dylan's DNA, which is what all the small print PUB MED documentation say. Dylan's T-Cells, a vital component of a healthy immune system and response, we were soon to learn were also damaged to a fault.

Very proudly and with personal determination, Dylan did learn to read and write a little better with one-on-one assistance from his distance education teacher, just weeks before we lost his poetry in life forever, aged 8.

In the months prior to Christmas 2009, Dylan had been to what we thought was his last hospital check-up ever. He was given a clean slate of health, it had been two years since remission was declared and statistically, we were told he should be fine… to grow old with the rest of us. Usually if 18 months remission has been maintained, the all clear is given.

So, what happened? Chickenpox went through his primary school just before Christmas, my husband and I separated by agreement also at that time.

In the new year of 2010, I felt free of an unsupportive partnership, I had good employment, the children seemed happy with life and school holiday activities…

Upon reflection, I have learned that environment is everything, and stress, while invisible creates inflammation in the body. Stress of illness, change, dietary, relationships, it all adds up. Alpha and Omega, association and empathy, children mirror naturally.

Just prior to Dylan's second Acute Lymphoblastic Leukaemia sufferance, he had participated in a summer camp run by Camp Quality. He loved these camps and usually had a great time. However, his new camp buddy, made an independent, unusual decision to take Dylan with him while accompanying another child to the local major hospital. Not protocol. During his visit, Dylan made friends with a child with cancer in the ward they visited, and was later told at camp that the child had died… Such was his news to me, as he spoke of his experiences on the way home. I looked at him seriously, lovingly, saying "Know how lucky you are!"

I felt outraged that my child, a sensitive empath, was taken to this place of pain and memory, for him, a cellular memory!

So instead of a happy child, Dylan was sad and empathized deeply. What a terrible Camp Quality experience to take away?!

I have often wondered if his empathy that week affected his health as a trigger.

Depression of the Portal Valve?

So, I picked him up on Monday, on Tuesday he was running around the yard with neighbourhood kids and having a great time, bare chested, fit looking. I noticed a rash on his ribcage and treated it as one would a scratch or allergy. Each day it seemed a little bigger. On the Saturday, after trying a few things to get the rash to leave, I took Dylan into the Hospital Emergency for them to see.

I was not prepared for the news. They took me to a small room, sat me down and said....

"I'm really sorry, but Dylan has Leukaemia again." My mind and time stood still. A whirring of what? How? Why? All running their own programmes... The Oncologist said, "The odds are like winning first division Tatts-Lotto two weeks running." But with none of the joy... just horror...

I only picked him up from camp on Monday, and now they were telling me I had 4 hours to pack some belongings and be on the Angel flight to Melbourne.

His T-Cell count was dangerously high, and emergency responses were initiated.

In Melbourne, Dylan did not achieve remission with the renewed round of intensive chemo drugs and was given a less than 5% chance with a bone marrow transplant.

Only one sibling was tested for compatibility, and years later it was discovered his half-sister to my first husband, had a match in blood group, a rare blood group that could have provided life-saving donations...Unfortunately, the doctors did not think her to be close enough genetically, as half-sister? So, she was never tested. So, with the not so good news, we recommenced with the Entelev Supplement, stayed positive and made a focus on quality of life, with palliative options at a later date...if ever.

Dylan's health and cell count seemed to improve remarkably up until May 2010. He had his birthday, and we went on a Make-a-Wish trip to the Queensland theme parks. Here we learned of the mistake in choosing an external 'Port', a device implanted, to take bloods and deliver chemo, directly over the heart.

The internal port Dylan had the first time, was restricted to delivery, and cannulas were placed for bloods. Our decision was intended to reduce his pain; however, the externalized 'port' was open to infection... So here we were in and out of wet and wild, and hotel swimming pools. I was fearfully attentive to cleanliness, but this was out of control. The theme park turned out to be heaven for the children and hell for myself, attending with my 'asset focused' ex-husband. I was facing the loss of my home as well as my middle child.

The last theme park day at Wet n Wild was exciting and exhausting, and that evening, Dylan looked tired and had an unexpected neutropenic event, presenting with pinprick bleeding. Life again went into overdrive...

We rushed to the Gold Coast Hospital, only to spend hours in emergency where I had to educate staff about the functioning and access of the 'port' and Hep-lock procedures… Wow!

This being the hospital that all the Make-a Wish children go to if there is a problem, I had assumed staff would be aware of the technology and treatment protocols? A terrifying time…

Once on a ward, it was close to 2 weeks before he was stabilized sufficiently to fly home. Blessings to all the amazing staff.

Poor little man, Dylan hated to be restricted physically, he was such an active boy we referred to him as Crazy Horse, being born in the year of the horse, and Dylan had an incredibly special relationship with our family horse of 18 years. He was very happy to get back on a plane and return to our home state, however, devastation struck when we arrived and he had to go straight back to hospital for a further 10 days, missing out on the limousine ride home, as was arranged by Make-a Wish. He suffered and endured, but depression was a real thing when restrictions apply to living, running, being outside. Outside hospital he was a different boy, alive, engaged, and joyful. Athletic, competitive and creative.

A day that sticks in my mind, beautifully, a few weeks before… It was after Easter, Dylan wanted to attend the local school cross country event. And he did. Looking normal, healthy and strong as any of his classmates. He ran second all the way but was pipped at the post by one of his best mates, so Dylan ran third over-all. The look of determination in the photos is priceless.

That day, he looked invincible to me…

Now June and we were driving home from the hospital, and out of the quiet, Dylan asked me if he had been in hospital for chicken pox/shingles, for which he was also being treated?

I wish I had lied, or changed the subject, instead, I laughed at his innocence and said "No mate, the Leukaemia came back, and that is what you have been staying in hospital for". "Don't worry my love, we'll beat it again." "You're going to be ok". I sounded strong, determined, but inside something felt wrong, like I should not have told him. Sometimes ignorance is bliss. Particularly, for the very young and very old, sensitives.

He was quiet for a while after that, contemplative. Unfortunately, his health deteriorated rapidly from that day. Just like he got tired of it all…In May, before the Make-a-wish trip, everyone was excited. Dylan was looking like achieving remission on Entelev. However, after he learned the truth of his condition at the end of June, his cell counts worsened. Dr John said he had suddenly produced four different populations of Leukaemic T-Cells and this was not good.

July was the month nightmares are made of. I begged the oncologists to use intravenous Vitamin C – they refused saying there was none on the premises…?

Dylan had a nosebleed, while at his dad's place, that started at midnight and remained untreated. It was 8am by the time I took delivery of my limp boy and raced to the hospital an hour away. He had lost so much blood and was drifting in and out of consciousness upon our arrival. Choking on giant blood clots that just seemed to keep coming… The hospital staff managed to stabilize his bleed in an hour or so and four bins full of blood-soaked cloth later. It took 4 days of HB (haemoglobin) transfusions to bring his count back into balance. It was the 10th of July. Dylan was noticeably weaker after losing so much blood, and the donation products, are routinely 'radiated /irradiated', making them un-alive/ toxic, if you need a lot of transfusions.

Studies conclude radiation/irradiation destroy healthful vitamins and minerals in vegetable foods, so why would radiated/irradiated blood products not show similar correlation?

The Doctors Kaali and Lyman blood electrification technology may have been more beneficial in cleaning national supply blood products, that are to go into sick people, without harming cells and adding, unnecessary radiation.

It was later in 2011 that I discovered Mr Smith's story done by 60 Minutes New Zealand in 2009. The story focused on the effects of Vitamin C, in high doses, saving a man's life from swine flu and Leukaemia… And how the Auckland Hospital reacted! I remembered my own request for Intravenous vitamin C in Dylan's final weeks, and now I felt outraged, knowing the hospital I had attended with my son, had strong and clear links with the hospital Mr Smith attended in Auckland New Zealand… I refer to the ANZECC Study that controls the treatment of Leukaemia and cancers in Children… That get funding from lobby groups and fur fey foundations.

Intravenous Vitamin C, beneficial right down to the electron exchange, could have saved my sons life… But rules of oncology would not permit the use of harm free vitamin C.

I wish I had known about Liposomal Vitamin C at that time.

The spirit of my son visited me a couple of years later, "Don't worry mum" he said, "It's not your fault, the system is rigged."

The bubble with its strength of Pi and perfect form,
Is as fragile as a newborn,
Perfect as a rose.
Its fragility, like the life of our children…
Surface tension, once broken, the bubble
Once shining proud against the sky… Pop!
Now invisible to the eye.

It's gone… No longer,
Its shell of light reflecting pearl-essence
Preserving the integrity of the physical form.

The building blocks of healthy life do not come from corporate conglomerates, but
From the gardens of the world…
To Protect Life in perfect form, do not pollute nor poison.

July 28. After a fantastic fishing trip in the bay with family and friends, where they caught more than thirty Flathead, Dylan woke up with a headache.

We had a lovely evening prior, he and his mates had built a fire in the fire pit and were playing around, they all loved toasted marshmallows, but Dylan seemed quiet and tired. He just wanted to sit close with me by the fire, and later we did some work on a jigsaw puzzle inside, while all the other children played outside.

This day was to be the birthday party day of his best mate and neighbour. Dylan was not usually one to complain about pain, but this morning he was complaining of pain in his head. I had been given morphine to deliver, and in my haste, I gave him too little to have any effect. His pain worsened and I decided to take him to the hospital, where they rigged up a morphine pump. Staff insisted he remain in hospital until dosage was stabilized, 24 hours they said. The headache was a potential bleed.

The extreme nosebleed Dylan had two weeks earlier had weakened him physically.

I stayed with him, holding him through the night, praying for miracles that everything would be alright.

He complained in the night that the headache was intense, and morphine seemed to just dull senses but not the pain.

At 5am on July the 29th, his little body lying next to me jerked and he could no longer talk.

I kept talking to him and found that he could hear and answer me with squeezing of my hand in his...

One for Yes and Two for No... Grandparents, his father and siblings, uncles, aunties and cousins came in to give him love and support.

I begged for him to be transported home without further delay, and thankfully a few hours later, hospital staff made it happen.

I sat kissing him and holding him in the ambulance, he looked like not making it home, but he did.

After arriving home, the ambos set Dylan up in the lounge room on his mattress on the floor, and the family again gathered around him... It was only 10 minutes later that he gasped aggressively and was gone... I know he was pleased to have made it home.

It ruined his mate's birthday. Our family lost its man in the middle.

We spent the night in the lounge-room with Dylan's body, watching a movie he had picked out called 'Nine9'... It was like he was still there with us but happy and free.

I have a lot of love for all the hospital staff that attended Dylan. He was a shining personality. More than 100 people, young and old, friends, medical staff, family turned up to his funeral. Anyone would have thought it a celebrity funeral. Dylan was a Star for us.

I sought to make his last public appearance a moment that focused on being a tribute to his short but powerful life and sparkling personality. A slideshow and video were shown, the crowd laughed and cried.

It was comic relief that showed his character perfectly. Many people came up to me at the end and said it was the best funeral they ever went to, and shockingly it was for a child. That is my Dylan, Humour right to the end...

If his story, our story, brings greater understanding and less suffering to other children, like him, he would be proud of that. The suffering of these children need not be so toxic, extreme nor tragic.

I cannot bring my son back nor ease his past sufferings but perhaps I can assist through his story, to bring back choice in medicine and ease the need of future sufferings of children and adults.

Make choice sacrosanct. May that be Dylan's legacy.

Freedom of choice, that more children survive illness and endure less cyto-toxic inefficient conscription of the World's Biggest Psychopath, 'medical division'.

Dylan was only here for a short time, but he provided me an education that no university could…

A degree in 'how the system is rigged'… with honours.

Many details remain unsaid, as I feel it counterproductive to transfer my experiences of pain to others, too much, but rather to stick to the purpose of 'Understanding' the pathways of a deliberately unsupportive system.

I have a lot of love for the hospital staff that cared for my son, however, I have lost respect for their idea of "unquestionable" toxic, inefficient medicine. They are paid to do a job, and discouraged from questioning, themselves. They follow the rules, of a flawed and toxic system that fears free choice, or the methodology would be debunked.

On the foundation of foundations, is it enough to encourage donations to find cures and then spend the money on patient transport to chemotherapy that can never be a cure, always it remains a 'study'…of inefficient cyto-toxins on children and now everyone, supporting zero progress away from WW2 chemicals, controls and protocols? This is the HOAX that the status-quo hope the mass diversionary therapy will keep hidden away.

But while adults still have legal choice, children are doomed to false laws and forced toxic protocols that produce high mortality rates, within 5 years.

'Environment is everything' and in an environment of economic product protectionism, medicine cannot be trusted to support wellness.

I spent many years prior to this time in government jobs, not unlike 'Yes Minister'. The result of this illness experience is that I have learned that not all is equal, and the World's Biggest Psychopath (WBP) is not only active in government's outsourcing power and lobby group manipulations, not only in agriculture and trade agreements, promoting harmful chemicals as efficacies… but the WBP is active in medicine as well, and has been for some time… lurking in a toxic eddy of the medicinal stream's 'management of disease division'.

When threats and fear are employed to mainstream consumer compliance, Ethics has long since flown, out the proverbial window.

Cigarette science maintains economies and comfort with lies. Science, once noble questioning of the nature of reality, now shackled as a prostitute to the pimp of mainstream corporate realty.

I look forward to the day where sympathetic resonance vibrations are used mainstream to smash leukemic cancer cells. The 11th Harmonic is now known, two frequencies applied between 100,000 Hz and 300,000Hz have been shown to shatter unhealthy cells like in Leukaemia while healthy cells are undamaged.

The day when Vitamin C is the first line in defence and repair, as a harm free alternative in cancer recovery, or cannabis oil which is more efficient by 100,000 times than chemotherapy in killing cancer cells of many types without harming healthy tissue. This would be a better investment in health than current protocols.

So much research is routinely hidden if it is found to be competing with grandfather business profits, doctors, researchers thrown to the wall to maintain the status quo. Do not believe me, do your own research.

Just one year after Dylan left this world, I discovered that the Worlds Annual Endocannabinoid Conference had been running for six years... Why is it that none of our Doctors or Oncologists were aware of these healthful discussions and discoveries surrounding Cannabis? Why is there a push for synthetic substitutes when the "Entourage" effect has been found true?

(Entourage effect concludes that the whole plant/herb is of greater benefit than any single part in isolation)

Questions

- Can an intelligent population that are sold on the globally interconnected information and economics, suddenly be told to ignore international senior scientists, immunologists and The Centre for Disease Control (CDC) "whistleblowers" regarding the risks of the multitude of inoculation products forced upon the population today?
- Were not, the injunctions "not to speak" laid by product manufacturers and government investors? And Why?
- Is it not a clear conflict of interest for any Minister of Public Office, to be calling for 100% vaccination, which directly supports his/her personal investments?
- Did not, Dr. William Thompson Senior CDC Scientist and whistleblower, drop many thousands of documents on USA Congress – in full public view in 2016 – confirming an internationally agreed fraud and cover-up regarding Vaccination Risks? YES!

- Did the Australian Media report on this? NO!
- Is the CDC whistleblower, Dr Judy Mikovits video interview of November 2015 vimeo, worth a look at as it is now proven TRUE? De-engineering genetics, she explains, brings consequences of existing natural suppressions being undone.
- Should Doctors and Citizens beware, the contracts for product take-up that bind civilian choice, and be educated of the risks and contraindications?
- Is it right that the next generations genetics are maimed by toxic overload and blind trust? No.

Faulty "chemical insurance" of immune modulation is a risk, my family genetics cannot take. Having been through the rigors of childhood cancer twice already... Acute Lymphoblastic Leukaemia, now in epidemic proportions comparatively since the 1970's. Such disease is linked with one of these products, and confirmed by the CDC, themselves.

- Are not the first 8 sections of the Australian Constitution said to give freedom of choice to citizens as to what substances go into theirs and their children's bodies? Yes.
- Is this a government that supports the first 8 sections of the constitution? Or
- Ignore the first 8 covering civil rights and adopt, just the 9th section that gives power, to dominate and subvert civil rights to cooperate contracts and fake, lobby-group/corporate laws?

Hmm, the Judges are out to lunch? Swearing allegiances to the corporations rather that The Peoples Constitution?

- Has not the CDC already published a quiet admission (copied from their website before it was removed) that 93 Million Americans have been infected with a 'Green Simian monkey virus, SV40' from contaminated polio vaccines? YES. This Virus manifests as various blood cancers in people and in particular Acute Lymphoblastic Leukaemia, which now affect Millions of young children.

Hmm looks like Mr. Turnbull got on the Clinton Investment bandwagon, too late, and fatefully now can watch the tower of trust, falling.... Falling.

- Should not Doctor Education be influenced by more than just the economic product peddlers of the day?
- Perhaps a read of Ph.D. Viera Scheibner's book 'Vaccination 100 years of orthodox research shows that vaccines represent a medical assault upon the immune system' published in 1993.?

- Should not, 'Choice' be allowed for liability purposes and scientific 'controls'?
- Will Assault on the immune system be litigated, by future generations? Thalidomide babies come to mind, from a so-called harmless nausea medicine, blind trust, many innocents were maimed?
- Is it not every Australian Citizens right under the constitution to be able to say "NO Thanks" to any 'product' regardless of WHO peddles it? Yes.

Trust is blown in my family line, having years of hospitalization and study behind me…Living is more than believing.

- Should expertise be ignored? Leading immunologist and ex CDC researcher, Dr Judy Mikovits states in her interview that babies, pregnant women, teenagers and the elderly are already 'immune suppressed/compromised' and these groups should avoid the immune modulating products, as these are the groups most at risk from toxin injury and 'cytokine storms' that vaccinations produce.
- Is it acceptable to have such products, now multitudinous as conscripted/compulsory to whole populations? Or
- Should family, knowing their own, have choice in these products that are classified, 'non-medical'?

Be careful with Future Genetics.

The Proverb arises; 'One often meets his destiny on the road he takes to avoid it'.

The truth of this can be observed over time, that many things that start as 'good intent', end up Bent.

The efforts of any industry or government to hide a truth, erodes trust, forever… As

Truth is always revealed, eventually…

As examples: Banking deregulation, mining, electricity power brokers, forestry/chip industry, the party system of government… All were introduced as a Savior for the future that backfired or ripped off the future generations. Sold Out resources, and civil rights for profits overseas…

- Has anything changed, or is this pattern of overt control via trade deals continuing?
- Vaccines are 'chemical insurance products', where risks should be fully disclosed and above all, civil choice respected and honoured, beyond the economic drone of the day. Is this Happening?

- Dr Fiona Wood's safe, non-toxic, spray on skin will not be available for 25 years or more I was told by the Head of Oncology, but vaccines are developed and marketed within weeks. Not medicine, so no regulations as such upon vaccination products. No trials lasting years, as expected with cannabis or spray on skin? Why?
- Are they using whole population trials on an unwitting public.? Yes.

Sold just as an insurance product, they predate upon FEAR and rely upon Total Trust of the Consumer, with little known, if any benefit... Until something goes wrong... Big business does what it does... Cover Up... Media Blackout... Dollar speaks in hundreds and thousands of silent, ignorant choices – They profit, keeping it that way.

- The protocol for dealing with unwanted Truth teller's is, First Ignore, if it cannot be ignored, discredit, if it cannot be discredited, destroy it.... Or so a State newspaper Chief Editor once told me... There is a formula for every control imaginable. Should we take careful note of everything said by a Whistleblower? As a miner watches his Canary for danger.
- Weigh it up... Your genetics or Their Profits?

Big P.S - Since writing this piece, 2018 legal actions in America against manufacturers of these immune modulating products saw $3 Billion US dollars paid out for victims of "Iatrogenic Injury" directly attributable to these products. Then legally termed, "unavoidably unsafe".

My last questions...

- Was this news, of the previous point, reported upon and broadcast in Australia? NO. And Why not?
- Is it to prevent litigation and choice of citizens being swayed?
- Is it ETHICAL to NOT report on this FACT and other CDC whistleblower admissions?
- What role should the AMA play in having a public voice to influence a population other than Doctors? Did the AMA do anything to alert the public or doctors to this clear admission of Fraud by the CDC, who gives them directives?
- Are the AMA ethical in influence? Have they been peer reviewed, or do they review themselves? Have they made Doctoring more ignorant and less efficient, by the directives of dependence on information they control? Look only at sanctioned information or be deregistered as a health professional...very unscientific.
- Do the AMA actively discourage research outside the favored existing pathways? Western Australian Dr Hope could not get anyone to take over his successful microwave treatment, reported on by Ray Martin in 60 minutes. Why are the AMA involved in controlling

people's choice in medicine? Look at cannabis, the AMA wish to ignore and discredit any research, done anywhere? And no mention of cannabis as a Cancer treatment is permitted? Conspiracy Fact. Follow the money trail. Beware the Wolf you feed.

- Should pre-existing media/government agreements regarding 'blacklist' topics, adhered to by media be abolished and reviewed in favour of Truth?
- How is it so that beneficial research and new health technologies are routinely hidden from public view and practical use is prevented?
- How is it that a control drama economy takes precedence over public wellness?
- How is it that families must deal with entrapment" within closed system medical fields as well as manage the conditions of a terminal disease in the modern world?

I rest my questions in your capable awareness.

Constitutionally speaking, Choice in any medical or associated products should be Personal and Private, not a matter for States or Big business to hold unethical, profitable, sway upon innocent peoples.

Have a good day.

Chapter 2

In modern medicine's management of disease, every intervention necessitates further interventions. Biology operates on open systems, not a closed loop. In open system modalities, healing of the body occurs, with less intervention and intrusion.

Why Not?

Why not present the people with a new solution of greater choice?
A new protocol for Cancer Trials including Childhood Cancer Trials,
Specifically modelled to cater to multiple modalities and
Alternatives, to the more damaging current protocols,
Which should be the Last resort.
Instead;
Using Vitamin C, Cannabis Oil, Gastro Nassene's 714X, and
Entelev/Protocel, found to be especially effective on those inoperable brain tumors,
Dissolving and lysing the tumor away without harm to healthy cells.
Ojibway Indian Tea/ESSIAC, Paw, Mangosteen and Graviola among others...
This would create a boom in research and diversity in understanding.
This would create a new respect and freedom in medicine, for researchers and patients Choice.
The current system is likened to a passive aggressive Nazi entrenchment, that has poor results and
Refuses questioning.
Good people work their asses off to help, but are prevented from doing anything but
Placating the system, of psychopathic population statistical protocols from World War Two.
A wise man once said, "One man's medicine is another man's poison", this is
True in a world of diverse genetics.
The current system of forced protocols and population statistics,
Ignores this diversity and dignity of choice.

Lobby groups, lies and farcical foundations.

As a parent and citizen who has endured the rigors and protocols of childhood Leukaemia twice, I would like to ask Australian citizens to 'think twice' about supporting foundations and lobby groups of Lies...

They perpetuate their own existence by ensuring, there will be no
Publicly available Cures!
I have witnessed the influence of the Cancer Council and Leukaemia Foundation...
Follow the money trail...
These black holes of public money and support, for which I have lost all respect.
Clowns and sugar coated diversionary entertainment, covering for a plethora of economic lies,
All the while, our children and loved ones die.
End the Foundations of Death, to let the real Cures publicly circulate.
Follow the money trail, to discover that
Diversionary entertainment and patient transport to chemo, does not count as a 'CURE' and
Never Will!
Let us have – 'The Purple Heart' for choice in treatments and protocols...
Follow the money trail...
Cures end the need for LF or CC... Get the picture? It's Real!
When you shave off the emotional sycophantry LF truth is as thin as the razor they use.
Keep your hair on and turn out the Light on LF, instead
Wear a Purple Heart for freedom of choice in medicine.

Children are harmed each day by compulsory chemotherapy and compulsory immune modulation products. While Big Pharma spends Billions of dollars in Doctor education on product and simultaneously Billions of dollars on the Prevention of Natural or Herbal competition... 714X, Protocel/Entelev, Cannabis Oil, Iodine and Vitamin C... to list a few, known to cure cancer and auto-immune diseases.

A perspective - A recipe from which bakery?

So, everyone agrees that the Banking industry was/is corrupted and needs an overhaul, and guess what?

Both the Banking system and modern medicine system were set up and funded by the same elite family companies... So perhaps Banking and Medicine industries have been tarred with the same brush? YES.

Beware the 'Products' forced upon the collective. Rothschild's efficiencies are often public disasters, they bank on it.

Did anyone in Australia report on Dr William Thompson's expose in US Congress 2016, of International Fraud and cover-up regarding vaccination danger findings?

NO, the Aussie media is so controlled by gag agreements and now so Americanised...

Aussie pollys are suckers for U.S investment and have kept up with the Jones's, Nixon's and Bush's, at the Public's expense… In defence, in banking, in medicine, in compulsory agricultural poisoning and toxic water management…

Sold out to big industry in the name of efficiencies, has left the Aussie Battler with naught but natural disasters to manage.

So much for the Eureka Star and Australian Constitution, a complacent, entertained and kept ignorant, Australia, 'Sold Out' from underneath…

Like taking candy from children, but with trade deals.

Children forgive and forget if you give them water of neuro toxin contaminate fluoride, sugar and entertainment…

A couple of generations later, look, Foreigners, Foundations and Lobby Groups, run the country- for a profit that is always in arrears… while their feeding on fear is so profitable.

Next time you attend a World's Greatest Shave, or Light the Night, wear a Purple Heart and give 'voice' to Choice in Medicine.

Harm free choices are REAL – see "Outsmart Your Cancer" by Tanya Harter Pierce.

It will not cost 'civility' anything to support Choice in Medicine.

Too many are dying from Toxic Therapies of 'No Choice', and the 'LIE', that, "that is all there is"!

Any perceived Cure or threat/rival to chemotherapy, also threatens the existence of the

Leukaemia Foundation and the Cancer Council…

Who are sellers of 'Products' that are dependent on Cancer maintaining its status as being an 'incurable'?

Wear a Purple Heart to end the FARCE...

Call in the Auditors on Fake Foundations.

That which arises, so too must pass away, such as

The great corporations/foundations that hold

Too much sway.

Time to make LF, CC disappear and Make Cancer History

By 'Allowing' citizens and Doctors the use of Therapies that Heal, more than harm.

Note: NA Defender Doctors for Choice, may like to check out the suppressed studies around

GCMaf. A Natural human enzyme that heals brain damage, fully reversing Parkinson's, Alzheimer's and Autism… Worth investigation? Studies were shut down, mysteriously and violently, possibly due to GCMaf's effect on politician owned big pharma profits in the USA. 15 natural health doctors in the USA, who were documenting the healthful effects of GCMaf, on Parkinson, Alzheimer's and Autism patients, mysteriously died all within a few months of the European manufacture plant being closed. Was this for the public good?!

An excellent read, the book 'Pawns in the Game'. Telling of the Agreement in 1776 and Rothschild's Plan for global domination… Population control via disease and starvation, control of youth via abuse, sex and drugs… Hmm plan seems to be in place.

And too, the never publicly shown in USA documentary video "Conspiracy of Silence" telling of illuminati and media agreements/controls…

And note that not one word of the CDC fraud admission viewed publicly in the USA Congress was mentioned in Australia… Agreements in train… The gravy train.

But this is our children, and future genetics they are poisoning?!

So, the Media is not your friend, unless you are selling something…

The whistleblowers are your environmental canary, listen up...

They are silencing the birds, and your family's DNA may need to hear their words.

100 years since our young men lost their lives in the great Con of Gallipoli, fighting against Tyranny…

A time when most men were honest and sane, Sovereign and True Blue…

When Steiner predicted the multitude of new diseases that would offend Man as a result of de-mineralisation from chemicalisation of our soils and food supply...

Australia is young, malleable but no longer sovereign and free, sucked into a psychopathic chemicalised economy.

A subtle generational vehicle," The Law of Graduation", saw it **sold to us as Progress in Medicine and Competitiveness in Agriculture**, we allowed powerful, slick and persuasive Multi-National chemical companies to move in, on the promise of economic boon and delivery from colonialism.

They were given power in our educational institutes, regulatory institutes and service institutes, our governing institutes. These chemical conglomerates, control much of our food and medicine industries systemically and directly, overtly and covertly.

Before our soil profiles and food profiles were destroyed by chemicalisation,

Before our children's immune systems were destroyed by chemicalisation,

Before sugar addiction motivated big business and made the western world insane, and acid with disease,

Before Multi-National Big Agro and Big Pharma owned our Institutes,

our servants and our children's futures,

Before our children's opposable thumbs, and brains were hijacked by anti-human life/anti-sensory technology...

Life was simply more sustaining on all levels.
We rejoiced in creativity, and had time for family.
Cancer was rare, as was insanity, only war and famine a threat to humanity.
Now the threat is the daily grind, the enslavement of all your money and
All your time,
The children, sick and unhappy, mother too stressed,
Extended family has died and elderly, not valued, are sent to be opiated.
Divided we fall... And within this sick structure...Isolated are we all.!

Dependency on this fake economic overlay has eroded our skills, our joy and our sovereignty.
Would a person give away their legs and the joy of jumping for the convenience of wheels?
And yet convenience is the reason we have to blame...

Let our constitution shine again,
Let not a Multi-National interest have any rights above our own to grow our food and cook our food within the home.
The right to choose harm-free medicines like cannabis or vitamin C over harmful chemotherapy.

Our constitution was created to prevent FALSE OVERLORDS, whether they be of religious or commercial nature. Lawyer and Doctor politicians with powerful lobby groups behind them, on both sides of politics, have been instrumental in creating False laws by stealth to undermine your constitutional right to choose, health products, and soon, basics like; your right to grow and cook your own food.

The right to choose to buy Natural medicines, herbs and even Vitamin C over the counter is under threat. Labelling laws have changed already in Australia and all Natural and/or Harm free treatments, relating to cancer, previously sold by non-Pharma natural health outlets and/or cancer clinics, have been removed from sale across the country, swiftly and without a public vote.

Products like Entelev/Protocel, the harm free, great brain tumor dissolver and cancer killer, have not been outlawed due to zero toxicity, but points of sale have been shut down permanently, so to speak.

The 'underground' wellness movement, is the only place to move beyond the, "management" of disease (to death), to wellness and cancer free life. Pity the Doctor that discovers his own enslavement into a system of systemic disease and death management, that fly's in the face of Hippocrates oath. One such person, Dr Peter Baratosy M.B, B.S, wrote the book titled "There is always an alternative" published in 1995.

I may just be one person, one voice of the hidden many, that have shared in the enlightening and terrible experiences that formed these insights and consistent with many others that have walked this path.

Let the veil of illusion fall away from the mega-industries that are killing diversity and hijacking our health, our choices and sovereignty, in the psychopathic pursuit of profit via overt and/or subtle control.

Diversity is essential to the balance of life, in nature and in human evolution within nature.

Imagine giving away thousands of years of evolution of cooking, the spices, the flavours, the different textures and varieties of recipes developed so there would be no waste...the diversity of many cultures... to the convenience of letting a multi-national corporation cook your food? McDonalds, or other chemically enhanced, sugar enriched, starchy, zero nutrient food product.

A couple of generations of such consumers are showing the world that this multi-national chemicalised food and agriculture regime does not grow healthy cells, healthy bodies nor high intelligence. It promotes disease, dependency and skill loss in less than 2 generations.

Is this a smart governance strategy for our genetics? Or just a good economic regime to handball good governance to multi nationals and avoid responsibility for agricultural and health management unless it pertains to a large trade deal with another multi-national... McDonalds is the food provider in a Melbourne Children's Hospital!?

Must be about money not diet!. Is that 'Die' with a T?

"Small is Beautiful", is probably the most intelligent economics book ever written and common sense dictates that, things in moderation are not offensive to mind, body or spirt.

The first sign above the temple of Delphi reads – "Know thyself", the second reads – "Nothing in Excess".

Sir John Maynard Keynes famous quotes: "Capitalism is the astounding belief that the most wickedest of men will do the most wickedest of things for the greatest good of everyone."

"The difficulty lies not so much in developing new ideas as in escaping from old ones." ...

"The decadent international but individualistic capitalism in the hands of which we found ourselves after the war is not a success. It is not intelligent. It is not beautiful. It is not just. It is not virtuous. And it doesn't deliver the goods."

And

"The social object of skilled investment should be to defeat the dark forces of time and ignorance which envelope our future." Sir John Maynard Keynes was the British delegate to witness the inception of the new global economic model, and he was unimpressed. In fact, it could be seen as 'the Bretton-Woods Curse'.

Read more at: http://www.brainyquote.com/quotes/quotes/j/johnmaynar152044.html

Australia, the land milk and honey or the land of a thousand foundations, but no choice in health care.

I am a 7th generation Australian, from free settler stock, an educated bunch with a love of this country and good hearts. As an honest law abiding and generous citizen, I expected to have choice regarding all areas of health care for myself and my children. It is written into our constitution, right? Well now that false laws that the public did not vote upon have overwritten our constitutional rights, you are considered criminal if you decide to choose an alternative, something other than the inefficient outmoded chemotherapy protocols or radiation in the treatment of cancer, or refuse the poorly trialed inoculations, immunity bombardments, foisted upon all families without proper consideration.

It is all about selling products and protecting market share. If you can manage to get your products supported by government, you have a captive market, for wrong or right.

I was forced against my free will to allow my child to be subjected to highly toxic, DNA damaging agents, in the name of the ANZEC Study Protocol, which is an agreement between Aus, NZ and Big Pharma USA.

Only in Australia, Britain, Canada, NZ and the USA is no choice given to people wishing to choose alternatives to the harmful WWII modalities currently used on people with cancer.

Why, because it was the American Industrialists that set up the Global Economic platform through a war bribe at the Bretton Woods conference in 1944. The USA contingent at that conference held Great Britain to ransom, they would provide ships if the British delegate would ratify the American model for our Global Economy. The rest is history. It is very interesting to read the comments of John Maynard Keynes, British Genius mathematician, at the Bretton Woods conference, as he clearly explains the outcome of the American model was descriptive of the next 70 years of history, big business raping poor countries of resource, creating conflict and war to perpetuate economic gain, world starvation and disease, widening gap between rich and poor, and the expediential indebtedness of the poor countries would doom them to enslavement of rich countries. The American contingent then agreed to add safety measures like the World Health Organisation, which has become just another vehicle of diabolical chemical control and marketplace for Big Pharma, Giant Agro chemical businesses.

The Birth of this economic model in the 1940s, I choose to call the World's Biggest Psychopath, and since that time it has infiltrated everyone's lives, rich consumers or poor consumers alike.

Like a wolf in sheep's clothing, it stealth's its way into our world by playing on our comforts and desires, for growth and pleasure. An easy task in the 1950's when people all over the world were tired of war and were hungry for progress and change out of pain and difficulties of the depression and war years. Women were employed and targeted in this first stage. Who works harder than a woman, who cares, who wants the best for her husband and children...Women are suckers for comfort and convenience, as their backs were breaking, who could blame them?

I am not against progress or technology, what has gone on is Excess, and slick psychological marketing that renders most people "undiscerning" because an addiction has occurred, and that produces lack of sovereignty, and there, is easy prey for any psychopath. Like giving lollies to children, to hop in a vehicle they have no idea where it is going but they are enjoying the lollies and plush upholstery. Well, the car has just pulled up and the driver is a psychopath, and its desire is you get no choice, just consume and become dependent, so that the Psychopath can do what it likes, and you won't complain...because you're an addict.

Fractal geometry, where you can look in at the small, and it is the same pattern as the macro, large picture pattern... This is a snapshot of modern western life...and soon with the de-humanising technology, the neural pathways of our children and their enslaved opposable thumbs will be the new generation of consumer prey. The world's biggest psychopath is all about dependency and enslavement. .. Of our land and agriculture, our food and water supply, our education, our health care and aging, free will is only an option if there is a codex approved product on the shelf.

I would prefer my children to have the rights of our constitution, to be free to choose who they want to be, to eat bio-dynamically farmed food, to use harm free medicines, and be natural if they wish it. Our constitution was set up to protect the peoples of Australia against false overlords. Specifically, the King James Bible was used as a reference point for the past persecution of Protestants by Catholics of the day, crimes against the Great Spirit's humanity then surely equaled the madness and slaughter going on in the Middle-East at any time in the past 30 years.

However, our constitution and our personal choices about how we live and what remedies we take has been hijacked by plebiscites that have given "industry" corporate rights over the people's choice.

A classic example of Wolf in sheep's clothing, is the Compulsory Immunisation Register. This is Compulsory chemicalisation of an entire population. Immunisations are made by multinational Chemical companies, and one of these companies was convicted in Poland by International Courts of attempting to start a pandemic of bird flu N1H1 in 6 eastern bloc countries 2004. Convicted, proven guilty of sending live virus to these countries with poor health conditions and poor economies. No oil but good black soil...?

The Varcerella vaccine is on the Australian Register, and yet its chief researcher published papers after 25 years of research stating that not only was this vaccine not effective at reducing complications from adult form of chickenpox known as shingles, but the vaccine receivers over this period had greater complications than if they had not had the Varcerella vaccine.

The Meningococcal vaccine on the register, was brought on with in a fortnight of an outbreak of Meningococcal amongst teenagers in Tasmania, Australia. The vaccine was un-trialed and for a different strain of Meningococcal, the vaccine would not have assisted any of the teenagers that died from that outbreak.?

The massive evidence coming out on the Gardasil vaccine, and its dangers, begs the question as to how these heavy metal/foreign protein immune modulating agents get on to the Compulsory register so quickly in Australia? Are we truly the 'Cooee' nation, a testing ground of Guinee pigs for Big Pharma interests?

Why I would not even question it if I had not seen so much damage from blind acceptance of chemical products, because your doctors are more manipulated than educated by the medical Vatican, AMA.

My son came down with Leukaemia just a few weeks after a catchup immunization protocol, the offending product being, according to research of independent others was the Polio Vaccine. My GP mentioned at the visit in question that the previous batch of the Polio vaccine had been recalled as faulty, even though my son had it, he would have to have another...

Here is what Dr Robert Mendelsohn, MD writes; that we appear through the use of immunisation products, containing heavy metals and foreign proteins, we are swapping manageable childhood diseases for a new set of diseases, like epidemic proportions of Autism, Cancer and Auto-immune diseases, for which there are not cures, nor ease in management.

Dr Viera Scheibner Ph.D. wrote the book: Vaccination 100 years of Orthodox Research shows that Vaccines Represent a Medical Assault on the Immune System.

Or the book by Dr Judy Wilyman – Vaccination Australia's loss of health freedom. Critical analysis of government's actions.

Headlines: Court Awards $137,500 After 8 Vaccines Kills Infant, Peyton Leigh Krause-Blocker, in just 12 hours. "The medical experts found the evidence that proved the DTaP, Hib, Hepatitis B, PCV, IPV and Rotavirus vaccines were the cause of her death in 2008. Compensation was paid through the National Vaccine Injury Compensation Program (NVICP).

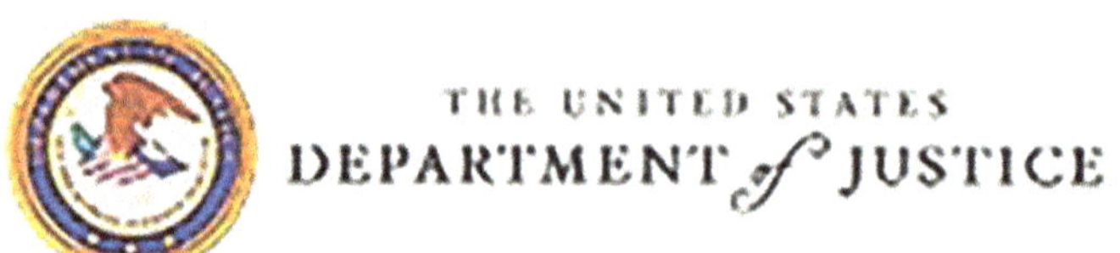

Home » Office of Public Affairs » News

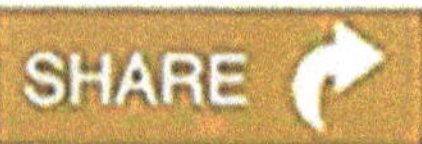

JUSTICE NEWS

Department of Justice

Office of Public Affairs

FOR IMMEDIATE RELEASE Wednesday, September 2, 2009

Justice Department Announces Largest Health Care Fraud Settlement in Its History

Pfizer to Pay $2.3 Billion for Fraudulent Marketing

WASHINGTON – American pharmaceutical giant Pfizer Inc. and its subsidiary Pharmacia & Upjohn Company Inc. (hereinafter together "Pfizer") have agreed to pay $2.3 billion, the largest health care fraud settlement in the history of the Department of Justice, to resolve criminal and civil liability arising from the illegal promotion of certain pharmaceutical products, the Justice Department announced today.

"PEOPLE ARE LETTING CONVICTED CRIMINALS INJECT THEM WITH DANGEROUS EXPERIMENTAL PRODUCTS. (The following list was circulated by The Concerned Lawyers Network, together with the U.S. Justice Department 2009 picture of notice, above)

Pfizer Lawsuit 2012 – Pesticide ViolationPfizer Lawsuit 2005 – Environmental Violation
Pfizer Lawsuit 2009 – Health ViolationPfizer Lawsuit 2004 – Environmental Violation

Pfizer Lawsuit 2012 – Health ViolationPfizer Lawsuit 2002 – Safety Violation
Pfizer Lawsuit 2006 – Environmental ViolationPfizer Lawsuit 2010 – Environmental Violation
Pfizer Lawsuit 2009 – Unapproved Promotion Of Medical Products
Pfizer Lawsuit 2016 – False ClaimsPfizer Lawsuit 2004 – Drug Safety Violation
Pfizer Lawsuit 2008 –Product Safety Violation
Pfizer Lawsuit 2009 – Kickbacks And Bribery
Pfizer Lawsuit 2013 – Safety Related Offences
Pfizer Lawsuit 2008 – Unapproved Promotion Of Medical Products
Pfizer Lawsuit 2012 – Medical Equipment Safety Violation
Pfizer Lawsuit 2018 – False Claims / Kickbacks And Bribery
Full List: Pfizer Violation Tracker"

Online you can watch lectures of medically educated people like Dr Suzanne Humphries, who uses the research of our very own Linus Pauling, Nobel Prize Winner, relating to Vitamin C and its use in curing any cancer or auto immune disease.

The 60 Minutes NZ story of Mr Smith, admitted to Auckland Hospital in 2009 with Swine Flu and Leukaemia, on life support, his family arranged Vitamin C intravenously. Mr. Smith recovered so well that the Hospital Dr took him off the Vit c, and he relapsed. His family administered Liposomal Vitamin C orally, and Mr. Smith made a full recovery in his 60s. The Drs at the hospital according to the film footage of the family on the internet, wanted to switch off life support, and were hostile at the use of Vitamin C, especially after recovery was achieved. Alarm bells people.

I wish my Oncologist had been sincere enough to offer my son intravenous vitamin C. Apparently if it is requested the standard response is there is none available. Now products are made that put the Vitamin C inside a fat lipid, which is quickly assimilated, as efficient as intravenous delivery, and does not attach to water molecules in the gut, causing diarrhea.

Big Pharma hates anything it cannot make money out of…Nature. Graviola and Mangosteen have been studied in relation to cancer, and both were found to be 10,000 times more effective at killing cancer cells than the Very Toxic and common chemo drug, Cyclophosphamide, this drug has many nasty side effects and will give you cancer again…

Our Choice is our only Sovereignty, and it is the World's Biggest Psychopaths only economic supply. All the media, advertising, propaganda, is all about controlling your choices, and not for your benefit, but the benefit of a Psychopathic Economy that is playing the field.

If Fear is used, question it. If Guilt is used, question it.

Someone else is benefiting if either of those passive aggressive power plays is in action.

If a foundation is set up, and it is all about comfort, transport, sugar coatings and clowns, you bet it is supporting the status quo. No Cures Allowed! Foundations are the bluff that allow people to think they are helping with their millions of generous dollars, but the modalities of treatment have not changed, choice has not improved, in fact if you ever enquire about something other than Chemo through the Cancer Council or Leukaemia Foundation you will be met with ridicule and excuses as to why you should not think about doing anything different, just do as the Dr says. The foundations have no answers, their researchers are only paid to look at Cyto-toxic research, they pedal patients to and fro and they window dress the industry with sugar and all things nice.. It is fake. Especially disgusting when you discover like I did that it was in fact the Cancer Council of America that actively prevents competition to chemotherapy, by requesting competitive cures are thwarted through the FDA in America, and like the TGA they complied.

I am going to share with you the shocking truth of how one treatment, that saved my son's life the first time he got cancer, has been suppressed from the public domain, and you will see that the same thwarting pattern has been applied to an Australian Researcher and Cancer Cure champion Dr Hope and his Microwave treatment.

Also, worth discussion is the organisation Codex Aluminataris/Alimentarius, and World Trade Organisation, which from 1995 started peddling toxic chemicals banned by the western world to third world nations, like china, and the consumers of the west were poisoned through trade agreements. Free Trade Agreements allow for restriction and regulation outside Australian law, not voted on by our people, and through trade loopholes, chemicalisation of agricultural soil and food supply are continuing.

Only the wise education of Farmers and Doctors can keep our resources safe, and in sovereign hands. Such an education in biochemistry should be devoid of chemical company sponsorship or direction. Discernment of product usage is then enabled, and less waste and toxicity produced.

Tobacco is taxed in accordance with its harm, alcohol is taxed also, perhaps all agricultural and pharmaceutical products should be taxed according to their ongoing dependency and/or harm?

Funny how you can be put in jail for smoking around your kids, or in the car, and authorities will throw you in jail and make your child a ward of the state if you refuse chemo for your child.

Basically, I was not allowed to say no, I was threatened with court action and jail, I was threatened that my child would be made a ward of the State, if I refused chemotherapy for him, regardless of efficient alternatives available. I was supposed to sit by in this Nazi death camp, and watch him, support him to be chemically tortured, and damaged. This was a horrific nightmare to me, especially when I had the use of a harm free treatment that worked. Protocel/Entelev as it is known in Australia, effectively removes cancer and auto-immune cells from the body.

I went underground, but not before I faced many Drs and Oncologist with my case. Many agreed with me but said their hands were tied, they did not want to lose their jobs. The AMA is a Nazi Priesthood, according to most Drs, and unless they prescribe the approved cocktails on their list they will be struck off. My Doctors were not able to assist.

The False laws that were put in place to prevent Religious folk from refusing blood transfusions, is now applied to all parental choices that are not in alignment with AMA regulations and or investor profits.

My son was tortured and murdered slowly by inefficient, ineffective, DNA harming chemicals, delivered by ignorant, frightened doctors, who are beholden to a Chemical company Guise called the AMA and the ANZECC Study Protocol. I would have been put in jail for using anything other; any natural system of healing, that according to all "Indoctrinated" Drs are a HOAX.

It would be preferable to all real humans, that Doctors have available to them the full gambit of healing modalities available, personal choice will keep a healthy market. A smarter Doctoring as we have seen occur in Europe, greater choice, better health outcomes, less chemicalisation. Do not let Australia be shepherded toward the American Drug management modality of Doctoring, which is against nature and against human rights.

My constitutional, human rights and the life of my son were hijacked by forced/conscripted chemicalisaion.

Until Doctoring in Australia recognizes modalities that include nature, and greater choice, I will be steering clear of all AMA controlled medicine. FIRST AID is the one area of medicine you can trust.

Emergencies only.

Nightmares Dressed in White

My nightmares come dressed in White,
Ara-C Screams in broad daylight…
Long hospital corridors at night,
Daily waking to dreaded fear,
Another chemotherapy session near…
Where No, means Yes and no one hears…
No way to save my child from this?!
Foundations of Fun and Good Will
Fill Peoples ears with the accepted Drill…
Now so Accepted,
No one hears our cries…
Our children being killed in front of our eyes!
Banned from choosing another less harmful path,
We should be grateful for all the
Pomp and Pampering, the Wishes and Camp Qualitying…
All amount to NOTHING but diversional therapy. Masking Death.
A guise in the continuance of useless suffering by
A closed minded system of
Medical Nephitism, that is
Better protected than 'Oil'.
Another 'Outmoded' Technology.
So much for progress?
That may spoil, profits of old…
What was the point of all the years of Toil,
If not, to save our children from this Foil?
Those who wish to maintain the status quo…
I am not taking your choosing from You!
And you should not 'Assume',
Chemotherapy is for everyone.
'Assumptions' are fallible, not scientific, you know…
Observably true, there are as many reasons for
Wellness, as there are for disease…
People should be happy with whatever therapies they choose.
Life without Sovereignty of your health, is a cruel ruse.

Life offers no guarantees of the win, or lose.
So at least Return,
Sovereignty in Health, to the People,
The Right to Choose.

Aunty Wendy

My Mother told me the story
Of how her sister passed away…
Wendy was a Down's syndrome child, whom
Are susceptible to Leukaemia we are informed.
I got curious to know what treatments they had back then, in 1957?
The standard was chemotherapy then, I was told.
Painful and terrible, then as it is now,
Aunty Wendy did not last long…
So how, in that 60 years, has treating Leukaemia evolved?
It is piled high with more and more
Cyto-toxic therapy, attacking the cell cycle…
Still the children affected, do not get to grow old…
Such is the entrenched ANZCC Study Protocol.
I was shown 30 years of statistics in one page,
Detailing success, an up to 82% remission rate…but
That statistic is Another painful ruse, because
It only applies for 5 years… and
To children less than 5 years of age (due to rapid cell replacement).
Then relapse occurs…In too many cases.
These statistics I was shown, 'one page'… are
Held in such high esteem by Oncology, and
Advertised, as
'Reason' for every-one to go with an
Unquestioning chemotherapy protocol…Are we all toddlers now?
Surely as a community we are mature enough to let something else in,
To the medical system, that will deliver Real Healing and better results than...
The same Ole, Same Old, disenfranchising treatment protocols.
Profits and Losses are clearly, not affecting the same people's pockets.
Like Thomas the Tank Engine stories…

Devolved and Exclusive, the Protected Siding of a Medical Systems, Cancer contribution,
Becomes Toxic in its Isolation, and
Harbour's Priestly delusions of medical grandeur...
Such 'strongholds' exist, vested and systemic, they
Do not wish, to allow, a
'New Health Station' in service of the current economic Gravy train.
Protectionism? Avoiding Natural Medicine...
Because they cannot dismantle all the research foundations that
Make Billions perpetuating 'No Cure' economies?
Progress? Supporting Natural Medicine in 'multi-modality' 'pro-choice', Doctoring...
Because they love the people and are focused on wellness and
Desire better health outcomes and less cost in health care?
Natures Medicine Combined with
Positive medical pharmacology and technology is
The Evolution of Good Medicine.
Better: That good doctors have more success in their days and
Access to useful tools of healing to promote wellness and
Save us when we fall. And
The ability to ask Reasonable Questions,
In an environment of 'Transparency',
Without being, professionally assaulted, by their 'Union', The AMA.
Too bad the Investment choices of 'Big Business'
Are not the same as the 'Peoples Will'.
Let, "Doctors for People,
Choice and Wellness" Prevail.
Image of: Newtonian Medicine giving way to Quantum Healing and Wellness,
A New Era has arrived.
Newtonian Physics could not stop the truth of Quantum Physics joining with it,
As partners in the underlying and greater reality,
Serving the fabric of existence...
Pointless effort, trying to stop Gravity. Life has its own way...
Falsehoods in economies or science, by their very nature, in time, all fall away...
This too is Change.

Poem "Anzac Spirit"

It's been 100 years since Gallipoli
Where our young folk sacrificed their lives fighting Tyranny over the sea
For Our right, to live Sovereign and Free...
And yet children diagnosed with cancer have no rights
And parents watch in helpless horror or be criminalised
As our youngsters' lives are sacrificed to barbaric WW2 chemical Tyranny,
Right here on our shores.
State Approved, False Laws and "Trade A-Greed,"
AMA Approved Death by Oncology Gestapo Creed.
Threatened Parents Silently Plead! God Help Me!

Think of the death of our soldiers and our children too,
We tell their stories, so the future knows better what to do.
Remember the Anzac lives lost and the Constitutional Freedom
They fought to uphold.
And Why are parents of TODAY told?
They must adhere to a deadly toxic WWII medical protocol!?

Follow the money trail...
Under the guise of progress, and
Applying the Law of Graduation...
Four generations hence.
The Psychopathic Machine is in place.
Cigarette Science and sucrose coated lies with multi-national dollars invested;
Contaminated soil, food, water, medicine and marketing the choices you're permitted...
A silent scourge, and toxic harvest.
The health of our soil, our water, our bodies now
At the Limit!

So many Anzac lives lost indeed, but
Our inheritance appears to be a la system "Economics of Greed"
Where our constitutional rights, be omitted?
Where no Sovereign right to choose HARM FREE MEDICINE can be allowed to succeed, not
Over Multi-National Codex and the Trade/A-Greed....
So much for a Constitutional Creed!?

Whether it be in Trenches of Gallipoli or Hospital Corridors,
Too many lives are still lost in the quest
For Sovereignty of Choice and
Truth in Medicine Right NOW!
Would be Best.

So spare a thought on commemoration days,
For the young warriors
Walking the trenches of today,
Of long white corridors..
And the drip trolley, always an arms-length away...
Children fighting for life and the opportunity
Just to have their day... And maybe to play...
All for the want of True Medicine,
Vitamin C or Cannabis Oil, that would give life and end pain.
Sadly, these little troopers have no rights, no say,
In the protocols of their toil each day.
All for the want of True Medicine, that;
Does not fit, the "Against Life" Codex Machine, It's
Chemical Empirical favoured Doctrine, and
Its' desire for overwhelming rule, nor
Ethics Committee Insanity of the ANZCCSG "Study" Protocol...
Sugar coated marketing,
Commonly known as Cyto-toxic CHEMO.
Hijacking our Health choices thus
Condemning our Young and Elderly to lose.
A Crime Against Humanity, they will call this "Study" one day;
This Chemical Rouse,
ANZCC Study group
Cunningly Legitimised as Whaling Science does,
And in the same way.
Outmoded excuses for
Evil/Against Life, trials of toxic abuses,
That do more harm than good.
ANZCCSG Study Protocol - Agreed between Nations
It kills our young and influences our old,

Plying danger, outmoded war-time chemicals
Cyto-Toxins and Radiation,
Solely to behold!
And be witness to investment pathways, that
Don't want competition and have vowed,
Never to let Nature's 'harm-free' medicine into the fold,
As told by the Oncology Mould...
A Population problem could unfold, if people
Were cured and/or allowed to grow old....
"Managing" Disease is a $150 Billion
Cyclic economy of Ease.
No Money they say, in the cure of Disease, and
This is an economy of which I would wish to be Free!
Just between You and Me...
Truth in Medicine, for ALL People, for Humanity.

With Love to My lost boy Dylan,
He endured Cancer diagnosis twice!
"Go the Anzac Spirit!"
Dylan Lost his life at 8 years old.

Due to a Lie about the ANZCCSG 'Study' being Law, and the only legal path, despite other successful treatments being used around the world. We were threatened, by court action, and removal of our child, if we did not comply with the Protocol...of death.

Children fight for their lives in the modern trenches with no defence and no rights.
Want to know Pressure! Try Saying No to Forced Medical Treatment...
Bring in the Clown Doctors... No!
A Choice in Medicine, Harm Free Preferred. And
End the unquestioning and binding use of the Australian and New Zealand CCSG ALL "study"!

End Chemical Barbarism.

The ANZCCSG "Study" is not a Cure nor healing modality, it's a crime against humans, that has been allowed to continue with poor success beyond 5 years, with damaging/dependency side effects.

The continuation of this damaging chemotherapy "Study" should be a Last Resort not a first response, and should be recognised as a crime, as coercion, under the guise of a "Study".

Alternatives exist and are acknowledged outside Australia.

Citizens should have the right to choose Harm Free Alternatives to damaging Chemo or Radiation treatment, especially in First Instance Response. Leave the Damaging Science to the Last Resort!

ANZCCSG Study is No better than Whaling Science in the net result. I know, I lived with the effects!

For the good of our future. Be Well.

Make Laws that Ensure Oncologists can allow Harm Free Treatments to be available at patient discretion. NOW!

Politicians VS Penis Wraps

We consider politicians as an 'integral' part of our system of governance..
So what is Good Governance? – Managing public services of the group.
Why do we need politicians at all?
Politicians in the role of good governance, are as needed as penis wraps, of
Cultural significance in Melanesia.
This garb, has become accepted, as culturally necessary, yet it serves only vanity,
A lot like politicians assisting in any Good Governance.
If you take away the penis wrap, the organ it dresses up,
Still works just fine.
As with politicians and good governance, when the Vanity of politician, after politician passes,
Seasonally, the public servants of public services, continue good deliverance.
Politicians come and go from the lime light glow, but
beurocrates and public servants keep the civil services flowing.
If the vanity culture of politicians, were removed, one would find they are superfluous to the work 'people' do supporting 'people'.
Politicians are mere puppets of hidden economic overlords these days.
Many incapable of decision making for themselves let alone others, or future generations...
Penis Wraps are more Functional and Protective of Melanesian tribesmen, than
Politicians are, of the population of Australia.

Chapter 3

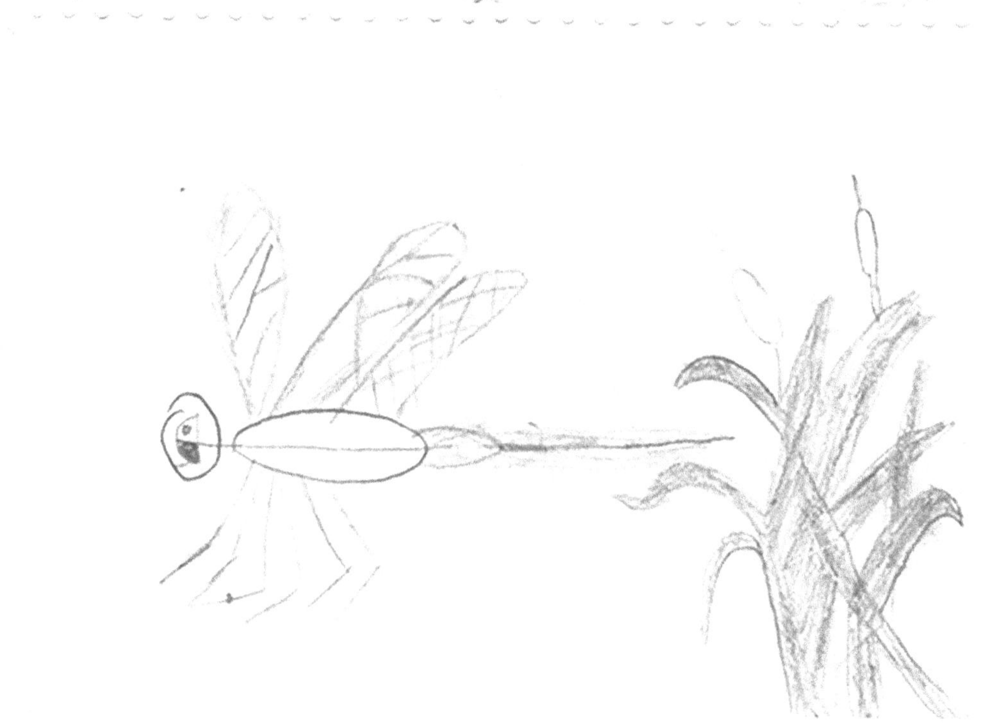

The System – behind the veil

A rigged system is a racket.
If you knew there was a giant pothole hidden in the road of modern life, a
Road the masses travel… would you tell your friends and neighbours or
Stand by and watch them Drop Right In!?
Note to Self: The system is rigged,
If Dr Dishwater can choose that exclusively only cyto-toxins are ever, ever to be
Researched in the Melbourne Children's Hospital Cancer Research facility?!
He said "Alternatives will Never be trialled here" …. Alternatives to chemo poison and death?
A children's Health facility that chose McDonalds- processed food, to be sold on the premises?

The system is rigged, if medical cannabis is only available to epilepsy and pain sufferers, no mention of it as an effective treatment for Acute Lymphoblastic Leukaemia (ALL) a terminal illness that is in epidemic proportions comparatively since the 1970's.

The system is rigged, if all natures cures and medicines, proven effective as treatments, in other areas of our world, are called a Hoax by doctors educated in Rothschild investments, oops universities, in Australia, New Zealand, Canada, UK, USA...

Is it not a Hoax in and of itself to promote chemical management of disease without curative health?

The system is rigged by the ANZECC Study, treaty, which is not only associated with supporting pointless and harmful wars, but also pointless, harmful WW2 cyto-toxic medicines and radiation experimentation on uninformed populations.

The Lie of NO "CURES".
The system is Rigged to perpetuate public ignorance, fear and
The blind choosing of toxic products recommended.
The system is rigged so you won't ask too many questions...
Market share is everything.
The system is Rigged to keep you hooked in to your
Domestic screen, and consuming, consuming, consuming.
The system is rigged to perpetuate dependency on a false economic overlay,
That is encouraging you to give all sovereignty away, blindly.
The system is rigged to continue the Game; Club of Rome – Where
They build a machine in your lounge room, bit by bit, nice and slow,
So no one ever suspects, loss of freedoms at all...
Slowly carefully, catchee monkey.
The system is rigged, when conscription is brought in to
Assist the Zombie Nation.
New technology and vaccinations forced upon unwitting populations,
Too comfortable to see, the hijacking of civil rights.
The new Nano-weapons of mass destruction could be in the form of vaccination, against Life.
The system is rigged when a country's constitution and governments recognition, responsibility and management are not aligned or in unison.
Civil responsibilities and rights are not real possessions of
Big Business, Might is Right.
Call for the restoration of civil rights, healthy food, clean water and shelter;
Of personal choice, as the proper human order. Not to be monopolized!
The system is Rigged when the most effective, most promising
Treatment for cancer, seen in decades, Cannabis, and

our lawmakers' intent in Australia, renders it only available
to epilepsy, nausea and Pain conditions? If at all?
A fur fey upon constitutional citizens, to perpetuate
Big Pharma control of our failing Doctors and failing health system.
All the while, flawed products and treatments that kill, are given mainstream "compulsory-ism".
A virtual Red Carpet investment deal.
The system is Rigged my friends, when Big Pharma, owns
Our doctor's educations, careers and the 'rights' to "manage" every disease...
Over-riding civil rights, upon individual's bodies, and health choices with ease. Why?
It is good for foreign relations treaties and the economy.
No civilian got to vote on this 'Erosion' of civil rights, via
Economic 'might is right'?
The system is rigged squarely for hijacking and slavery.
The system is rigged my friend, and to this I lost my son.
No Avenue to complain – Freedom of speech is black-banned
In the public media domain.
Whenever cancer cures are mentioned, where are the flock being driven?
Can anyone else see the pathway toward the zombie machine...?
Herd immunity, compulsory, the only death acceptable is via radiation or chemotherapy?
The system needs tweaking if it is to support people rather than a psychopathic economy of harm.
Iatrogenic injury just cost the manufacturers of Vaccines 3 Billion dollar in the USA. Legally coined "Unavoidably unsafe" ... 2018. FACT.
OOPs, did not the Australian Media run that story? ...Wonder why?
When you see the EVIDENCE in these cases, you too, may insist on the 'Right to Choose' your medicine or your poison.
Compulsory-ism is an unjust economic ploy, not for the good of the people's health at all.

The system is rigged, no worries about elections, but daily life,
now in the West... Choices and assistance, streamlining and efficiencies?
Right down to foods and medicines, homogenized and pasteurized,
raw foods and raw milk, demonized? After thousands of years of humans working with raw dairy...
But plastic foods are ok? Not for public safety of 1% but an economy of 80%.
More sense to pay debunkers, with all those shareholder dollars at stake.
Big business monopoly on food and medicine is good for economy but
A disaster for the Human Body.

Sovereignty of sensory experience of Life on Earth, Human Avatar, put at risk
By robotizing and de-generation.
Choose wisely, what you join your body with.
The so-called New World Order diabolical care protocols, do not suit me, or
My children's children.
A civil nation should stick to the commitments of a CIVIL constitution.
Right now, Civil Rights in Australia sit in sections 8 and below, within the Constitution.
The governments reign and recognition are exclusively within section 9, of the same constitution?
There is a glaring delusion of 'Good Governance', right there!
Fiddling with a second set of books, created in the year 2000.
The Australia Corporation.
Not a level playing field, as little Johnny pretended at the time, but a vehicle to sell our nation out, and citizens' rights, in big business deals and get a seat on the UN.
Who are the Shareholders? Who do the Judiciary swear allegiance to?
The People or the Corporation? Who are the Directors?
Some talk of Treason against civilians of this peaceful nation?
Whatever, "It's just not fair Cricket".
The difference between a machine and human is LOVE.
I objected to animal cruelty, battery hens, pigs, whatever, and
I object to humanity being treated as livestock to support fake overlords.

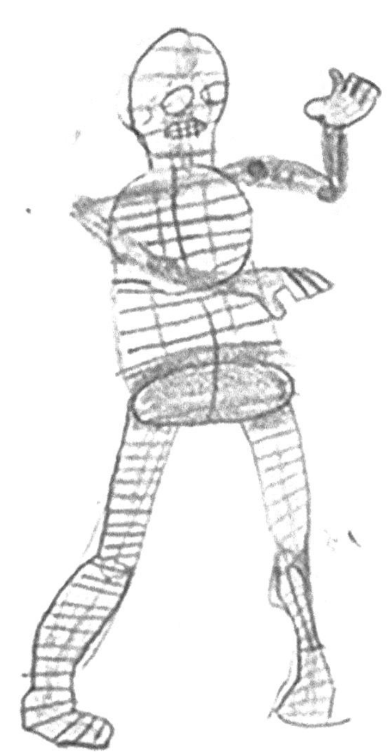

Contraindications

When medicine and marketing combine,
Two powerful threads entwined, now
Predator upon humanity made blind.
Fear supporting trillion-dollar industries, protected
By false laws, and manipulated
Statistical flaws.
When fear and guilt are employed the sales pitch is
Fraud, and 'Truth',
Sits in the balance, well below the priorities of
Shareholder profits.
Truth sits with freewill and human dignity, while
Conscription ignores the needs of diversity.
When medicine and marketing join hands a
Human health calamity takes the stand.
Preventative medicine's new legal label, now;
"Unavoidably Unsafe".
Three Billion dollars paid out in 2018 for
Iatrogenic Injury...

This is the Fact they try to hide.
Toxic medicine, maintained, by removing
"Freewill" and the right to litigate, in economic owned
Courts of law.
Civility and personal decision making,
Made a Whore to industries of chemical control
By ignorant and greedy politicians who have never
Given consideration to seven generations hence…
Four years is the limit of their focus,
So easily bent.

Hmm, Cancer Council appear to have invested billions of dollars,
Not on research to finding cures but in legal injunctions,
To prevent 'alternatives' to their preferred modalities, from
Ever competing in the public medicinal domain.
The Deeds of the Cancer Council have sought to monopolize treatment and
Make a cancer of themselves by default.
To support an Empire…
Not actions of an organisation interested in "Cures" but
In "preventing news", of alternatives from ever
Reaching public ears or that of your Doctors.
Puppet masters of the FDA and TGA they have
The support of Big Money and
"Your Choice"
In medicine is what they seek to Monopolise.
Propaganda patterns, the same as
War mongering governments… Passive aggressive, fear mongering
Lies, of purpose;
Economy.

The Cancer Council got fat on
Desperate people's good will to cure 'ILL'.
Not an authority, or voted in as a controlling body?
This Fundraiser has developed exceptional marketing habits and
Has become habituated in Western lives.
However, the Cancer Council has developed other
"Patterns" of survival/self-perpetuation that

Are unhealthy to every Nation...
"Patterns" would indicate something that is done again and again...
Over decades to perpetuate economic health, to
The detriment of human health, and dignity in every ANZAC nation.
Lies and Conscription...
The economy of Cancer cannot continue in the presence of "Cures".
So many effective alternatives have been falsely tested, demonized and made illegal...
At the 'request' of?
The Cancer Council, no less.
As Tanya Harter Pierce reports in her book, Outsmart Your Cancer,
The Cancer Council have been caught out influencing the FDA/TGA,
Objecting to any treatment that was not paying their bills...
Vitamin C, Amygdalin, Protocel/Entelev, Gaston Nassene's 714X, Dr Hope's Microwave treatment, and recently, studies on Iodine's curative properties they suppressed, among others such as Graviola, Mangosteen and Cannabis.
This is the Hoax on Health, they have themselves become
The Council of Cancer.
No cures ever to be delivered, just your loved ones to the
Chemotherapy gravy train, a few treats and a warm hand to hold
Everything will be ok. Right?!
Wrong!
Make it legal, once more, to choose differently.
Let Constitutional civil choices in health treatments be restored,
Along with respect and dignity.
Shame on the Fur fey fundraising bodies that
Have done naught but sweep alternatives to
Death by chemo, under the carpet and out of sight.
Put out the Light on toxic conscriptions and protocols of poison,
Forced upon innocent children.

CANNABIS
is MY
MEDICINE
And it CURED
MY CANCER
Brave Mykayla!

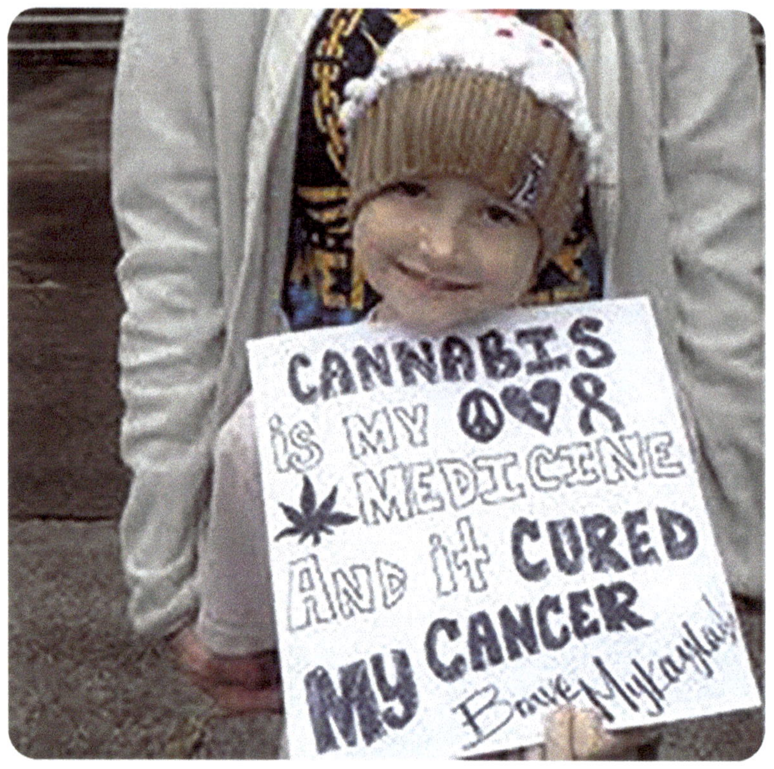

Here is my prayer:

The machine of Entrapment and Slavery upon civil humanity,
Has already begun to crumble, to fall…
A quickening now in awareness,
Psychopathic tendencies, lose power and are left behind, or
Die by their own 'hidden-hand'.
Protecting Innocents, a wiser humanity, respecting
Sovereign choice and cultural, genetic diversity,
As Key;
To the future children and diverse human population,
Develop more care and balance in servicing needs of
The People essential, before economies of trade.
Freed of the need nor deeds of conflict as a tool of control.
Poison and weapon economies are dismantled and gone.
Biological Farming, Natural Medicine and Regional creativity bloom, anew.
Happiness and fulfilment of good creations ensue,
BE Well.
Know that each and every one is treasured,

As golden thread in the Great Tapestry of Life.
Brains behind the weaving of the World Wide Web, try to shut the 'Gates' on the Web of Life.
Population control by W.H.O a promise of the
Bretton woods in 1944, now paid for by
B&B Gates, masters of philanthropy, wealth and power.
Now new masters of population control via chemical management and economic bastardy,
Having overreached themselves in arrogance, thinking their wisdom as great as their wealth.
These people who used stealth and were later found guilty of stealing the "windows" environment from Apple Mac...
Now they are stealing a biologically sound environment from the people...
Those that rely on supermarkets and are addicted to the domestic screen,
Do not have eyes to see!
Natural forces of Millennia are the cleaners...
Naturally catching modern living unaware,
The callous and the ignorant, suffer and pass away.
Those meek and close to the earth, who live with respect for balance and fellow man, who make their own bread by hand... It is such folk were intended to remain after the change...
Not the selfish and the wealthy, or those responsible for poisoning of land and sea,
The reverse engineering of humanity, funded by the Gates Corp, and W.H.O be damned for
Their influence in stealing health from future generations.

Do Gooders be warned.

The road to Hell is paved by the best intentions of those inconsiderate of real consequence.

A Chinese proverb:

"One will often find one's destiny on the path one takes to avoid it."

If actions are made in haste, without due consideration for consequences, problems can be created that are bigger than those one first sought to address.

I.E Weapons and War manufactured by bankers, Westinghouse whitegoods and LG domestic screens. Masses hypnotised by overt and subversive controls.

G.M Mosquitoes, sent to alleviate one disease only to deliver a worse disease. Zika.

Deregulation of banking and industry brought more problems than benefits to the general populace. Profits and foreign ownership...

Pasteurization and heat-treated fats... Dr Joanna Budwig got sacked by Margarine king, her boss for publishing papers contrary to his, now her findings are valued and found to be true.

Cane toads and other introduced biological vermin, pest control becoming pest problems, Fluoridisation of water supply, does nothing for cavities but keeps governments safe from rebellion, enabling mass marketing unquestioningly... Profits for players supreme.

Toxic herbicides and pesticide used on mass, sees bio accumulation grow, now a major threat... To whole food chains!

Monoculture and streamlining agriculture, are the cause of many land and health degradation issues.

Combined with the conscription of medicine, chemotherapy, vaccination overload, brings a Toxic Harvest for future genetics.

Opiate addictions galore... yet more pain in the population than ever before.

Government funded Drug Testing Initiatives for cannabis, as a flow on effect, created an ICE epidemic in high income working class. See the Australian Mining/Construction Industry.

Fake Foundations, fully funded, peddle chemical protocols of wartime experimentation. NO Cures allowed!

Big business nuked family business, as corporatization supersedes the constitution.

The 1944 Bretton Woods model of Global Economy was not a solution but

A psychopath. The Wolf dressed in Sheep's Clothing.

A red-carpet investment, for conflict, perpetuating profits, of waste and obsolescence.

This was sold to the people as a solution.

For their and our, own Good?

Convinced to support the economy of the Dollar$$$$ -

Not an economy supporting humans, 'The People'?

Psychopathic economies are unnecessary and can be discarded and replaced,

Individually and collectively at community levels.

Regional economies with the "Small is Beautiful" modelling will succeed for this Future's need.

- "small is beautiful – a study of economics as if people mattered", by Ernst Friedrich Schumacher is an economics book that is relevant today as it was when it was written decades ago in 1973.
- Professor George Monbiot of London- provides an excellent resource on economic history and the Bretton-woods economic curse that was born of a war bribe.

Removing the blindfold

Journalism of Truth displaced by sales management.
Monsanto paid Google to cut unfavourable content.
Modern media is bought and sold by big business.
Finally, the journalists are taking note,
Media moguls have supported the "blacklist" of publishing for years.
No truth or good journalism is permitted on many topics of human interest, that
Have powerful lobby groups… In war, health and food.

A well-respected journalist of many years was prevented from publishing an article detailing links with bowel ill health and pasteurization of milk in the 1990's. She advised me that the dairy industry was a powerful lobby group that prevented unfavourable journalism to protect their profit margin.

Pity so many people have become intolerant to this food stuff. Is it the pasteurization or the glyphosate in the feed of cows? Bowel Cancer has become an epidemic, is there a connection?

Writing about Cancer is also 'blacklisted' unless it is a favourable story on Chemo or Radiation therapy…

Alternative treatments and Natures medicines are propaganda fodder and treated as economic enemies.

The powerful lobby groups around the trillion-dollar pharmaceutical industry prevent public discussion on Vitamin C, as a curative, and attempt to outlaw words, like

"Cure" for use in any public discussion other than their own, exclusive social license, to themselves given.

That media is the ASS of business is plain to see, with the human rights travesty of West Papua, the Solomon Islands or Norfolk Island, Minerals Mining and Economic Fishing Zones deals rule overall, to the detriment of the dignity and 'will' to self-rule.

Most Australians would not even know, what has gone on in the name of business supported by governments and propped up by greed.

The 'blacklist' of the unreportable and media has played a large role in preventing truth where powerful lobby groups exist...

For they do not want 'the public' to Resist.
So, Truth in Journalism is threatened again and again, like
Tele-tubby programming for innocent minds, trained to be dazzled by the screen flicker,
Continuously, encouraged to look away from reality, not seen.
Rose coloured glasses presented for addicted viewing, while
Truth wears the 'block out lenses'.
This is where Big Media and Big Business blend....
And deals are done on what to say, what image to present...
Product sales and Programming as a 'Diversion' from Reality.

The Kraken and Tinkerers

Interesting to observe how the things everyone complains about in the world, as a problem...
Seem all to be linked with the platform of 'economy'.
The Kraken of Economy, as an image, has many arms...
All individual complaints about the system, whether speaking of
Energy or Medicine, are just flags flapping in the wind...
Nothing will come of seeing issues in isolation, when
Economically, people created the root cause...
A big adaptive psychopathic economy,
Driving and supporting its' own perpetuation.

Going back to the beginning and isolating elements,
Wealthy families of banking, oil and diamond mining, of chemicals and invasive medicine.
Dupont poisons, plastic, and the nemesis of Hemp.
Industrialists wanting to exploit and explore new markets.
WW2 Brittan requiring warship, wheeling and dealing.

A new world order of economic management was the deal of favoured American Zionistics.
Disasters were foretold correctly of this economic model, by genius mathematician John Maynard Keynes, so
W.H.O was invented as a safety mechanism, to protect the people, but in actuality,
W.H.O is being used to do unwise biddings of 'foundational industrialist policy'.
Now the Number 1 product distributor, of chemical management, for the Corporations of 27 ruling members.
They play the world like a Monopoly Game, and as such,
Conflict is the acrid taste in the mouths of babes.
Maintaining the status quo, on every stage.
Image: Problems as likened to sails flapping in the wind
On a noticeably big pirate vessel – ship of Economy.
People are all looking up at the sails, when
The problem is in the bilge below...
Time for a vessel refit, so it will float,
Smooth water sailing again an aid to human lives and trade.
The basis of the global economy bears far too much resemblance
To the Dutch 'Tea' trading co... Turned delegates of tyranny.
The current ship of economy has been rigged to fail Humanity.

The Kraken of economy has many arms my friend, and
Soon it will be plugged into everything...
Unless we choose again... differently.

This ship was built to carry the human economy from shore to shore,
After eighty years of plundering every port for resources to,
Sell, sell, sell.
The crew of admiralty realized whenever they attempted to
Correct the plotted direction of sailing,
Into a storm they would go, always,
Weakened into submission to continue the plotted course.
One day the cabin boy discovered,
A tendril of the Kraken in the Hull.
The Kraken had made itself into the rudder of the ship and
Had been steering humanity, unaware,
Towards the edge of the world of oblivion,
For some time...

If disturbed, watch out for
Crackdown...
Rule by fear, scare tactics for submission, and
Any who would seek to alter economic direction?
Kraken forbids.
Abandon ship, for steadier shores.
Like heretics of the bounty, mutineers of
The new religion of economy are
Feared by 'Kraken Control', who's
Arms are oceans wide, sensitive and stretch across many industries...
Be aware, be well, and be sovereign in your choices.

Removing the False – Non-Essentials

Take back your bombs, one cannot eat weapons, yet
They are traded as Supplies?
Once upon a time, weapons denoted warrior skill or improved hunting prospects,
Now they are made to destroy the world, whole cities, towns, non-economic global parties, governments and man, woman and child.
Most modern weaponry is not associated with food provision, 'nor skill
Nor intelligence, just ill will.
Senseless destruction, because they can.
Senseless destruction, to maintain weapons as a tool in an economy of fear.
No less than to perpetuate the value of the dollar, blind mass production and
Mass waste, of consumer driven economies.
Convenience making 'dumb' terminals of men and women,
Drones in their contribution, to a culture of waste and haste.
Creating the wastelands of wasted man.
Nature and Humanity await, with tapping foot, in the wings... for
The vultures of war culture,
The stupid and garish performance of the modern drama queen to end...
Back to the continuum.

Exposing the medical priesthood

A child dying of thirst is given a cup of sand,
That is how oncology treats our children.
Not allowed to choose, against rigged population statistics and a
Treaty of medicinal control, the ANZECC study protocol.
Not allowed to question?
Threats of jail, and loss of freedoms, even to visit the child.
Psychological torture applied to force compliance.
Alternatives that work overseas, denied?
Is this not organized murder, legalized?
Constitutional freewill of health choices, in diverse gene pool,
Access denied?
May these words of close witnessing be as a cytotoxin on the
Industry of chemotherapy in Oncology of zero cures.
These people are trained in 'passive aggressive' persuasion and
Ignorance of industries dictation, such that,
They do not know what they are doing.
Any professionals, that ask questions are demoted or removed from this loophole of Medicine.
They spend more energy on defending their toxic "manslaughter" strategy
Than saving lives of our children.
Cytotoxic Medicine with tragic and predictable reoccurrences, of
Cancerous conditions. 80% may survive initial treatment but
1% get to live life beyond 5 years, subsequent to treatment in
This protocol of law and medicine, gone insane...

They window dress, applying sugar and clowns, a
Diversion to prevent complaints or questions of care?
They kill children using pointless poisons, poisons
Guaranteeing genetic destruction of future cells...
They are supported in continuance by powerful foundations as lobby groups,
Funded by Big Pharma and public sympathy...
Our doctors are educated by pharmaceutical companies that fund university curriculums and build new hospital wings...
Transport and accommodation provided for recipients.
A closed system loop, locked up, with
A $150 Billion economy to defend.

Whether it is individual ignorance or systemic in the system?...
Is it not still Murder, of which no one is allowed to question?
They are sanctioned to kill your loved ones too.
No choice, just diversional therapy...
Once ensconced in the feel-good family, they hope you will refocus and
Forget what it is they do...
Perpetuate toxic dead-end protocols of lasting consequence, with
Religious reverence and fear of questioning procedure.
This is why there are no cures allowed, and
Natural medicine is treated as the economic enemy.
Look up the research done on graviola and mangosteen,
Laetrile, or 714X, for evidence of this truth.
**See appendices 10 and 11*

Portrait of Pathways

The World's Biggest Psychopath is set up like a giant corporation.

There are controlling parent companies and child companies that are the arms and do the work of the psychopath, feeding back to a central point.

The Bilderberg club/Club of Rome oversee the IMF World Bank, Bailiff System of finance, at the central core.

Arms of 'control' are;

- Education,
- Power/energy
- Appliances LG/weapons manufacturing/conflict control,
- Health and W.H.O as agents for Big Pharmaceutical pills of dependency and vaccines/ population control,
- Agricultural giants which are managed along with W.H.O by C.O.D.E.X (conglomerate of Agricultural chemical manufacturers and pharmaceutical manufacturers) controlling imports and exports, and
- Media/information control/Murdock power/1956 USA memorandum of understanding blacklist topics not to discuss, with global compliance from media ownership/editorials.

How is humanity to navigate safely, its children, from the clutches of the WBP without awareness of the Guise it wears and the pathways it treads?

Psychopaths are clever, camouflaged as chameleons, as in nature, if you did not know what to look for, you would not even realize what you were looking at…

And so, the predator, the psychopath, remains hidden in full view.

Without eyes to see and ears to hear, humanity is enslaved unwittingly. Manipulated beyond belief to support a few rich family businesses and their dollar god.

The rest of us are pawns in their play – and be sure not to get in their way!

Ted talks: 27 people run the world – Mathematician talks about statistics from public companies globally, all leading back to; all global decisions being made by 27 people.

In observing patterns of nature, it teaches one about the patterns of life.

Life breathes, in and out, trends, fashion, our bodies' vessels, the seasons, the earth's tides, the universe, expansion and contraction, movement in and out.

The tides of the World's Biggest Psychopath have moved and the high has now passed, its tide is on its way out.

Change is the only constant that anyone can rely upon. DO NOT PANIC!

Everything is change and the psychopath is breathing its last breaths – sometimes erupting like a boil, to help us heal our addiction to deadly dependency and control by fear.

Upon observation for themselves, people discover the insidious and systemic nature of this psychopath – it is natural to feel foolish and possibly angry at the great deception that is upon us All. However, be grateful for having open eyes – you will be able to read the signs and avoid the gas chamber that others will walk blindly into.

Teach the children to stay sovereign.
Take responsibility for releasing/letting go of personal hubris/emotions of fear and pain.
Do not pass hubris on to others, especially children.
Teach children the guises and patterns of deception and control used by psychopaths, that rob sovereignty of the self.
Teach children how to move beyond fear, to do what is right, no matter what.

Teach children that a smart brain is of no service without a good heart.
CHOICE IS OUR POWER.

Life's givers, give with love, life's takers, take with fear.
Each person has the responsibility to discern this and align themselves with either,
Life enhancing choices or life depleting choices – choice is OURS.

Teach our children to question, question. If something cannot be questioned, it needs to be! Whether authority or education, if it cannot be questioned, it is a control drama, not a truth.

Teach our children to consider the effects of choices (consequences) on Seven (7) generations hence, so to avoid repeating the patterns of destruction, of food supply, peoples and places in the past 1000 years.

Corporations/businesses and bodies that have 'no beating heart', should have no say or influence in our Governance or basic services that are supposed to be provided by good governance.

Teach our children that all religious conflict is an excuse for a control drama via fear and to Remember, all the Masters of every creed have all the same basic message, simple truths for humanity:

Respect the Mirror of One -Treat others as you would have yourself treated... All eyes are the eyes of GOD/ALLAH/YAHWEH, having its personal experience in form.

Do not take, that which is not yours.
Unconditional love is the highest law and compassion is its expression.
In the heart and mind, truth sets us free, lies bind and create confusion...
Remember, that which cannot be questioned, should be questioned, vigorously.

The Separation Principle

Is and always has been, a furphy upon Humanity.
Kept in place by religious or political control dramas.
I.E the Roman Catholic Church at its origin, sought domination and control.
A tad diabolical, they melded parts of the book of WAR with Sacred Scriptures...
Turning the Love of GOD and sacred teachings into expressions of Fear and Guilt.
Bizarre indeed for a religious creed, as
On the spectrum of emotional responses in this perfect template world,

Fear and Guilt are furthest away from Godly emotional experience of Nirvana, Bliss and Love.
Fear and Guilt has served the purposes of those who seek to OWN GOD, and the power that comes with such narcissism or megalomania... The ownership of Public Will.
The tools of focus were set to profit, ill will.
Divided people Fall.
The Truth is Unified and Whole.
The Truth is Love is the Law.
Let Love now underpin 'will' as was written, hidden and intended from the beginning.
Peace Love and Creativity for All.

Love under Will is sustaining the most important element, Free Will...
The 'Will' of all healthy people is basically 'Good'.
This is the enemy that the separation principle sought to kill, or
Harness for its own purposes...
The 'Will' of Man, Woman, Child
The sacred Triune experience, of
The Great Omnipresent Divine.

The sacred template remains
Perfect, whole and complete for
Man-Woman-Child to work creatively and play, with
Love and Light in the most Sacred Geometry of 'Life'.
Living Light. Living Geometry, frequency, patterns of perfection everywhere.

In the precision move of the Club of Rome dynamic, the
Most sacred Gems of Truth and fractal life teachings, were
Thrown from the quarry of gatherings, that were to form the biblical matter.
Gnostic and Essene teachings, cast out and hidden, for they promote
The sacred union with All of Life.
Here is a refresher for humanity...
The Sacred and Saving Teaching of the Tree of Life.
From Enoch to the Dead Sea. By Dr Edmond Bordeaux Szekely. Transcriptions of the Essene contemplations and connectivity. (further described in chapter 8, page 137)
One can learn from contemplation, without the need of loud preaching.
In working consciously with the elements as described, one can drink of the refreshing Stream of Life.
Following the Truth of All Masters, letting Love underpin 'will'...

For your 'will' becomes your world.
Let the past creations based on fear and diabolical control, be gone.
With the One True Love, as Love is the Law,
All Eyes are the eyes of GOD.
Communities responsible for their own services have no requirement for governments, and Good Will Sovereign Humans have no requirement for dogmatic religion, the control drama of pain, fear and guilt is merely distractive, away from divine focus...
Healthy life discipline is of daily choosing, and for this one must consider, essentially "A man either lives with the pain of discipline or the pain of regret". (quote check, who by)
Life is filled with consequence. Be the Master of your own consequence.

The study of Consciousness, eventually, will render far more benefits than all the expenditure on space and war.
First, 'know thy self'
Living out of Living Earth – Sons and Daughters of a Living Light.
Quantum Physics has already rendered any lesser description, as rubbish.
We are all the dust of old starlight.

Cleaning house...an individual and collective responsibility.
A reminder, to do away with waste and wastefulness, in this regard, again
'Carelessness' has been the only enemy.

The multiverse/many halls/rooms of Odin/Thor/Amenti/God or whatever name you care to use...
Understanding the Mandala effect will prevent its abuse.
Understanding of the Mandala effect will help humanity to see how living life via a domestic screen is a dead end for humanity, and a falsehood developed to keep consciousness entrapped.
Transcendence of Craving and Aversion is the maturity of Man-Woman-Child,
The freeing up and falling away of past restrictions and controls, to
Allow true creativity and flow.
Respect and Love for Diversity renewed, as lifeblood for the continuance of All.
Gotuma The Buddha provided an effective technique that remains true to this day.
Vipassana meditation, frees the consciousness from the binds of Craving and Aversion, while strengthening one's ability to focus, on life as it really is, without the lenses of craving or fear.
Shamanic and Shambhala teachings also enable the work of the Soul.

This word is being put out there to thwart oppressive technologies and systems that threaten the evolutionary sovereignty of Mankind and would seek to continue to Harness the Freewill of Man for worse than dead, purposes.

Let not the Freewill given to Mankind, be used against itself again!
The shackles held by Fear, Jealousy and Greed are weakened by new frequencies.
Once out of the proverbial fishbowl, and into the ocean, human spirit thrives.
Man-Woman-Child, need only apply consistent Loving Focus to anything for it to improve…
Adjustment by Adjustment.
Human focus and intent are a Force.
This force is measurable, and inventions like the 'Mind Switch', intended for invalids, was developed due to this measurable force of "intent". (Australian Science show- Beyond 2000)
Join together in likeness of mind, to focus Love and help your best projects to blossom.
Help your brothers and sisters feel fine…
All are One. Evolution of thought.
Keep Love underpinning one's 'will' and rejoice in the beauty and perfect functionality of one's creations in the sacred geometry, organic template of Life.
Love this Space. This Now! As a newborn…
When treading lightly with one's feet and Heart, the
Hands can work miracles of Love and Light.
Master.
May your heart be light as a feather, lifting your feet to dance,
Your voice to sing,
Allowing the frequency of Joy to come up from within.
Blessing to all Beings.

SOME BIG LIES OF MONEY, MEDICINE AND SCIENCE

A tenured Canadian physics professor, fired for his dissidence, breaks ranks by asserting that established orthodoxy in economics, medicine and science is intended as a web of lies to shield and maintain power structures.

by Denis G. Rancourt, PhD
© June 2010

Blogsite:
http://activistteacher.blogspot.com/

[T]he majority of politicians, on the evidence available to us, are interested not in truth but in power and in the maintenance of that power. To maintain that power it is essential that people remain in ignorance, that they live in ignorance of the truth, even the truth of their own lives. What surrounds us therefore is a vast tapestry of lies, upon which we feed.

— Harold Pinter, Nobel Lecture (Literature), 2005

The maintenance of the hierarchical structures that control our lives depends on Pinter's "vast tapestry of lies, upon which we feed". Therefore, the main institutions that embed us into the hierarchy, such as schools, universities and mass media and entertainment corporations, have a primary function to create and maintain this tapestry. They include establishment scientists and all service intellectuals in charge of "interpreting" reality.

In fact, the scientists and "experts" define reality in order to bring it into conformity with the always-adapting dominant mental tapestry of the moment. They also invent and build new branches of the tapestry that serve specific power groups by providing new avenues of exploitation. These high priests are rewarded with high class status.

The Money Lie

The economists are a most significant example. It is probably not an accident that in the United States at the end of the 19th century the economists were the first professional analysts to be "broken in" in a battle that defined the limits of academic freedom in universities. The academic system from that point on would impose a strict operational separation between enquiry and theorising as acceptable, and social reform as unacceptable.[1]

Any academic wishing to preserve her position understood what this meant. As a side product, academics became virtuosos at nurturing a self-image of importance, despite this fatal limitation on their societal relevance, with verbiage such as "the truth is our most powerful weapon", "the pen is mightier than the sword", "a good idea can change the world", "reason will take us out of darkness", etc.

So the enterprise of economics became devoted to masking the lie about money. Bad lending practices, price fixing and monopolistic controls were the main threats to the natural justice of a free market, and occurred only as errors in a mostly self-regulating system that could be moderated via adjustments of interest rates and other "safeguards".

Meanwhile, no mainstream economic theory makes any mention of the fact that money itself is created wholesale in a fractional reserve banking system owned by secret private interests given a licence to fabricate and deliver debt that must be paid back (with interest) from the real economy.

thereby continuously concentrating ownership and power over all local and regional economies.

The rest of us have to earn money rather than simply fabricate it, and we never own more when we die. The middle class either pays rent or a mortgage. Wage slavery is perpetuated and further degraded in stable areas and installed in its most vicious varieties in all newly conquered territories.

It is quite remarkable that the largest exploitation scam (private money creation as debt) ever enacted and applied to the entire planet does not figure in economic theories. Economists are so busy modelling the ups and downs of profits, returns, employment figures, stock values and the benefits of mergers for mid-level exploiters that they don't notice their avoidance of the foundational elements. They model the construction schedule while refusing to acknowledge that the terrain is an earthquake zone with vultures circling overhead.

Meanwhile, the financiers write and rewrite the rules themselves, and again this process does not figure in macroeconomic theories. The only human element that economists consider in their "predictive" mathematical models is low-level consumer behaviour, not high-level system manipulation. Corruption is the norm, yet it does not figure. The economies, cultures and infrastructures of nations are wilfully destroyed in order to enslave via new and larger national debts for generations into the future while economists forecast alleged catastrophic consequences of defaulting on these debts...

Management tools for the bosses, and smoke and mirrors for the rest of us: thank you, expert economists.

The only human element that economists consider in their "predictive" mathematical models is low-level consumer behaviour, not high-level system manipulation. Corruption is the norm...

The Medicine-is-Health Lie

We've all heard some medical doctor (MD), interviewed on the radio, gratuitously make the bold proposal that life expectancy has increased thanks to modern medicine. Nothing could be further from the truth.

Life expectancy has increased in First World countries thanks to an historical absence of civil and territorial wars, better and more accessible food, fewer work and non-work accidents and better overall living and working conditions. The single strongest indicator of personal health within and between countries is economic status, irrespective of access to medical technology and pharmaceuticals.

It's worse than that because medicine actually has a negative impact on health. Medical errors (not counting misattributed deaths from correctly administered "treatments") are the third leading cause of death in the US after heart disease and cancer, and there is a large gap between this conservative underestimate in the number of medical error deaths and the fourth leading cause of death.[2] Since medicine can do little for heart disease and cancer, and since medicine has only a small statistically positive impact in the area of trauma interventions, we conclude that public health would increase if all MDs simply disappeared. Think of all the time and stress that sick people would save...

One of the most dangerous places in society is the hospital. Medical errors include misdiagnoses, bad prescriptions, prescriptions for medications that should not be combined, unnecessary surgery and unnecessary or badly administered treatments including chemotherapy, radiotherapy and corrective surgeries.

The lie extends to the myth that MDs anywhere near understand the human body. This well-guarded lie encourages us to put our faith in doctors, thereby opening the door to a well-orchestrated profit bonanza for Big Pharma.

The first thing that Doctors Without Borders (MSF) volunteers need to do in order to contribute significantly in disaster zones is to "forget their medical training" and get to work on the priority tasks at hand: supplying water, food and shelter, and preventing disease propagation—not vaccinating or operating or prescribing medication... Public health comes from safety, stability, social justice and economic buying power, not MRI (magnetic resonance imaging) units and prescription drugs.

Bonehead MDs routinely apply unproven "recommended treatments" and prescribe dangerous drugs for everything from high blood pressure from a sedentary lifestyle and bad nutrition to apathy at school, anxiety in public places, post-adolescence erectile function, non-conventional sleep patterns and all the side effects from the latter drugs. In professional yet nonetheless remarkable reversals of logic, doctors prescribe drugs to remove symptoms that are risk indicators rather than address the causes of the risks, thereby only adding to the assault on the body.

It's unbelievable the number that medicine has done on us: just one more way to keep us stupid (ignorant about our own bodies) and artificially dependent on the control hierarchy. Economically disadvantaged people don't die from not having access to medical "care": they die from the life constraints and liabilities directly resulting from poverty. How many MDs have stated this obvious truth on the radio?

Environmental Science Lies

Exploitation via resource extraction, land use expropriation and wage slavery creation and maintenance is devastating to indigenous populations and to the environment on continental scales. It is therefore vital for the exploiters to cover up their crimes under a veil of expert analysis and policy development diversion. A valued class of service intellectuals here is composed of environmental scientists and consultants.

Environmental scientists naively and knowingly work hand in hand with corporate and finance shysters, mainstream media, politicians, and state and international bureaucrats to mask real problems and to create profit opportunities for select power elites. Here are some notable examples of specific cases.

It is therefore vital for the exploiters to cover up their crimes under a veil of expert analysis and policy development diversion.

• Freon and Ozone

Do you know of anyone who has been killed by the hole in the ozone layer? The 1987 Montreal Protocol banning chlorofluorocarbons (CFCs) is considered a textbook case where science and responsible governance led to a landmark treaty for the benefit of the Earth and all its inhabitants. How often does that happen?

At about the time that the DuPont patent on Freon™—the most widely used CFC refrigerant in the world—was expiring, the mainstream media picked up on otherwise arcane scientific observations and hypotheses about ozone concentration in the upper atmosphere near the poles. There resulted an international mobilisation to criminalise CFCs, and DuPont developed and patented a replacement refrigerant that was promptly certified for use.

A Nobel Prize in Chemistry was awarded in 1995 for a laboratory demonstration that CFCs could deplete ozone in simulated atmospheric conditions. In 2007, it was shown that the latter work may have been seriously flawed by its overestimating the depletion rate by an order of magnitude, thereby invalidating the proposed mechanism for CFC-driven ozone depletion.[3] Not to mention that any laboratory experiment is somewhat different from the actual upper atmosphere... Is the Nobel tainted by media and special-interest lobbying?

It gets better. It turns out that the DuPont replacement refrigerant, not surprisingly, is not as inert as was Freon. As a result, it corrodes refrigerator cycle components at a much faster rate. Where home refrigerators and freezers used to last forever, they now burn out in eight years or so. This has caused catastrophic increases in major appliance contributions to landfill sites across North America, spurred on by the green propaganda for obscenely efficient electrical consumptions of the new appliances under closed-door (zero-use) conditions.

In addition, we have been frenzied into avoiding the sun, the UV index keeps our fear of cancer and our dependence on the medical establishment alive, and a new sunblock industry *à là* vampire protection league has been spawned. Of course, star university chemists are looking for that perfect sunblock molecule that can be patented by Big Pharma. I predict that as soon as it is, there'll be a surge in media interviews with skin cancer experts...

• Acid Rain on Boreal Forest

In the 1970s, it was acid rain. Thousands of scientists from around the world (northern hemisphere) studied this "most pressing environmental problem on the planet". The boreal forest is the largest ecosystem on Earth, and its millions of lakes were reportedly being killed by acid from the sky.

Coal-burning plants spewed out sulphides into the atmosphere, causing the rain to be acidic. The acid rain was postulated to acidify the soils and lakes in the boreal forest, but the acidification was virtually impossible to detect. Pristine lakes in the heart of national parks had to be studied for decades in attempts to detect a statistically significant acidification.

Meanwhile, the lakes and their watersheds were being destroyed by the cottage-building industry, agriculture, forestry, mining, overfishing and tourism. None of the local and regional destruction was studied or exposed. Instead, scientists turned their gaze to distant coal-burning plants and atmospheric distribution, and postulated chemical reactions occurring in rain droplets. One study found that the spawning in aquarium of one fish species was extremely sensitive to acidity. Long treatises about cation charge balance and transport were written, and attention was diverted away from the destruction on the ground towards a sanitised problem of atmospheric chemistry that was the result of industrialisation and progress rather than being caused by identifiable exploiters.

As a physicist and an Earth scientist turned environmental scientist, I personally read virtually every single scientific paper written about acid rain and could not find an example of a demonstrated negative impact on lakes or forests from acid rain. In my opinion, contrary to the repeated claims of the scientist authors, the research on acid rain demonstrates that acid rain could not possibly have been the problem.

This model of elite-forces-coordinated exploiter whitewashing was to play itself out on an even grander scale only decades later with man-made global warming.

• Global Warming as a Threat to Humankind

In February 2007, nearly three years before the November 2009 Climategate scandal burst the media bubble that buoyed public opinion towards acceptance of carbon credits, cap and trade and the associated trillion-dollar finance bonanza which may still come to pass, I exposed the global warming co-optation scam in an essay[4] (as well as in an interview[5] and in earlier essays[6]) that Alexander Cockburn, writing in *The Nation*, called "one of the best essays on greenhouse myth-making from a left perspective".[5]

My essay prompted David F. Noble to research the question and write "The Corporate Climate Coup" to expose how the media embrace followed the finance sector's realisation of the unprecedented potential for revenues that going green could represent.[7]

Introductory paragraphs from my essay "Global Warming: Truth or Dare?"[4] are as follows:

"I also advance that there are strong societal, institutional and psychological motivations for having constructed and for continuing to maintain the myth of a global warming dominant threat (global warming myth, for short). I describe these motivations in terms of the workings of the scientific profession and of the global corporate and finance network and its government shadows.

"I argue that by far the most destructive force on the planet is power-driven financiers and profit-driven corporations and their cartels backed by military might; and that the global warming myth is a red herring that contributes to hiding this truth. In my opinion, activists who, using any justification, feed the global warming myth have effectively been co-opted, or at best neutralised."

Other passages in the essay read this way:

"Environmental scientists and government agencies get funding to study and monitor problems that do not threaten corporate and financial interests. It is therefore no surprise that they would attack continental-scale devastation from resource extraction via the CO_2 back door. The main drawback with this strategy is that you cannot control a hungry monster by asking it not to shit as much."

"Global warming is strictly an imaginary problem of the First World middle class. Nobody else cares about global warming. Exploited factory workers in the Third World don't care about global warming. Depleted uranium genetically mutilated children in Iraq don't care about global warming. Devastated aboriginal populations the world over also can't relate to global warming, except maybe as representing the only solidarity that we might volunteer."

"It's not about limited resources. ["The amount of money spent on pet food in the US and Europe each year equals the additional amount needed to provide basic food and health care for all the people in poor countries, with a sizeable amount left over." (UN *Human Development Report* 1999)] It's about exploitation, oppression, racism, power and greed. Economic, human and animal justice brings economic sustainability which in turn is always based on renewable practices. Recognising the basic rights of native people automatically moderates resource extraction and preserves natural habitats. Not permitting imperialist wars and interventions automatically quenches nation-scale exploitation. True democratic control over monetary policy goes a long way in removing debt-based extortion."

"Recognising the basic rights of native people automatically moderates resource extraction and preserves natural habitats."

The essay is a thorough critique of the science as bandwagon-trumpeting and interested self-deception.[4] Climategate only confirms what should be obvious to any practising scientist: that science is a mafia when it's not simply a sleeping pill.

Conclusion

It just goes on and on. What is not a lie?

Look at the recent H1N1 scam—another textbook example. It's farcical how far these circuses go: antiseptic gels in every doorway at the blink of an eye; high school students getting high from drinking the alcohol in the gels; outdatedness of the viral strain before the pre-paid vaccine can be mass-produced; unproven effectiveness; no requirement to prove effectiveness; government guarantees to corporate manufacturers against client lawsuits; university safety officers teaching students how to cough; etc.

Pure madness. Has something triggered our genetically ingrained First World stupidity reflex? Is this part of our march towards fascism?

Here is another one. Educators promote the lie that we learn because we are taught. This lie of education is squarely denounced by radical educators.[9, 10] University professors design curricula as though the students actually learn every element that is delivered, whereas the

Continued on page 82

Some Big Lies of Money, Medicine and Science

Continued from page 42

truth is that students don't learn the delivered material and everyone only learns what they learn.

One could dramatically change the order in which courses are delivered and it would make no measurable difference in how much students learn. Students deliver nonsense, and professors don't care.

Obedience and indoctrination are all that matter, so the only required skill is bluffing. Students know this and those who do not don't know what they know, don't know themselves.[8,9,10]

Pick any expert opinion or dominant paradigm: it's part of a racket. We can't know the truth because the truth is brutal. ∞

About the Author:

Denis G. Rancourt, PhD, was a tenured and full professor at the University of Ottawa in Canada. He was trained as a physicist and practised physics, Earth sciences and environmental science—areas in which he was funded by a national agency and ran an internationally recognised laboratory. Dr Rancourt has had over 100 articles published in leading scientific journals. He developed popular activism courses and was an outspoken critic of the university administration and a defender of student and Palestinian rights. He was fired for his dissidence in 2009 (see http://www.academicfreedom.ca).

Dr Rancourt can be contacted via his blogsite, http://activistteacher.blogspot.com.

Editor's Note:

Dr Rancourt's article was first published as "Some Big Lies of Science" at http://tinyurl.com/2cq2gqa.

Endnotes

1. Schrecker, Ellen, *No Ivory Tower: McCarthyism and the Universities*, Oxford University Press, 1986
2. Radio interview with Dr Barbara Starfield, CHUO FM 89.1, Ottawa, 21 January 2010, http://trainradio.blogspot.com/2010/01/health-care-in-united-states.html
3. *Nature* 2007; 449:382-383, http://www.nature.com/news/2007/070924/full/449382a.html
4. http://activistteacher.blogspot.com/2007/02/global-warming-truth-or-dare.html; http://climateguy.blogspot.com/
5. Jay, D.O., "Questioning Climate Politics: Denis Rancourt says the 'global warming myth' is part of the problem", interview in *The Dominion*, 11 April 2007, http://www.dominionpaper.ca/articles/1110
6. http://www.counterpunch.org/cockburn06092007.html; http://climateguy.blogspot.com
7. http://activistteacher.blogspot.com/2007/05/dgr-in-my-article-entitled-global.html
8. http://activistteacher.blogspot.com/2010/01/canadian-education-as-impetus-towards.html
9. Freire, Paulo, *Pedagogy of the Oppressed*, Continuum, New York, London, 1970, 1993, 2000
10. Rancière, Jacques, *The Ignorant Schoolmaster*, Stanford University Press, Palo Alto, 1991

82 • NEXUS www.nexusmagazine.com OCTOBER – NOVEMBER 2010

Chapter 4

Bio-Accumulation: Our toxic Harvest

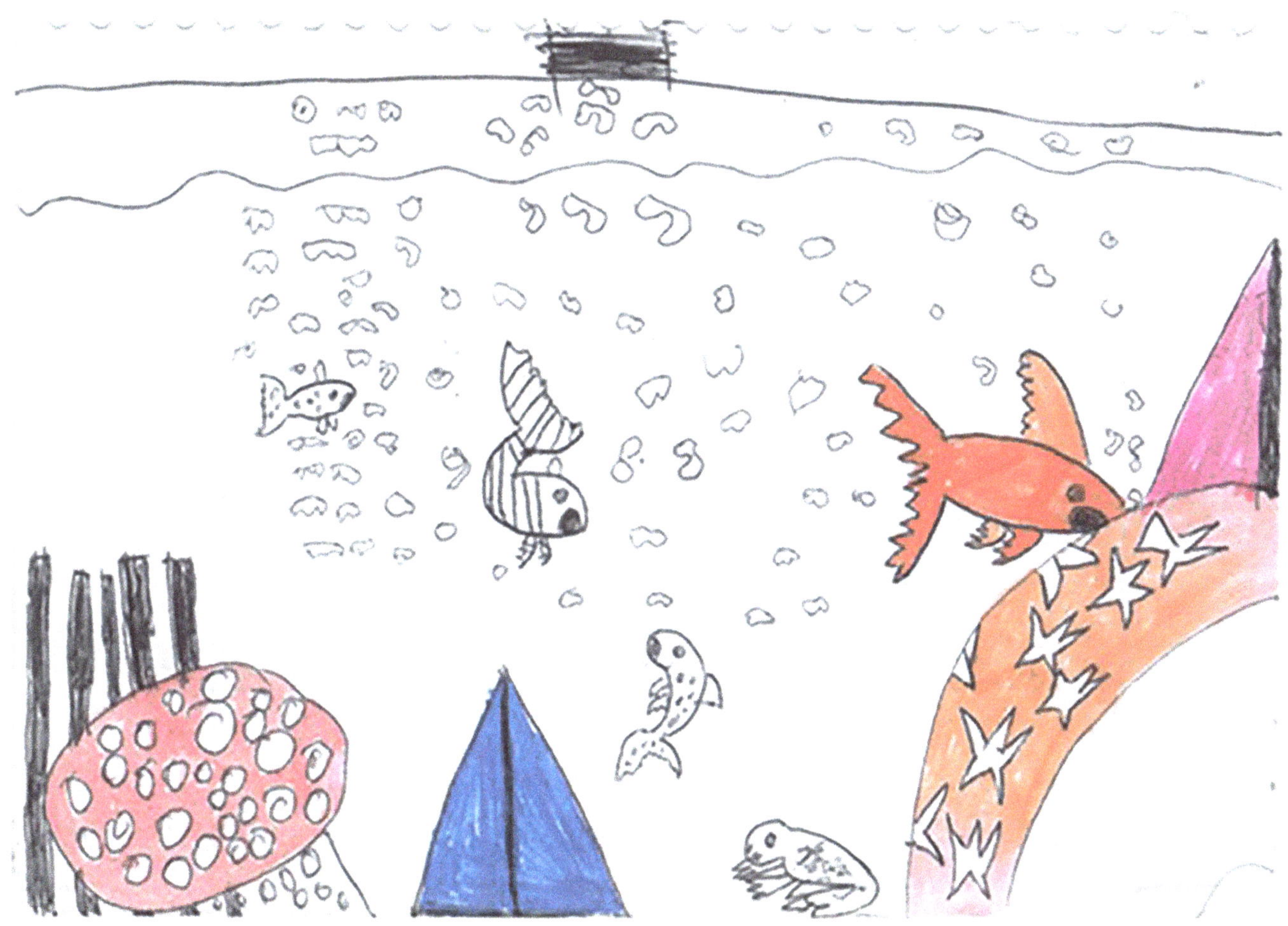

Baby-boomers spray with glee, profits from

Bayer/Monsanto, Merk and DuPont go on a killing spree, of

The whole food chain.

Generating fragmentation, weakness and disease in every family.

Sold as "Progress for your country and the world",

Whole populations now medicated and influenced daily by the domestic screen,

Drinking the sleeping waters,

Drinking water that makes rebellion and discernment sleep, the fluoride sleep of sheep.

To trick a population into poisoning themselves, with complacency consumerism and lies.

'Weed n Feed' products on every lawn, the pill, chemotherapy and medicines flushed down every toilet.

.02-micron filters cannot remove hormones, chemotherapy or steroids, from filling our waterways and fish nurseries.

Human consumption now harming the oceans food chain. Toxic Algae blooms and viruses wipe out

Aquaculture industries... Do the maths on 22 Million Aussies peeing six times per day – Bio accumulation and gob-smacking toxicity!?

The consequence of commercial chemical management of Soil, foods and human biology, is the consequence of politicians sold on a psychopathic economy. Thanks to Monsanto, Bayer, DuPont and Merk to name a few, and your pee, for the family's genetic downfall and the general wellness poverty, across the biosphere.

Reverse the trend? Boycott companies that commit crimes against nature and humanity for product profit.

To give the future a chance at good health...Do it today.

Ask those rich corporations to pay for remedial steam distillation of all urine and liquid human and farm animal waste made toxic by their products.

Find a way to dispose of these surplus products in a way that never again harm our soils, waterways or biology.

Our children's futures and Pesticide/Herbicide use cannot co-exist safely.

So, who is it that deserves popular support? Multinational profits or

Your lifeblood and natural genetics?

Jobs for the big boys, Bayer/ Monsanto/ Dupont directors, CEOs and employees –

Community service… Service back to Nature, to humanity…i.e., steam distillation of your Pee, and micro filter plastics out of the Sea.

Replace all plastics with Hemp products and Nature's balance will be restored, 'harm-free'.

Replace toxic, inefficient chemical medicines with Cannabis Oil, Vitamin C and Herbs,

And Nature's balance will be restored in the human biosphere, 'harm-free'.

Embrace "Small is Beautiful" economies and communities, trade, only in equity beyond self-sufficiency; and consider seven (7) generations hence… for consequence of futures beyond today.

A news announcement in September 2016 chimed that Australia is the world's most allergic Nation…

Our farmers use chemicals and pesticides to fulfil trade agreements of old, now

Agricultural Departments managed law…

Organics rules have been watered down to allow the use of herbicides like systemic Glyphosate used

'routinely' prior to harvest to provide a "Clean Crop Kill".

All the grains and legumes that animals and people consume, have by the nature of systemic poisoning, taken up some of the herbicide used in this way. Could this be the answer to the question of wheat and dairy intolerance that has grown exponentially in the past 40 years?

A Bio-Accumulation and intolerance of natural biology to toxic herbicides, pesticides and fungicides?

Then there is, Compulsory Vaccination with many containing peanut oil, foreign animal proteins, aluminium, mercury and detergent. Add this to a culture that eats sugar rich, plasticized fats, chemically enhanced, coloured, flavoured, rancid, mass produced products… Voila, an Allergy Nation.

A canary for the whole biosphere.

Is it wise, trusting corporate Blathe,

That seeks to make the population a Slave?

Without commercial impetus, herbicides and pesticides would not be used... Full Stop.

Introduced by industrialists with commercial interests in the 1930's to manage biology for efficiency, on larger crops, than ever before were seen. A new global economy was set up to support exploiting business interests of industrialist money... Sold to innocent folks as a service to feed humanity...After the War that was needed to create desperation and less questioning from the herd.

Instead, the new economy, bringing slow destruction to soils and water ways, note the orchardist families of that time were heavily hit by Polio and Cancers, these people were the first users of the new world order chemicals of pest and weed control... These people's genetics damaged, to further a controlling economy.

Monocultures that defy sensibility, fragment natural systems violently, arrogantly... Creating

more pests, more weeds and more degradation of soils and water quality.

Streamlining agriculture created massive profits for a few, while food and mineral deficiencies effect whole generations. This streamlining removed Millet from the human diet, a high nutrilicide alkaline grain that inhibits cancer cells naturally.

High Nutrillicide grains have vitamins B17 and B15, known cancer inhibitors.

In the pursuit of profits and ease, the population has shot itself in the foot, pulled the wool over proverbial eyes. Helping poison manufacturers to control the food supply and production, effectively killing the food chain from the soil up.

The fix? Obvious... Break the cancerous chemical habit and begin again with healthy soil microbes that build carbon and produce mineralized fruit and vegetables, to benefit healthy biology.

Naturally, in harmony with 'all biology'... Look up: 'Natural Korean Farming' practices on YouTube to see, how simple and beneficial it can be.

Look up: Companies supporting regenerative agriculture such as Nutri-Tech Solutions (NTS) in Australia. Soluble seaweeds, soil testing and Wood Smoke Vinegar, replacing herbicides and pesticides, also decreasing the need of chemical fertilizers, by 60% or more.

Emotional and Chemical Bio-Accumulation

The motive of media, propaganda and dogmatic religions in perpetuating emotional controls, is the management of mass emotion to 'divide and conquer'.
Using force; of violence and war as the tool of fear control, to cripple free will.
Creating situations; of dependency and doubt, in self-sustainability.
Fear is a divided place where sensible decisions have no basis.
A population maintained under fears controls, is fractured into dependence, and creativity is stifled.
An un-natural state for human existence and thus some western governments allow Nazi fluoridation, a known neuro-toxin…
Sleeping waters for whole populations, pituitary and hippocampus suppressed, enabling acceptance, of anything… preventing rebellion, from the un-natural economic management of populations.
The benefits: Blind acceptance supports blind consumerism. People are more susceptible to propaganda or advertising.
Creativity beyond fear, this is where 'Nature in Humanity' breaks through the cracks in the concrete pathways to grow again. Beyond fear.
Emotional control dramas over whole populations must end.
Living begins where fear ends.
Choose love now, because you can.
Respect and love bring the harmony, an essential ingredient to life's future.
'Harmony' can be viewed as a harmonic frequency that is brought into focused balance with love and respect.

Sugar and spice and all things nice,

Leukaemia Foundation and Cancer Council
Don't want anyone to think twice.
Chemotherapy Kills our children thrice.
Multi-National products and prejudice,
Infiltrate our education and law,
Removing our choices and making health poor,
See health costs Soar!
Taxpayer dollars supporting a tort,
Toxic Agriculture and Medicine Galore
And Governments ignore
The disaster that befalls us all…

Allowing unelected lobby groups to run the country's show puts an end to diverse futures we could know, in preference for their own monoculture continuance. Does this make good health sense or is it just a perpetuation of a toxic status quo? We allowed the lure of progress and comfort to blind us and our Governments,

We allowed Multi-National Chemical Companies control of our Agriculture, and they
Poisoned our soil and food supply;
We allowed Multi-Nationals to cook for us, and they
Poisoned our bodies and created unbalanced consumption and disease;
We allowed Multi-Nationals control of our Health and Medicine, and they
Poison our children, promote untreatable disease, and begin a war on all natural therapies.
Our system and bodies are overloaded with too much toxic product, in soil, food, medicine and media...
Environment of absorption, to the detriment of discernment and the cost of loved ones lives.
Bring back the senses, bring back sensibility.
Our children are being robbed of diverse experience through the senses, as they are tied to their electronic contraptions too many hours a day.

In dealing with children who have a terminal condition, the one thing that stands out more than anything is how Alive they are when in Nature. They soak up every aspect of sensory delight, the smells, sounds, feel of the breeze on the skin, the warmth of the sun, the sand between the toes and water on the face.... Brings you back to basics and being in the Now!

Gardens of life assist people to come back to their senses and feel alive. The Great Mother is our supplier, regardless of money. Being connected to the local garden, or your own, gives more to the body and soul than any government or other so called service provider.

Every effort you give to the garden is something you later reap, which is a natural energy exchange. The more you give to your garden the healthier and more discerning/sovereign you become.

A Garden gives Life its continuum.
A Government if Not the true servant of a Sovereign people, becomes its oppressor, enslaver and executioner.
A Sovereign backlash is revolution, Thought, Words, Action...
Creativity of desperation and innovation, put on hold to continue the old?
Buying power at Grass Roots level,
A simple and empowering way to put an end to the toxic economy.
Renaissance and creativity ensue.

This too would be the case if Good Governance were employed by our governments, today however, the energy exchange with this man-made-structure is so depleting, and sucks too much out of the poor, while supporting the rich…that engaging in the system today is exhausting, ourselves and our children's futures. A black hole of excuses for progress to only apply where old profits do not suffer, old alliances maintained at the expense of people, kind of Governance.

Government today is more about supporting big business and its endpoint "slavery", and less about service provision and serving sovereign citizens.

A new party The Constitutional Service Party, with a plan of good governance to ensure service supply to the sovereign population, would be a vote winner right now! Existing parties will sell our Australia to foreign interests, allow foreign multinational organisations to provide all our health care and agricultural support. Then when there is no manufacturing or processing in Australia, we will have to import all the things we would have grown ourselves.

Survival tips:

KISS principle to good governance
Provide the services that people pay taxes for….
Encourage innovation and self-sufficiency of our Island Nation
Don't import anything we can make or grow ourselves.
Don't invest in foreign economies without a fair return to the People of our Nation.
Ensure that no business entity or product is above the law of harm reduction, nor above sovereign choice.

The Sacred Temple.

The human body is 'The Sacred Temple' and
No credence should be given to acts of defilement.
The famous healer and wise man Hippocrates clearly stated: First, Do No Harm!

Just a few weeks before it was discovered that Dylan had Leukaemia, we attended the local doctors' clinic for a second round of catch-up vaccinations. The Doctor said, "There was a product recall on the last batch of Polio vaccine that we gave Dylan, so we had better deliver it again, just in case?" I asked why the recall had occurred and he said, "a fault?" he did not know, "perhaps something wrong with that batch? we have a new one now…" One year after Dylan's death someone sent me a copy of a document that had been put up on the Center for Disease Control (CDC) website, it was removed a few days later. The document is an admission of vaccine contamination with an animal virus, the Green Simian Monkey Virus SV40, and this virus which had been said to have contaminated 93million Americans. The virus mutates and becomes blood and bone cancers in some people....!!! Is this why the rate of Acute Lymphoblastic Leukaemia in children has skyrocketed since the 1970's? Is this how my son and other children became ill?

CDC Admits 98 Million Americans Received Polio Vaccine Contaminated With Cancer Virus

CDC Admits 98 Million Americans Received Polio Vaccine Contaminated With Cancer Virus

Jul 17 • Articles, Big Pharma, Vaccines • 1698 Views • 1 Comments
64849 152 687 49 56 Share68376

Vaccine The CDC has quickly removed a page from their website, which is now cached here, admitting that more than 98 million Americans received one or more doses of polio vaccine within an 8-year span when a proportion of the vaccine was contaminated with a cancer-causing polyomavirus called SV40. It has been estimated that 10-30 million Americans could have received an SV40 contaminated dose of the vaccine.

V40 is an abbreviation for Simian vacuolating virus 40 or Simian virus 40, a polyomavirus that is found in both monkeys and humans. Like other polyomaviruses, SV40 is a DNA virus that has been found to cause tumors and cancer.

SV40 is believed to suppress the transcriptional properties of the tumor-suppressing genes in humans through the SV40 Large T-antigen and SV40 Small T-antigen. Mutated genes may contribute to uncontrolled cellular proliferation, leading to cancer.

Michele Carbone, Assistant Professor of Pathology at Loyola University in Chicago, has recently isolated fragments of the SV-40 virus in human bone cancers and in a lethal form of lung cancer called mesothelioma. He found SV-40 in 33% of the osteosarcoma bone cancers studied, in 40% of other bone cancers, and in 60% of the mesotheliomas lung cancers, writes Geraldo Fuentes.

Dr. Michele Carbone openly acknowledged HIV/AIDS was spread by the hepatitis B vaccine produced by Merck & Co. during the early 1970s. It was the first time since the initial transmissions took place in 1972-74, that a leading expert in the field of vaccine manufacturing and testing has openly admitted the Merck & Co. liability for AIDS.

The matter-of-fact disclosure came during discussions of polio vaccines contaminated with SV40 virus which caused cancer in nearly every species infected by injection. Many authorities now admit much, possibly most, of the world's cancers came from the Salk and Sabin polio vaccines, and hepatitis B vaccines, produced in monkeys and chimps.

It is said mesothelioma is a result of asbestos exposure, but research reveals that 50% of the current mesotheliomas being treated no longer occurs due to asbestos but rather the SV-40 virus contained in the polio vaccination. In addition, according to researchers from the Institute of Histology and General Embryology of the University of Ferrara, SV-40 has turned up in a variety other tumors. By the end of 1996, dozens of scientists reported finding SV40 in a variety of bone cancers and a wide range of brain cancers, which had risen 30 percent over the previous 20 years.

The SV-40 virus is now being detected in tumors removed from people never inoculated with the contaminated vaccine, leading some to conclude that those infected by the vaccine might be spreading SV40.

Soon after its discovery, SV40 was identified in the oral form of the polio vaccine produced between 1955 and 1961 produced by American Home Products (dba Lederle).

Both the oral, live virus and injectable inactive virus were affected. It was found later that the technique used to inactivate the polio virus in the injectable vaccine, by means of formaldehyde, did not reliably kill SV40.

Just two years ago, the U.S. government finally added formaldehyde to a list of known carcinogens and admitted that the chemical styrene might cause cancer. Yet, the substance is still found in almost every vaccine.

According to the Australian National Research Council, fewer than 20% but perhaps more than 10% of the general population may be susceptible to formaldehyde and may react acutely at any exposure level. More hazardous than most chemicals in 5 out of 12 ranking systems, on at least 8 federal regulatory lists, it is ranked as one of the most hazardous compounds (worst 10%) to ecosystems and human health (Environmental Defense Fund).

In the body, formaldehyde can cause proteins to irreversibly bind to DNA. Laboratory animals exposed to doses of inhaled formaldehyde over their lifetimes have developed more cancers of the nose and throat than are usual.

Facts Listed on The CDC Website about SV40

- SV40 is a virus found in some species of monkey.
- SV40 was discovered in 1960. Soon afterward, the virus was found in polio vaccine.
- SV40 virus has been found in certain types of cancer in humans.

Additional Facts

- In the 1950s, rhesus monkey kidney cells, which contain SV40 if the animal is infected, were used in preparing polio vaccines.
- Not all doses of IPV were contaminated. It has been estimated that 10-30 million people actually received a vaccine that contained SV40.
- Some evidence suggests that receipt of SV40-contaminated polio vaccine may increase risk of cancer.

A Greater Perspective on Aerial Spraying and SV40

The Defense Sciences Office of the Pathogen Countermeasures Program, in September 23, 1998 funded the University of Michigan's principal investigator, Dr. James Baker, Jr. Dr. Baker, Director of Michigan Nanotechnology Institute for Medicine and Biological Sciences under several DARPA grants. Dr. Baker developed and focused on preventing pathogens from entering the human body, which is a major goal in the development of counter measures to Biological Warfare. This research project sought to develop a composite material that will serve as a pathogen avoidance barrier and post-exposure therapeutic agent to be applied in a topical manner to the skin and mucous membranes. The composite is modelled after the immune system in that it involves redundant, non-specific and specific forms of pathogen defense and inactivation. This composite material is now utilized in many nasal vaccines and vector control through the use of hydro-gel, nanosilicon gels and actuator materials in vaccines.

Through Dr. Baker's research at the University of Michigan; he developed dendritic polymers and their application to medical and biological science. He co-developed a new vector system for gene transfer using synthetic polymers. These studies have produced striking results and have the potential to change the basis of gene transfer therapy. Dendrimers are nanometre-sized water-soluble polymers that can conjugate to peptides or carbohydrates to act as decoy molecules to inhibit the binding of toxins and viruses to cells. They can act also as complex and stabilize genetic material for prolonged periods of time, as in a "time released or delayed gene transfer". Through Dr. Baker's ground-breaking research many pharmaceutical and biological pesticide manufacturers can use these principles in DNA vaccines specific applications that incorporate the Simian Monkey Virus SV40.

WEST NILE VIRUS SPRAYING

In 2006 Michael Greenwood wrote an article for the Yale School of Public Health entitled, "Aerial Spraying Effectively Reduces Incidence of West Nile Virus (WNV) in Humans." The article stated that the incidence of human West Nile virus cases can be significantly reduced through large scale aerial spraying that targets adult mosquitoes, according to research by the Yale School of Public Health and the California Department of Public Health.

Under the mandate for aerial spraying for specific vectors that pose a threat to human health, aerial vaccines known as DNA Vaccine Enhancements and Recombinant Vaccine against WNV may be tested or used to "protect" the people from vector infection exposures. DNA vaccine enhancements specifically use Epstein-Barr viral capsid's with multi human complement class II activators to neutralize antibodies. The recombinant vaccines against WNV use Rabbit Beta-globulin or the poly (A) signal of the SV40 virus. In early studies of DNA vaccines, it was found that the negative result studies would go into the category of future developmental research projects in gene therapy. During the studies of poly (A) signalling of the SV40 for WNV vaccines, it was observed that WNV will lie dormant in individuals who were exposed to chicken pox, thus upon exposure to WNV aerial vaccines the potential for the release of chicken pox virus would cause a greater risk to having adult-onset Shingles.

CALIFORNIA AERIAL SPRAYING for WNV and SV40

In February 2009 to present date, aerial spraying for the WNV occurred in major cities within the State of California. During spraying of Anaheim, CA a Caucasian female (age 50) was exposed to heavy spraying, while doing her daily exercise of walking several miles. Heavy helicopter activity occurred for several days in this area. After spraying, she experienced light headedness, nausea, muscle aches and increased low back pain. She was evaluated for toxicological mechanisms that were associated with pesticide exposure due to aerial spraying utilizing advanced biological monitoring testing. The test results which included protein band testing utilizing Protein Coupled Response (PCR) methods were positive for KD-45. KD-45 is the protein band for SV-40 Simian Green Monkey virus. Additional tests were performed for Epstein-Barr virus capside and Cytomeglia virus which are used in bioengineering for gene delivery systems through viral protein envelope and adenoviral protein envelope technology. The individual was positive for both; indicating a highly probable exposure to a DNA vaccination delivery system through nasal inhalation.

The question of the century is how many other viruses and toxins are within current day vaccines that we'll only find out about in a few decades?

Dave Mihalovic is a Naturopathic Doctor who specializes in vaccine research, cancer prevention and a natural approach to treatment.

Another angle:

Dr William Thompson exposing corruption of the Center for Disease Control (CDC)

(NaturalNews) Donald Trump is no stranger to controversy, including the vaccine debate. In a series of tweets and interviews over the past few years, the presidential candidate has stated that he strongly believes that there is a link between "monstrous" vaccines and autism. He has suggested that delivering vaccines in smaller doses over time could reduce autism rates among U.S. children. Despite being cast to the lunatic fringe by the mainstream media for his remarks, CDC scientist Dr. William Thompson has confirmed Trump's suspicions — namely, that the link between vaccines and autism is real.

Congressman Bill Posey from Florida helped expose the corruption of the Center for Disease Control (CDC). He recently read a statement on the House floor written by CDC scientist Dr. William Thompson. In the statement, Dr. Thompson admitted to omitting data from a study which showed that autism rates were higher among African American boys who received the MMR vaccination before the age of three. (1)

"Regardless of the subject matter, parents making decisions about their children's health deserve to have the best information available to them. They should be able to count on federal agencies to tell them the truth. For these reasons, I bring the following matter to the House floor," Posey stated. (2)

He then proceeded to read the statement provided by Dr. Thompson. The statement pertained to a 2004 study published in The Journal of Pediatrics. The doctor revealed that he and his colleagues intentionally destroyed data in the study which showed that African American MMR-vaccinated boys under the age of three had a 340 percent increased risk for autism. According to the whistle-blower, the CDC held a meeting of scientists to discuss whether they should destroy the evidence. The authors decided to scrap their findings. Fortunately, Dr. Thompson saved computer files and hard copies of the omitted data for legal reasons. (3)

"Mr. Speaker, I believe it is our duty to ensure that the documents that Dr. Thompson is presenting are not ignored. Therefore, I will provide them to members of Congress and the House Committees upon request. Considering the nature of the whistle-blower's documents as well as the involvement of the CDC, a hearing and a thorough investigation is warranted," Posey concluded. (2)

Because the report pertains to vaccines, the mainstream media continues to ignore these revelations. Meanwhile, they continue to parade Donald Trump as a kook for suggesting that there is a link between vaccines and autism. The double standard boggles the mind and sickens the stomach.

Trump hasn't backed down from the vaccine debate despite the mainstream media's backlash against his remarks. In 2015, he appeared on the conservative radio host Laura Ingraham's show stating, "I've known people that had totally magnificent children, functioning a hundred percent, everything beautiful, smart as a whip, and they go for this shot and get this shot of this massive dose, of everything at one time, and they end up with horrible autism."(4)

In addition, Trump stated on a Fox News television program in 2012, "I've seen people where they have a perfectly healthy child, and they go for the vaccinations and a month later the child is no longer healthy."(5)

Trump made similar remarks in a series of tweets in 2014, after a CDC report revealed that autism rates in U.S. children had increased by 30 percent in the last two years. (6)

The CDC report that coincided with Trump's tweets did not actually state what caused the spike in autism rates. Given Dr. Thompson's recent testimony, however, it's easy to think of at least one possibility.

(NaturalNews)

So, what is all the drama about, all the propaganda, all the worlds advertising...?

Directing your choices where, the World's Biggest Psychopath wants them?

The path to world peace and harmony for all, is in choosing products that do not support the economies of Weapons manufacturers, of weapons that are solely for human destruction, nor economies of past wars like, Radiation and Chemotherapy as harmful Medicine, and harmful toxins in agriculture.

Powerful industries and lobby groups seek to control the choices made by Farmers, in relation to what they use on soil and crops, and Doctors in relation to what goes into our bodies.

The job of CODEX Big Agro/Big Pharma chemical companies is to attend trade meetings and influence the managers of Soil and Health in every country. This multi-national group are responsible for selling China Agricultural Chemicals that were banned by 170 other countries, confirmed carcinogenic, and consumers in the West buy fruit and vegetables grown with banned hazardous chemicals dumped by Codex into China at a dollar profit then and health cost later.

Saving our children from the World's Biggest Psychopath, involves **re-engaging personal discernment** and responsibility, something that is given away by allowing outside influences to control your focus.

The Job of Television is to control your focus, hold your attention, with images and emotion. Fear and Guilt are hard core motivators, while sex and desire for good things is more subtle but a potent tool.

Our love of products and convenience has been used as a weapon by a system of economics that profits from dependency in a sick cycle of conflict and chemical enslavement to ensure the status quo never ends.

When Walter Nelson-Rees died in January 2009 at age eighty, Hooper wrote a moving obituary entitled "The Death of an American Hero" (available at www.aidsorigins.com). Hooper recalls: "Walter delivered an understated and yet powerful speech entitled 'Responsibility for Truth in Research', which pointed out that further cases of lab cross-contamination were still occurring, and went on to state that in his opinion there was no logical reason why chimp cells could not have been used to make the Congo vaccine, 'given the availability of these normal non-human cells and the prevailing custom in the 1950s of using cells about which little or nothing was known except that they could optimally support the growth of a given virus'."

The idea of man-made AIDS and contaminated vaccines is so explosive that it is routinely dismissed by the major media as "conspiracy theory". But the theory almost destroyed Barack Obama's bid for the White House in the 2008 election.

A Wikipedia entry on Dr Leonard Horowitz states: "On April 27, 2008, Barack Obama's former pastor, Jeremiah Wright, during questions and answers at the National Press Club in connection with the general controversy over his opinions, was asked by a moderator, 'In your sermon, you said the government lied about inventing the HIV virus as a means of genocide against people of color. So I ask you: Do you honestly believe your statement and those words?' Wright responded, 'Have you read Horowitz's book, *Emerging Viruses: AIDS and Ebola* ... whoever wrote that question?... I read different things. As I said to my members, if you haven't read things, then you can't ... based on this Tuskegee experiment and based on what has happened to Africans in this country, I believe our government is capable of doing anything."

For more discussion, view my article "Rev. Wright is right about man-made AIDS".

Due to their ability to replicate indefinitely... immortal HeLa cells are now considered by some geneticists to be a contemporary creation of a new species.

The creation of a new species

Due to their ability to replicate indefinitely (provided they are fed properly) and the development of a non-human number of chromosomes, immortal HeLa cells are now considered by some geneticists to be a contemporary creation of a new species. (A human cell has 46 chromosomes; a HeLa cell has a chromosomal number of 82.) The proposed name is *Helacyton gartleri*, in honour of geneticist Stanley Gartler, PhD, who, along with Nelson-Rees, called attention to the worldwide contamination of tissue cell cultures with HeLa.

Transformed by the cervical cancer–causing human papilloma virus 18 and more than 50 years of continuing culture, the various strains of Henrietta's cells reproduce and spread on their own. Growing like weeds in many labs, they now appear more like amoeba-type cells than cells derived from a human. Amoebae are one-celled protozoa. There are several varieties found in humans that are not considered to be disease producers.

Twenty years ago, in *The Cancer Microbe*, I wrote about Wilhelm Reich, MD, the unfairly maligned and persecuted cancer researcher who was sentenced to a Federal penitentiary in February 1957...and was found dead in his cell on 3 November that year. He firmly believed that cancer is intimately associated with bacteria, which he called "T-bacilli". In cancer tumours artificially produced in animals, Reich observed the animal's cancer cells transforming into monster cells that greatly resemble tiny protozoa and amoebae.

Reich, in his time, was widely perceived as a menace and a crackpot. However, I'm sure he would not be surprised to learn that Henrietta's cancer cells have taken on a life of their own, much like the amoebae that he studied extensively.

The lab creation of new forms of life has not escaped the attention of the military, always on the lookout for potential agents useful for biological warfare development. The Defense Advanced Research Projects Agency (DARPA) is an arm of the US Department of Defense. On 5 February 2010, Katie Drummond of Wired.com reported: "The Pentagon's mad science arm may have come up with its most radical project yet. Darpa is looking to re-write the laws of evolution to the military's advantage by creating 'synthetic organisms' that can live forever...

"...The plan would assemble the latest bio-tech knowledge to come up with living, breathing creatures that are genetically engineered to 'produce the intended biological effect'. Darpa wants the organisms to be fortified with molecules that bolster cell resistance to death, so that the lab-monsters can 'ultimately be programmed to live indefinitely'."

Henrietta Lacks: "The Godmother of Virology"

At the end of January 2010, reviews began to appear of a new book entitled *The Immortal Life of Henrietta Lacks*, by Rebecca Skloot. The author spent 10 years researching the billion-dollar industry surrounding HeLa cells and extensively interviewed surviving family members. Lacks's family did not learn of Henrietta's "immortality" until more than 20 years after her death, when scientists investigating HeLa began using her husband and children in research without informed consent. And though the cells have launched a multibillion-dollar industry that sells human biological materials, her family never saw any of the profits.

Eric Roston, reviewer for the *Washington Post* (31 January 2010), noted: "Nearly 60 years later, Lacks's tissue has yielded an estimated 50 million metric tons of HeLa cells. Scientific and medical researchers add about 300 HeLa-related studies a month to the library of 60,000 studies. Lacks's surviving family members have learned what was going on—and have become subjects of interest for researchers, too."

In a *New York Times* review (5 February 2010), Lisa Margonelli wrote: "After Henrietta Lacks's death, HeLa went viral, so to speak, becoming the godmother of virology and then biotech, benefiting practically anyone who's ever taken a pill stronger than aspirin... HeLa has helped build thousands of careers, not to mention more than 60,000 scientific studies, with nearly 10 more being published every day, revealing the secrets of everything from aging and cancer to mosquito mating and the cellular effects of working in sewers. 'Deborah [Henrietta's daughter] becomes the book's driving force, as Skloot joins her in her 'lifelong struggle to make peace with the existence of those cells, and the science that made them possible'. To find the mother she never got to know, she read hundreds of articles about HeLa research, which led her to believe that her mother was 'eternally suffering' from all the experiments performed on her cells."

To use HeLa cells as a foundation, a cornerstone, a template, upon which to base viral studies strikes me as viral voodoo.

Horizontal gene transfer: gene swapping among life-forms

While HeLa cells were spreading around the world and contaminating cell cultures, there was little appreciation of how life-forms related to one another. Scientists now have a better knowledge of how viruses can "recombine" with other viruses. Viruses can also infect bacteria as well as human cells.

Over the past two decades, molecular scientists have become more and more aware of the back and forth gene-swapping between and among various species of life, from the smallest forms up to the largest. The process is known as "horizontal gene transfer". We are familiar with "vertical gene transfer", whereby the offspring of an organism inherits genes from its parent.

Horizontal gene transfer in cancer and vaccine research is a serious hazard because genetic engineering experiments allow the spread of dangerous transgenic DNA from species to species. This has tremendous implications for theories of evolution, as well as for cancer virus research when viruses are moved between various species of animals and sometimes adapted to human cells. This is basically what scientists were doing in the War on Cancer throughout the 1970s, the period right before the AIDS epidemic erupted in 1981 (see my book *AIDS and the Doctors of Death*). For more information, simply Google the key words "dangerous lateral gene transfer".

HeLa cell research: science or scientific madness?

Having graduated from medical school a half-century ago, I am disillusioned with my chosen profession. I spent 40 years researching the bacterial cause of cancer and showing bacteria in cancer tissue, where, according to the cancer experts, there aren't supposed to be any. This research sparked little, if any, interest among my colleagues. I spent a quarter-century trying to alert people to the evidence that AIDS is a man-made disease, with no response from the AIDS experts who educate people about HIV coming out of the African jungle to cause AIDS.

What do I really think about HeLa cells? HeLa cells are cancerous cells (infected with a known cancer-causing papilloma virus) to which was added the blood from a human placenta, ground-up beef cattle embryo and chicken plasma extracted from the blood of a live chicken heart. This is a concoction that I would expect from someone practising witchcraft, not good science. To use HeLa cells as a foundation, a cornerstone, a template, upon which to base viral studies strikes me as viral voodoo.

How can an infected cell culture like HeLa possibly help in cancer and vaccine research? Except to spread the known and unknown viruses, mycoplasma, bacteria and God only knows what other potentially infectious agents are contained within Henrietta's cells and the new species *Helacyton gartleri*.

The legacy of Henrietta Lacks

In all my research for this article, the one bit of reading that made more sense to me than any other was provided by an anonymous blogger who posted comments on the *Baltimore Sun* website (1 February 2010; reproduced here with minor editing) regarding Rebecca Skloot's new book:

"A complete and total injustice was done to her family to obtain these cells, and now some crazy cancer cells that KILLED her are IN US ALL. That's right: if you have ever gotten a vaccine, you got a little HeLa in you.

Continued on page 80

Immortal HeLa Cells and Viral Voodoo

Continued from page 30

"The cancer killed her, and, anyway, these are not normal cells, they are CANCER CELLS; and if you ask a science dude HOW OR WHY her cells are STILL ALIVE, they don't know, but they kept it a secret because at the time whites would have objected to having cancer cells that killed a black woman INJECTED INTO THEIR CHILDREN'S BODIES. I am an African-American; to me, her story is fascinating and tragic, like many stories of people who have been ripped off.

"Look at it this way: if her family had to be paid every time her cells were used, there would be some record of who got them. The rates for cancer have gone through the roof in the last 40 years, her cells have been found in places where it was impossible for them to have been—and still the scientists do not know why her cells are 'immortal'...

"If her family had been informed, possibly more care would have been taken with these cells that KILLED THEIR MOTHER, and, for all we know, could be killing people now because we don't know how they work."

Postscript:

There is an excellent free video available on the Internet entitled *The Way of All Flesh*, produced by British television documentarian Adam Curtis. It tells the story of Henrietta Lacks as the "woman who will never die".

The film received the Golden Gate Award at the 1997 San Francisco International Film Festival.

HeLa cell research helped influence and originate US President Richard Nixon's War on Cancer, eventually causing chaos between American and Russian virologists during the Cold War in the 1970s when widespread laboratory contamination with HeLa was discovered.

The video is available at the web page http://video.google.fr/videoplay?docid=8448974573505946013#. ∞

About the Author:

Alan Cantwell, MD, is a retired dermatologist and a cancer and AIDS researcher. His books include: *The Cancer Microbe: The Hidden Killer in Cancer, AIDS, and other Immune Diseases*; *Four Women Against Cancer*; *AIDS and The Doctors of Death*; and *Queer Blood* (all available from http://www.ariesrisingpress.com, Amazon.com and Book Clearing House [tel 1800 431 1579] in the USA).

Dr Cantwell's previous articles in NEXUS are "Bacteria in Stroke and Heart Disease" (vol. 16, no. 5; also see Letters in vol. 17, no. 2), "The Prostate Cancer Bacterial Connection" (vol. 16, no. 3) and "Do Tuberculosis-Type Bacteria Cause AIDS?" (vol. 15, no. 5).

Dr Cantwell can be contacted by email at alancantwell@sbcglobal.net and via his website http://www.ariesrisingpress.com.

"From The Forensic Nurse – RACHEL CELLER RN

Speaking about the MRC5 Cell Line – Human Diploids – Immortal Cells = Cancer

Found in MMR, Polio, Rubella and Chickenpox, lab-based inoculant concoctions.

Identifying lab v*ccines with medical witchcraft. First published Nov 2019.

https://www.bitchute.com/video/V4YsEY96FHWn/

OR The Forensic Nurse.org

http://humansarefree.com/2018

Doctors Against Vaccines – Hear From Those Who Have Done the Research."

The Age of Mass Consequence.

Carried by the 'Aversion' reaction of poverty and the lack of
Awareness in Baby Boomer choices,
The industrialists delivered with glee
Products and profits in the new economy of
Convenience and ease.
A shift from slaves to enslavement of the workforce,
Progress delivers the mass production economy to new shores.
Propaganda and marketing cleverly lull humans into consumer enslavement.
Fear and desire the new economy's emotional tweaks.
Hungry consumers buy, buy, buy,
Obsolescence replaces Quality in
Profit making stakes of
Waste, waste, waste.
The mass consequence of DuPont investments,
Oceans and soils filled with plastic, micro and macro,
Inhibiters of healthy electrical charge essential in
cellular communication when consumed by biology.
The mass consequence of Monsanto's Glyphosate,
Killer of healthy soil biology, plants and linked with digestive disease and cancers,
Used as a clean crop kill, this systemic poison, goes into legumes and grains.
Is there a link between, glyphosate and the mass gluten intolerances and dairy intolerances?
Technology is delayed by companies that profit from Crude Oil, and
The war racket bleeds humanity, while weapons manufactures legally profit from
Civil toil and destruction, as well as, mobile phones, fridges and 'Life's Good' promotions.
Where ever war goes, the WHO follows bringing profits from disease-population-control, with
Vaccines paid for by the Richest families, publically intent on reducing populations...
Like kids in the candy shop
Baby boomers have consumed too much, made a big mess and
The next generation is standing at the door, with
Hands on hips and tears in the eyes...Foot tapping!?
What have you done, and what is left?!
Point the finger as did Sir John Maynard Keynes, make the industrialists
Clean up the mess, DuPont, Monsanto and Westinghouse, Rothschilds and Rockefellers,
Whom have profited over many decades, profited on resources that were the Future's, but

They took ownership anyway… Shareholder profits, their God.
Custodianship would have been less profitable at the time, but at least future generations are catered for more richly.
Crimes against humanity, not just with guns and poisons but
Consumerism and convenience, gone mad.
Compensation and class actions will
Clean up the profit margin, made at the futures expense.
Chin Chin and Tally Ho 'Old Boys',
Its time to GO!
You who have brought madness and excess to the limit…
Redress.

The economics of Fear cries, Vaccinate, Vaccinate.

A pathway away from normal childhood disease… ?
Dr Robert Mendelsohn, of "Confessions of a Medical Heretic" state that
The injectable procession is towards, 'untreatable' disease of "Toxic Overload"…
Cancer, Auto-Immune disorders and Autism… Hmm
Safe levels of Mercury (thimerosal), Aluminum Nano particles, foreign proteins, pesticides, herbicides, bromine contamination, NIL 0%... No Safe Levels.
Be Wise to Disease.
Most can be managed Naturally.
-Allow Doctor education to come from outside Big Poison/Pharma product guidelines…
-Allow Citizens to say "No Thanks" to toxic chemical management… If they wish.
-Protect future genetics from Reverse Engineering.

Chapter 5

Suppression Propaganda and Social License

"When you confront professional elites with alternative possibilities of 'harm free' or 'low profit', and are met with 'stonewalling', there is always a reason. Whether personal or professional insecurity or contract obligations pre-agreed, there is always something other than 'facts' influencing. Only ones committed to healing are willing to ask different questions, take different paths, from the toxic inheritance that wants to last and last."
- Dylan Inspired quote

In 2006 I was writing an article for the New Scientist magazine asking where has all the good technology gone? I chose a medical discovery to highlight my query. In the mid 1990's Medical researchers at the Alfred Einstein Medical School in New York announced a breakthrough in the treatment of the Aids virus. Drs Kaali and Lyman had patented 14 devices that, surgically implanted could clean the blood of patients with the virus. Their discovery was monumental in understanding boundaries of pathogens and the human cell.

What they found was that healthy human cells could withstand electrical current up to 100,000 times more than any virus or pathogen. They used micro ampules of electricity on the radial and ulna pulse points in a biphasic manner to successfully clean the blood of pathogens. This understanding of limits of cell wall strength, within healthy human cells, versus virus and bacteria enabled them to kill and immobilise many pathogens in vitro, including Epstein-barr, Ebola, and HIV, leading to their development of devices for implantation into patients. At this time in history, Bill Clinton was president and the Clinton family invested heavily in the pharmaceutical economy. It was with Mr Clinton's announcement of 3-Million-dollar injection to 'manage' HIV with pharmaceuticals that Kaali and Lyman's research was made to disappear. Only a retired navy physicist, Dr Robert Beck, kept the research going and he developed external devices to mimic the original patents delivery of micro ampules of electricity using a 9-volt battery (For more information see: www.toolsforhealing.com). Dr Beck could not believe that such a beneficial medical breakthrough could be hidden from the public need, in favour of not so successful chemical 'management' of HIV. Most sane, non-pharmaceutical investor people would agree.

In 2006 with the N1H1 bird flu pandemic being discussed as a problem, and common knowledge that antibiotics are for bacterial infections and have zero effectiveness on any virus, I thought it pertinent to write about where this potentially 'life saving' technology got swept to and why not resuscitate it?

I sent my article to the much loved, popular scientist, in Australia, thinking that his mind would be immediately impressed by the possibilities. His reply to my question of his supportive thinking were a complete and transformative surprise to me.

Not a reply by email pointing out any errors but a personal phone call, after-hours.

Far from supportive of the information I had found and wanted to write about, Dr K sounded fearful and overly insistent that I not write such an article. I spoke briefly of benefits given antibiotics were ineffective against viruses and he blurted about the fabulous history of antibiotics (irrelevant) and dangers of frequencies (now he supports 5G), and that I would need to be peer reviewed before writing an article about Drs Lyman and Kaali's discoveries, their invention and its medical implications? So many writers and journalist write about new scientific innovations, why was this one so different?

Was he telling me that I needed social license from some approved university to enable critical thinking? Was this a form of social tailoring of acceptable scientific thought, policing? I was more than a little unsatisfied with Dr K's unscientific approach to the information presented to him.

"The most dangerous man, to any government, is the man who is able to think things out for himself, without regard to the prevailing superstitions and taboos. Almost invariably he concludes that the government he lives under is dishonest, insane and intolerable, and so, if he is romantic, he tries to change it. And if he is not romantic personally, he is apt to spread discontent among those who are."
Henry Louis Mencken

A few years have passed, and it has been noted that Dr K is a powerful social influencer that inspired a spot of poetry.

Dr Popular, the indoctrinated.

He wrote a Facebook statement:

"There are not always two sides to an argument,

The Earth goes around the Sun, Humans are the cause of climate change and vaccines are overwhelmingly safe."

Hmm, the first statement is the obvious,

The second statement, the subject of conjecture and partial truths, and

The third statement is a trust manipulation to make a fool of questioning?

Scientific?

A truer statement may have been:

- The Nature of Climate is change.
- The Nature of Man's economy is callous exploitation and pollution… Wasteful obsolescence focused consumerism, ease replacing skill. Dependence encouraged by a sycophantic system, the keeper of herd mentality, of war and economy.
- The Nature of medicine is ignorance and arrogant economic protectionism, making natural remedies enemies… If this were not the case, there would be more 'Cures' than 'Foundations'.

If there were suppressed evidence, as has been seen, this affable showbiz professional spokesperson, may be the last to know.

If you want insight into the science straight from the researcher's mouth, see Dr Judy Mikovits interview, 11/22/2015, https://vimeo.com/146831570, and the subsequent CDC confessions of her boss, Dr William Thompson in front of Congress 2016.

Providing 'evidence' that fraud exists in disease 'management', internationally.

In 2018 3 Billion Dollars US, was paid out to victims of Iatrogenic injury… the inoculant products of compulsory acquisition were legally termed "Unavoidably Unsafe".

Think of the economic consequence of this being publicly known in Australia?

Brings understanding to public figure statements that seek to render 'Questioning' foolish.

Trusting mass production of anything is unwise,

Being prevented from questioning or discussing modalities, is 'Corruption', an economic priesthood maintains, against civil liberties and diverse genetics.

In Agriculture or Medicine, the monoculture favouritism is a blight on Life.

Heavily marketing 'fear of disease' is economic exploitation of the ignorant, for product consumption.

With insurance companies like these, who needs enemies?

"I'll take my chances with disease."

A phrase used by Dr Mendelsohn, author of 'Confessions of a medical Heretic'

A practical perspective and information on the safe management of normal childhood disease....

Another corruption eye-opener is the work of Dr Viera Scheibner, author of 'Vaccination 100 years of Orthodox Research shows that Vaccines Represent a Medical Assault of the Immune System'. The book published in 1993, was made unavailable at the time 'industry' was paying politicians to bring in the red-carpet investor-protector, the compulsory vaccination register legislation.

Or the brilliant Dr Suzanne Humphries, discussing research on Vitamin C therapy, including many Pub Med references, yet she was banned from speaking in Australia, no Visa allowed? (See the link in the "helpful links" section at the end of this book and also the lecture notes I took from attending this lecture, in appendix 1)

Suppression of information supports existing economic structures, rarely does suppression of information support 'The People'.

So, are you condoning the suppression of evidence Dr Popular? Is this the science advocate telling people, what to think, rather than educating on how to think?

As a science pin-up-boy and influencer, silencing critical thinking with social license? Has he just overstepped ethics of sovereignty of choice to support the commercially profitable status quo? A herding?

Are you aware of the international fraud admitted and committed by the CDC, Centre for Disease Control?

The 4-year legal injunction to 'gag' Dr Judy Mikovits, ended in 2015, hence her Vimeo video of 11/22/2015.

2016 and the Chief Researcher Dr William Thompson of the CDC, tables 100,000 documents in Congress as Admission of fraud and fault.

Findings were the MMR vaccine posed a health risk to many…Auto immune disease, Cancer, Autism.

Toxic overload and Toxic Harvest with Iatrogenic Injury, occurring in a known 6% of the population, with African American rates much higher.

Gee, I wonder why none of this information was permitted to 'Air' in Australia?!

Perhaps something to do with injury payouts and compulsory laws, or the huge ownership and investment of some politicians, in the vaccine industry?

The National Disability Insurance Scheme (NDIS) should take care of everything that industry won't, including responsibility? Is the NDIS being used as a scapegoat for ethics and faulty products in industry?

Do they feel it better to damage a percentage of the population, rather than support sovereign choice in medicine – Oops – Vaccines are not "Classified" as Medicine, which is how none of the important controls, and lengthy trials, apply to these 'Immune Modulating Products', owned by big business operatives.

"Why is it so?" That Dr Fiona Wood's discovery with skin spray is kept away from public use, but vaccines get immediate approval and a red-carpet investment once accepted for Australia's Compulsory Register?

Conscription by Prescription and no "control" has been allowed? (A control is an un-inoculated portion/group that would allow scientific comparative analysis).

So, it must be about money and unhealthy "control", hence the fear and removal of civil liberty, of choice.

Dr Judy stated clearly that immune suppressed populations should be avoiding vaccinations, these are, babies, adolescents, pregnant women and the elderly. Poly sorbate 80 is a detergent used to open the blood brain barrier, mycerinol is mercury and a known neurotoxin of no safe limits, peanut oil is used as a base, noticed any increase in peanut sensitivity?

Foreign proteins derived from animals are used and linked with an increase in auto immune diseases and some cancers.

Dr Judy referred to the cocktail of too many and too much as having a 'de-engineering' effect on DNA.

That is pretty serious statement from someone committed to many years of research at the CDC.

She also states that it is vaccinated children that 'gas off' the disease in the 10 days following vaccination, that pose a risk to the unvaccinated, not the other way around...

How can a non-vaccinated child infect a vaccinated child if vaccination is a protection?

How is it that researchers find that 80% of all outbreaks occur in fully vaccinated populations?

Dr Viera Scheibner published her independent "findings" in the 1990's that spoke of these 'products', as being an assault on the immune system. Her book has not been made available to GP's or the Doctor Curriculum? WHY?

Politician/Dr Ian Wooldridge was paid $600,000 AU to bring in the 'Compulsory Vaccination Register', by vaccine manufacturers and investors in 1990's… WHY? No Public vote, to remove sovereign choice?

Like animals on the farm.

So, while some fine citizens are struggling to get 'Truth redressed', printed or reported on, speaker's Visas for international immunologists wishing to enter Australia, have been banned. Clearly a control drama upon information that does not fit with the economic plan, is active.

Other influencers, may be likable characters, but are asking you to 'look the other way', or

Don't question, the toxic overload forced upon whole populations?

He is the one given 'social license', that is business as usual…

Not justice, not the truth of the whistle-blower.

Naked Truth, her clothes stolen, is a nineteenth century painting called "Truth Wears No Clothes".

Powerbrokers, liars and exploiters have taken her clothes and wear them to pretend, thus perpetuate power.

Truth may remain hidden, but it will be set free, always, eventually.

The naked truth may be a shock to many…

This is not Anti-vax, this is Constitutional Pro-Choice, supporting diverse genetics of diverse peoples' and human sovereignty.

Val's Story

Val was 73 years old when diagnosed with Aggressive Limbic Carcinoma of both breasts in 2013 and given just 4 months to live.

Val was given information on standard treatment options, of aggressive chemotherapy, radiation and surgery, which were strenuously recommended by her Doctor at the time.

After discussions with family Val decided to try her luck with Cannabis oil.

Val suffered none of the debilitating health conditions evolving from chemotherapy, radiation or surgery.

Val had 1 gram of oil per day for 2 months.

In 2014 Val was hospitalized for food poisoning and the attending Doctor seeing Val had a previous diagnosis of cancer, dosed her with multiple opiates, believing her to be riddled with cancer.

Val's health decline was frighteningly rapid on opiates. Upon removal of all opiates, Val rapidly recovered to full functionality, mobility and mental discernment.

Val's medical scans at that time revealed, NO Cancer of the bone, brain or blood and no aggressive carcinoma enlargement since first diagnosis, but a decrease from 16mm down to 10mm.

Later scans showed all cancer to be gone.

Val's health continued to improve, and she lived a happy, active life assisting her boyfriend with a firewood and honey enterprise in the North East of Tasmania.

No Cancer – No Death by Opiates – Cannabis Oil cured Val's Aggressive Carcinoma of the Breast.

In late 2018 Val, suffering age onset dementia and a newly diagnosed lung cancer, she went to live close to family in New Zealand. In May 2020 Val passed peacefully at age 81.

Val lived an extra 7 years, healthy and free of debilitating treatments. She will be missed by all that knew her. A Gutsy, no nonsense, fun loving woman.

Cannabis Oil gave Val more life and no pain, a far saner option than the toxic and debilitating options currently forced upon an unwitting population.

At a guess, big business pharmaceuticals and eugenicists can't make money out of 'Natures Medicines'.

Cannabis as 'medicine' should be allowed as a personal choice in medicine, especially where cancers are concerned.

Could it be that the Cancer Council is bought and sold by funding from the status quo? Just in case anyone wonders why only epileptic sufferers are allowed to benefit from the 'healing weed'... or speak about its benefits?

It should be noted that research confirms that Cannabis doesn't mend all cancers. The old US patents described at least 170 cancers known to be cured by cannabis. So, see your health care professional, who probably didn't know to attend the Annual Endocannabinoid Conference which has been meeting since 2006, to discuss the marvellous healing capacity of 'whole Cannabis' extracts with consideration to the known 'Entourage Effect'.

The 'Entourage Effect' is similar to synergy, where the whole flower combination is greater in benefit than any individual part, thus making the creation of synthetic cannabinoid components another 'farce'.

To Be or Not to Be

I have been told many times by many people that I have talent for assisting people and I should become a naturopath or doctor...

I reflect upon my reluctance to institutionalization and conclude as follows:

What is the point in being a health professional, in a non-genuine environment of medicine pre-made, AMA ownership and product protectionism?

No. I prefer modern medicine in its place of effectiveness...

As first aid and emergency medicine, yes, but not in

The 'management of disease' where it fails wellness, in preference of dependency.

The illness economy is maximized unseen, with products and draconian protocols that perpetuate disease and disinformation.

Doctors are not educated in healing, independent research or free scientific thinking, but

In products and protocols of prescription that promote dependence on

A poisonous economic system.

Where doctors become unwitting peddlers of dependency and toxic preventables,

Delivering a new population to the new incurables…

This is not for me. A medical heretic is better for one's health.

Robert S Mendelsohn M.D. wrote the book "Confessions of a Medical Heretic", published by Contemporary Books, and

Being a 'successful' much loved family doctor for 5 decades, it's well worth a read.

He is particularly good at explaining how to manage normal childhood diseases, without panic, but ease.

Man Trap Ahead!

Question?
If you travelled a popular path and found a 'man trap'
Would you put up a sign of warning to your fellow travellers, or
Having saved yourself,
Walk on by?
(Who are we to cheat others out of learning lesson?)
Not I – For the futures children deserve better.
My Love for fellow travellers on this path of life is
Shown in details of this sign – pages long...
A great love indeed… as a map is required in the modern world and
The man trap in the path has grown, to be
A mine field, amid many superhighways.

Saving our children from the world's biggest psychopath

A perspective.
Not all share the eagle's view; macroscopic,
A vast perspective as seen from above with horizons in view.

A swift refocus to allow vision of detail, in microscopic view.
May this token perspective,
Share with you and yours, the
'Hidden in full view', of
Potential's hue.
400+/- years ago, a Shaman saw,
Not the peoples view, of butterflies, but
Ships of mass destruction on the ocean...
A perspective that is now known as true in the Americas.

While the rip-off merchant and racketeer of modern economics rushes by,
Nature, our nurturer and supporter, waits and watches,
Like the jaguar hidden in the green,
Studying the movements of
Robotic peoples and machines.
Observation and timing are everything.

Humanity, some lost as sheep,
Addicted and asleep,
Now livestock for chemical management systems.
Those that hear Natures calls will be in the right place at the right time.
The cleanse at addictions end,
Madness acknowledged, is where
Sovereignty and dignity begins for humanity,

My mother's Fibroid: Her Surgeon wanted a total hysterectomy, but my mother chose to go and see a Chinese herbalist to treat her football sized fibroid on her uterus. She was given three months to return. Three months later, the tumour had shrunk to the size of a pea. Upon her return to the surgeon, he was not only unimpressed by her healing but angry that she had not chosen surgery. He did not even ask how she had managed the recovery? Today she is free of the fibroids that were caused by Hormone Replacement Therapy.

See appendix for information on what Dr Russel Balylock can help you understand? And Dr Suzanne Humphries on vit C.

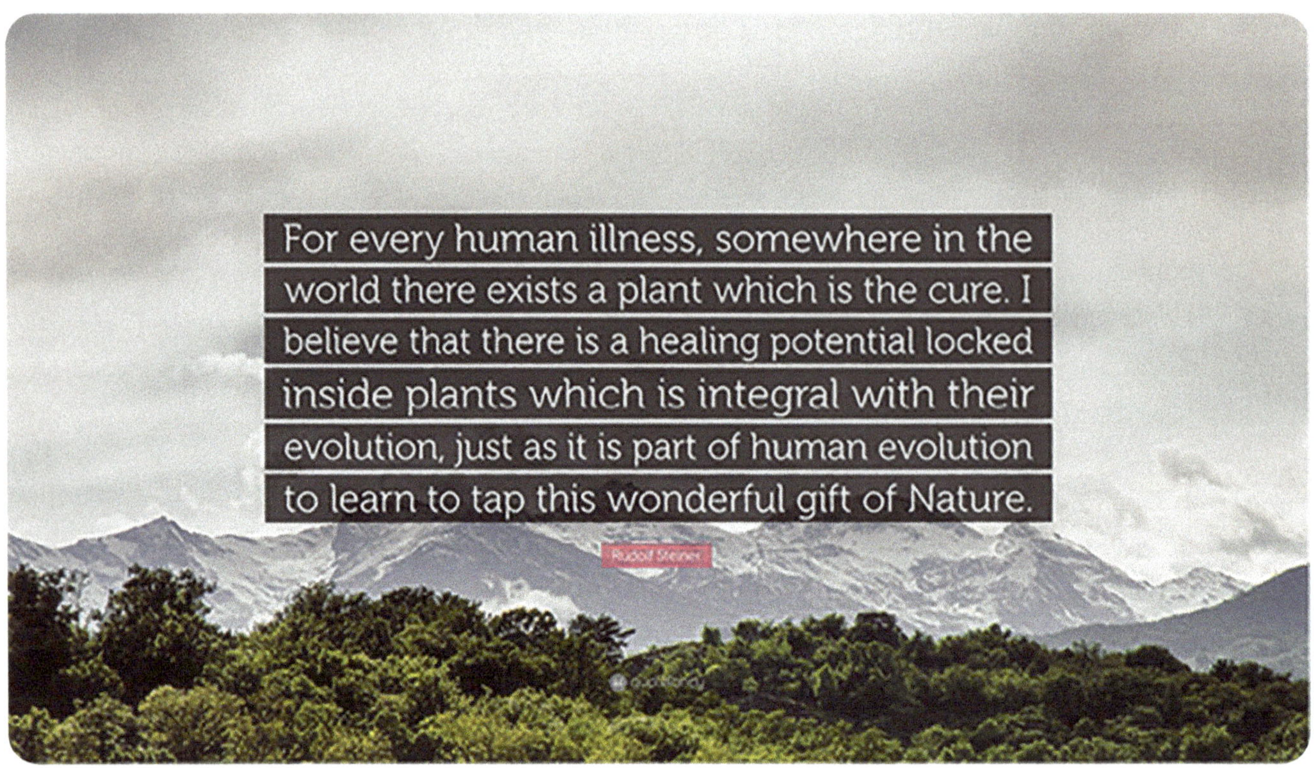

Science will save us

Was the catch cry of the 40's and 50's
Leading industries of consumerism and war.
Not great heart but great science has polluted the world,
Mechanized the world, rationalized away and destroyed 'family'.
Now humanity drones the same familiar cry..
"Science will save us…"
From What?
From our own poor, disenfranchised decision making?
From laziness or greed or the
Reek of isolation in economic dependency?
Only respect, Love and Willingness to change bad habits, can be the
Savior to the mess of carelessness, the mess of ignorance has made.
Welcome to Maturity, to the science of Life.
Cause and Effect human style.
Science will not, cannot save humanity.
All the best minds in the world cannot do the job of
Individual choices, daily.

Daily choices of individuals is
The sway they wish to control...
Daily choices of individuals is the Saviour of the World,
It is known.
E.g. My partner and I were in a lift one day in 2013, a World Climate Change conference was on the go.
The only discussion was around CO2.
As cell-culturists gasses are our game, in intensive culture environments.
We made a Methane comment, and watched their eyes widen in surprise. Until that moment, not one of them had factored 'methane' into the equation?! Yes... So...
Think Not, that elite science have the 'Answers', to
Problems they are yet to fully understand.
Where there is bickering over cause, there is an obvious lack of understanding,
A divided understanding, not a scientific consensus, for that is not the science of enquiry at all.

Daily choices, Yours and Mine conscious of consequences,
In the NOW..
That is truly important and influential!
Guard it well. Your Free-Will to 'Choose'.

Carelessness is the ONLY Enemy of Man...
Science of Oppenheimer...
Carelessness wrapped in Arrogance and
Managed by Great Fools.
Not 'Love', Only 'Will',
War Games... Just because they can?
Your choices change the world, focus and purchasing power
dictate more than you know.
Choose well Now, for the consequences will either Give to, or
Take from future generations.

The Digital Trojan

Through the Gates of wishing well, now Hell,
Computers control the world of
Domestic screens and weaponry.
Fake world demands attempt
New World Quo, in false
Techno planes and alternate platforms of experimental play,
No room for Real Living…
Flicker rate and marketing,
Forgetting and misplacing, the
True World and human gifts of 'doing'…
In the Earth Garden.
Hands, so many hands not busy, nor Minds.
Idleness as the body of couch potatoes, but focused on the 'un-real'?...
Hypnotized into unreality.
A new chemically managed zombie nation living in excess via
The domestic screen.
Through the Gates of Hell come, diseases unseen and plagues planned of consequences fully vaccinated, by W.H.O?
Controlling the health of the world for the Club of Rome economies, not
For the 'I AM that I AM" in you..!
Peace to the brothers and sisters of our shared garden.
From Humus to Humans, Life IS.
Be Kind to All.
Love is the Law.
Not chemical conscription that is a predicable bore.
Respect diversity of personal choice, as most intend only good.
$(z) = z^2 + c$ In fractal life,
All hangs elegantly from the Zero point, The Law of One is Love.

Chapter 6

"BE WELL" - Insights and recipes for wellness.

Thought, word and action are your artist palette,

For Life's Masterpiece – Let these things be not used against your sovereignty.

- Bring joy, sing, laugh, dance, love, create beauty in practicality.
- Tread lightly. Learn life skills beyond dollar worship.
- Be kind to all that you encounter, even the shadows of the self.
- Be genuine in all doings and sayings.
- Love and respect, yourself and others.
- Speak and act with honor.
- Do not Judge the path of another, for on a soul level, they do you a favor... your sibling doing a job you did not select to do.
- All eyes are the eyes of GOD (Great Omnipresent Divine).
- Pay attention, mindfulness in the now. You are recording life in Technicolour with GODs eyes, ears, smell, touch and taste.
- Know that the focus of your attention has power and is magnified by emotion.
- Every time the sycophantically driven domestic screen triggers an emotion, selling something – your power of focus and emotion are being used against you, in support of a marketplace.
- The Focus of your attention and love combined has the power of many minds joined.
- You will catch more bees with honey than vinegar.

Be Well, Be Aware

Nothing in excess...
Say "No" to fear.
It will happen quite naturally.
Each family will decide what is good for their genetics and there will be a movement away for the plastic fantastic culture and war.
Back to a more satisfying and sustainable way of living and growing healthy biology.
Our future looks good,

Old economic paradigms fall away, and
A more organic and creative management of society ensues...
Differences once seen as a riff, soon
Bridged by the evolution of understanding, will be
Seen as treasures of which to be proud.
Indigenous First Nation cultures of wisdom, balance and respectful,
Hold heads high.
We have learned through the patterns of life revealed, that
It is, the smallest things in our biological systems, that
Hold all the balances together...
Like atoms of matter and the space in-between, the
Phytoplankton in the oceans, the mycelium in the soil, the neutrophils of our immune systems.
Such single cell organisms and organisations hold all of life's biological systems together.
As with the creativity of the zero point, as a platform for the 'Mandelbrot Set' of life to exist.
So it is?

Bless your food

For all food comes with energy,
Likened to karmic debt...
How it was grown, lived and died...
Its region and handling,
Energetic qualities are taken on in layers
With its journey to your plate.
Grow your food with love,
Prepare your food with love, not poisons,
If biology is to thrive.
Is not biology of greater importance than toxic commerce?
Hunting – good hunters know
'The heart of the world' and seek to do no harm, but
A quick clean kill and giving thanks,
Honouring, every part of the creature in daily usefulness.
This approach brings no ill, but strength and value to the sacred chain of life.
Respect and balance... All true tribes,
Know this knowing.
'Know Thyself', and 'Nothing in Excess'...

Big lesson for little brother of the West.
"Simplicity is an advanced course" Sri Chinmoy once said.
They will get it, eventually...

Macular degeneration and Saffron.

Listening to a radio science show in 2012.
A researcher visiting from India gave an account of his work.
Saffron inclusion in the diet had the effect of reversing Macular Degeneration, even
In patients over 70 years of age... in a time frame of
Fourteen days or less.
An astounding breakthrough indeed, one would think...
Two days hence, on the same radio station, another science segment,
This time a Head of Research in the local State University medical facility –
And their discussion on their work on Macular Degeneration...
Which had little or no success, as yet.
It interested me to hear that no link nor acknowledgement of the
Indian Saffron research counterpart, on the airways just days before?
Instead the local expert managed a depressing expressing of
How far away any progress may be...
Hmm? A ruse to direct attention away from the Indian breakthrough story?
The game is to overlay the story of "Saffron Cures Macular Degeneration" with
The invested philosophy – Western Medicine's war on Natures medicine and cures, both
Seen as economically unviable to old investment grooves.
Our University research protocols are not 'invested', it seems, in economically dead end, Cures.

Australia has the highest rate of Allergies

Recommendations are no solids before 4 months of age, solids after 6 months and to include peanuts, eggs and fish. Don't avoid high allergy foods.

But what of the compulsory vaccination, products like nut oils, egg and animal proteins, heavy metals and aluminium nano particles, poly sorbate 80 a non ionic surfactant/emulsifier, not unlike detergent?

What of the herbicides and pesticides used routinely on food crops?

Australia has the highest rate of chemicalisation, particularly with foreign owned/managed farms.

Trans fats are still available in bakery and catering blends?

Chemicals used in dairy industry?

Systemic Herbicides used routinely as a "Clean Crop Kill" agent in legumes and wheat?

Did you know, Bromine replaced Iodine in dairy and bakery applications, two decades ago?

Bromine is in many pop cordial drinks... Bromine sets fat like concrete, inside the human body. It is linked with morbid obesity in teenagers and potentially insanity, due to fats in the brain being solidified.

The panacea is; including iodine, Lugols solution into the diet, effectively reversing the brominated condition.

What to use instead...

To raise arms against the said Evil (against life), business creed,
Is giving away energy to futility.
To empower your future,
Use buying power to avoid, such products that do
More harm than good.
In the same way one "starves a fever",
To restore balance.
Boycotts, starve business lines into evolution, towards
Naturally balanced wellness.
Make it a benefit to economics, for ethics to exist.
Follow the KISS (keep it simple) principle.

HERE ARE SOME HELPFUL HINTS FOR LIVING IN GREATER HARMONY WITH THE BIOLOGICAL ENVIRONMENT:

* Strong Vinegar as a foliate spray is an excellent herbicide without harming mycelium, biota of soil inter-connective bacterium.
* Extracts of Pelargonium, as a weed killer, are now used as well.
* Steam and Light block methodologies are also clean, weed removal systems.

* Wood Smoke Vinegar, used correctly, can reduce the use of chemical fertilizers by 80%.
* Regenerative agriculture products such as offered by Nutri-Tech Solutions (NTS) and Korean Natural Farming using mycelium, are excellent producers of balanced nutrition.
* Bicarb-soda and citrus combined are excellent grease cutting household cleaning agents. Great for your oven too when applied as a paste, and it will do no harm to your garden or waterways.

See the book: The Wonders Of Baking Soda by Amelie Laigneau published in 2005 by Willow Tree Press.

* *Micro fibre fabrics offer a useful cure for detergent addiction of the West, but may also contribute to micro plastic pollution.
* *Micro Ampules of electricity also kill many viruses and bacteria without harming healthy cells. See www.toolsforhealing.com for details on Dr Beck's support of Drs Lyman and Kaalis research of an AIDS cure.
* *In health Vitamin C – high doses, up to 6000mg per day, to flush toxins away and aid healing of many ills and connective tissues. Vitamin C is your body's collagen producer. As pure ascorbic acid powder, more than 6000mg per day can produce diarrhoea. Liposomal products bypass this effect to deliver as effectively as the intravenous delivery to the body. See Dr. Susanne Humphries link in "useful links" section.

A recipe from a chemist making his own zucchini liposomal vitamin C, is provided in the last chapter of this book.

Note: Magnesium supplements should be taken at the opposite end of the day to vitamin C, as the latter can inhibit the take-up of the former.

Here are some old remedies, tried and true, but not harmful to our life support nor genome.

Recipes for wellness:

The Golden Drink of Life

½ teaspoon of Turmeric,
½ teaspoon of Ginger powder
½ teaspoon of organic coconut oil

1 pinch of ground Cardamom,
1 pinch of ground cinnamon,
1 pinch of ground Nutmeg.
Mix ingredients in warmed Almond Milk or preferred alternate.
Enjoy the glow of good health every day.

~

Spicy Lemonade (for illness such as flu)

2 lemons fresh squeezed,
4 cloves of garlic, chopped finely,

Mix in 1 pint of water (400ml), and dessertspoon of natural honey.

Consume over a couple of hours just before bed....

You will wake up feeling much better.

Master Tonic (remedy for any infection)

7 Ingredients:

¼ cup finely chopped garlic,
¼ cup of grated ginger,
2 Tablespoons of grated horseradish,
2 grated turmeric roots,
¼ - ½ cup chopped onions,
2 chopped hot chili peppers,
700ml Organic Apple Cider Vinegar.

Fill mason jar 2/3 with chopped ingredients and fill the jar with Vinegar.
Close lid tightly and shake a couple of times.
Sit jar in a dark place for 2-4 weeks.
Strain through gauze and keep in dark glass jar.
Try a teaspoon in water first thing in the morning, daily as a general health tonic.
For illness, 2-3 teaspoons per day for children or adults mixed in water.
This is not too spicy when diluted in water.

For Speed healing of injury, collagen boost with Bone broth and organic gelatin. And Vitamin C.

Check list – Steps of understanding

- Mineral and trace element deficiencies? Magnesium, Zinc, Selenium
- Vitamin deficiencies? A, B, B15, B17,C, D, E and K?
- Diet and lifestyle?
- Water and salt? If active people do not get enough natural salt, they cannot make the bile to digest food efficiently, nor sweat. If any person does not drink sufficient clean water, their body cannot eliminate toxins, by-products of food or illness, efficiently. Our bodies evolved to be 70 percent water, as with much of the biological life on Earth. When clean water is taken into the body, it is recognized as water, the miracle molecule, not food. The body's recognition of water triggers a release of toxins from gut and lymphatic systems. Cordials and juices are processed by the body as a food despite their liquidity. If a person/child only ever gets to drink sweet and bubbly drinks the body does not get to do any regular toxin releasing, as nature intended. Water maintains the flow, coupled with correct levels of salts, acts like the Earth's own great ocean 'conveyors', both heat exchange and perpetual movement/flow.
- Environmental toxins, allergies and oxidative stress?
- Alkalinity Vs Acid factors? Sugar feeds cancer and creates acid in body. Bicarb soda in water as speed alkalizing.
- Parameters of conditions, time, acute or chronic, which bodily systems are affected?

A list of effective and inappropriately suppressed treatment options are listed in *appendix 2* to enable your further research.

In the act of suppression of all of the treatments labelled as alternative, no consideration was given to their effectiveness, nor harm free actions in curing cancer and autoimmune conditions. Deals were done behind the scenes, a high level thwarting protocol, to prevent competition with accepted, toxic and less efficient products and/or treatments currently used as standard practice.

Supplementation for health where deficiencies occur:

Cod Liver Oil – Vitamin D and A

Magnesium should be taken opposite end of the day to vitamin C. Transdermal application, sprayed on skin is the most bio available form.

Aloe Vera Juice aids digestion and reduces inflammation. Aloe correctly prepared, with gel washed clean of yellow sap, after skinning, is also excellent first aid for burns.

Colloidal Silver and Tamanu Oil from Calophyllum Trees, both demonstrate anti-microbial, anti-biotic, anti-fungal properties that remove infection and necrotic flesh. Both are excellent topical remedy for burns and coral cuts etc, preventing sepsis and promoting healthy tissue recovery. 100% Aloe Vera, Tamanu Oil and Colloidal Silver are all excellent inclusion to any Remote Area or farm, First Aid kit. So impressed with the performance of this oil I have included two Australian links for the little known Tamanu Oil below;

www.northerntamanuoil.com.au or northerntamanuoils@bigpond.com

www.ntshealth.com.au Australian owned and operated, Nutri-Tech Solutions Pty Ltd don't just support farmers with regenerative agriculture products but human health too, offering access to beneficial products... Like the Tamanu Oil, for skin regeneration and Probiotics for gut regeneration "Digest-EaseTM" etc. No kickbacks here, just impressed with efficacy of products, care and genuine service over the years.

Oxygenation of the blood is beneficial to keep the anaerobic lovers out. Viruses love anaerobic environments, i.e. environments that are depleted or lacking in oxygen.

Dr Joannah Budwig, her suppression story and research is relayed in Tanya Harter Pearce's 'Outsmart Your Cancer' book. Her studies on heat treated fats, trans-fats, is now well known but her boss, the King of Margarines, had her removed from her University Offices and through the courts attempted to prevent her research from reaching the people, for a short time.

Dr J Budwig's cancer recovery, Oxygenation recipe was a mixture of 3:1 ratio of cottage cheese (having a sulphur based protein) and Flax Seed Oil. Its combining creates a chemical reaction that enables the cells of the body to attach up to x6 more oxygen to themselves, achieving increased ability to eliminate toxins and for the body to heal. This simple remedy can be easily combined in a bowl and consumed daily.

Laetrile/Amygdalin, found in apple pips and apricot kernels is known as Vitamin B17. Do your own research of the function of enzymes within cancer cells and healthy tissue, behaving differently upon contact with B17. Beta glucosidase and Rhodanese.

Apple seeds and Apricot kernels, may be safely consumed, for an adult, up to equivalent of 6 whole fruit per day. It is best to consume pulp also, even if it must be stewed and added to protein to aid digestion. Stewed apple is also an excellent soothing, gut friendly, delicious food aiding the elimination of mucus. Most excellent with 'Kiefa Culture' too.

It is very interesting to research the Laetrile Cancer studies in the USA, last century, where Dr Morris Fishbein first perfected his model, for thwarting the truth regarding Research of a substance, that Big Pharma found to be an unwanted competitor. His Model of manipulating research to say what-ever industry desired, is repeated still, in every nation that has been influenced by US Health policy and investors. Australian ex Dr Hope and his very successful microwave-treatment, is a classic example of this research confirmation model, that I have expanded on earlier, in action. The treatment of Royal Rife would be another and the Canadian Gaston Nassenes 714X and more.

If it is legal for you to do so; the **'Sonication' of Hemp/Cannabis dried flowers to do a cold extraction of the beneficial bio-nutrients may be of interest. Grind dried flowers to tealeaf size particles and place into a clean, benchtop, jewellery Sonicator, up to the level indicated in device instructions. Pour MCT (medium chain triglyceride) 100% pure coconut oil over the ground herb. Fill up to the line as per instructions on Sonicator. Stir with wooden chopstick. Turn on Sonication device and leave for an hour. Can be treated for up to 8 hours, stirring occasionally. Time and quality of flowers will determine the strength and colour from golden to green.. Strain the contents through a fine hygienic cloth or mesh. Press on side of bowl or with press, to extract the majority of sonicated oil. Pour back into the Coconut oil bottle/s and store in cool dark place. One teaspoon, taken just prior to retiring for the evening, is said to aid health and restful sleep. It is now accepted and shown that, when certain endocannabinoids come in contact with cancer cells 'Apoptosis' occurs, death of the cancer cell, making this a most positive addition to any person seeking aid in; anaerobic cellular reduction. Harm free modalities such as this will one day be available and replace the toxic, long term damage, protocols currently 'prescribed' upon families and children with cancer.**

Cold extraction has no psychoactive effect, but the full benefit of the 'Entourage Effect'. Raw Cannabis is 800% better for health and rapid healing than the heated version, according the medical scientists and doctors considered, endocannabinoid experts, that have been meeting since 2006. *(See Rick Simpson Oil (RSO) ref on page 187)*

For further information, one can research the innate Endocannabinoid System.

"**A list of simple solutions** to combat viral disease.."

"**Anti Leukaemia herbs** as tea infusions or directly edible: Dandelion leaves and roots, Feverfew leaves and flowers, Nasturtium leaves and flowers, Pawpaw leaf, ground bark and roots, Cannabis whole plant, leaves, flowers, resin (see endocannabinoid system research). Fruit of Mangosteen and Graviola (Soursop)."

"**For TB and Avian Flu**, add Chlorine dioxide (ClO_2) to drinking water, for chickens or humans. This is a water purifying disinfectant that kills fungus, viruses and bacteria (see work of: Dr Pierre Kory). He also mentions the effectiveness of Xylitol nasal sprays, Iodine nasal sprays, Ivermectin, Vitamin D and Artemisinin."

"Purging Parasites and Cancer : new research shows using Ivermectin together with Fenbendazole is an effective treatment for removing parasites from humans and has an additional effect of starving cancer cells by preventing these cells from glucose uptake."

Shingles Remedy

10gm Chamomile, 10gm Lady's Mantle, 10 gm Meliot (sweet Clover) (or use Millet), 25gm Oak bark, 20gm Oats, 25gm Sage.

Four tablespoons of these well mixed herbs are put into 1 litre of cold water, in a saucepan bring to the boil and then taken off hotplate and infused for 3 minutes. Dab the affected areas gently with lukewarm infusion several times per day. The warm herb residue can be placed on a piece of linen and applied to affected areas overnight. This simple treatment removes pain instantly and reduces the time of infliction dramatically. Recipe from the book **Health through God's Pharmacy by Maria Treben**."

Dr Barbara Oneil – MD and Herbalist. A great teacher and author of many books on holistic human health and natural healing. Many video talks are available on-line. She is an advocate of the healing properties of Caster Oil using topical compresses. Her books include "Sustain Me," "Self Heal by Design," and a collection titled "Barbara O'Neill Natural Herbal Remedies Complete Collection". She also has books like "The Assassination of Barbara O'Neill" and "Back to Eden Health & Poultice Training Manual" (co-authored with Kaye Sehm).

Fate with Grace.

Each man or woman accepting their Fate with
Humble grace,
Finds a way to bring a spark of understanding, a
Glimmer, of the Love and Passion of Life, in the Eternal Garden.
Uplifting others and the focus of a new 'lens'
Bringing clarity and calm to hearts and minds,
Surfing the changing tides and
Turbulent surfaces of Man's folly in making.
This Too Is Change, and
That which was built on shifting sands, on
Neglectful understandings,
Fall away, Naturally, every day.

Image of Physics: Whether viewed from the microscope or universal consciousness.

Bubbles shifting between two panes of glass –
No matter how solid or fluid – bubbles of consciousness
Move and shift but continue to exist.
"The Lid of Heaven/Light and the
Base of Earth/Love -provide a place
In-between – for conscious play or
The play of consciousness in biology.
Love and Light are alive in all things,
In this creative space in-between.
A treasure to be seen in
Fractal diversity and perfection."

Chapter 7

WHAT IF?

Product Recall.

Send all the bombs, rail guns and mines back to the manufacturers for
Careful and Safe disposal.
Having consideration for no less than 7 generations hence.
A polite note will do:
Sorry guys, your products
Do not fit in with our Healthy World Protocol,
A Healthy World Protocol, relies upon respect and loving regard for all of life's diversity,
Not just the fear cultures, dependent on consumerism slavery.
Your products have NO place in our world market today!
War fear, as a controlling force on Earths populations is doomed.

Mandating Peace.

If Peace were mandated by law, who would be the customer of
The Weapon Manufacturer?

The biggest threat to world peace is the weapon manufacturer and their customers.
In the need to sell 'product', they profit from conflict, and its creation.
Generals have described WAR as a racket.
The gravy train leaves a trail of wounds and PTSD crossing generations.

Banker's economies manipulating the shifting sands of fortune, their armies
Predating upon economies wishing to base economies upon GOLD, by the new order of digitized
Numbers on the screen, not based on anything...REAL?

WW1 and WW2 were said, promoted to be the "wars to end all wars"?
Instead the newly chosen Bretton Woods global economy, has created more and more wars,
Everywhere...

Another arm of the economy grown up to a monster of manipulation by 'might is right'...
More inequity, starvation and disease... More PTSD!!!
Post-Traumatic Stress Disorder, as they now call it, afflicts more of the population globally,
Than ever before, whether war crimes, economic crimes or domestic crimes, that come with the new
Economic order... Innocent men, women and children suffer as victims of economic dependency and
Violent colonialism of planned psychopathic proportions...
By Men who would profit from the plan post WW2.

The economic GODMAKING is a false overlay, and within its initially corrupt basis, the cancer, the rot began...
Destruction as progress, and war as necessity, to continue the gravy train, herd the masses and maintain diabolical control for elites of their circles.
If one world consciousness is to coexist, peace would be paramount... Above economics.
Treasuring the great diversity of the 'Tapestry of Life', including humanity.
Allowing the military to assist the population in survival and recovery from natural disaster, instead of
Creating more pain, for each generation to pass on, again and again.
The 'Israeli Effect' must end, an eye for an eye makes the whole world blind.
It is an Insult to victims of the Holocaust that Israel has turned Nazi on Palestine.

Mirror of the universe and the patterns of pain are inescapable.
The Israeli Effect: When one party complains of an affect such as Nazism, and then
Effects that same Effect on another innocent party... or close neighbour, Palestine.
Israeli militarization is no different to Nazi militarization, nor is the passion, pain and Persecution.
In family violence, or paedophilia it is known that pain passes on the negative effect to Future generations, unless discipline and awareness are navigated for peace and Forgiveness.
Pain held on to, translates to pain, transference... A psychological fact.

Un-forgiveness is a toxic and dangerous disease. 'Man Made'.
Un-forgiveness and greed sell Weapons better than Peace..
To end the cycle of PTSD: End War as an Economic Tool.

Honourable governments could, by public demand, redeploy all troops to assist
The human plight of survival in changing times. As rescuers and rebuilders after natural disasters.
Take Responsibility! In the only time you can... NOW!

The military was always supposed to be 'The Peoples' Friend, and it can be again, once economic blindsiding comes to an end.
May Peace, Peace, Peace, Be Always, Everywhere.

So, what is all the drama about, all the propaganda, all the worlds advertising...?

Directing your choices where, the World's Biggest Psychopath wants them?

The path to world peace and harmony for all, is in choosing products that do not support the economies of Weapons manufacturers, of weapons that are solely for human destruction, nor economies of past wars like, Radiation and Chemotherapy as harmful Medicine, and harmful toxins in agriculture.

Powerful industries and lobby groups seek to control the choices made by Farmers, in relation to what they use on soil and crops, and Doctors in relation to what goes into our bodies.

The job of CODEX Big Agro/Big Pharma chemical companies is to attend trade meetings and influence the managers of Soil and Health in every country. This multi-national group are responsible for selling China Agricultural Chemicals that were banned by 170 other countries, confirmed carcinogenic, and consumers in the West buy fruit and vegetables grown with banned hazardous chemicals dumped by Codex into China at a dollar profit then and fail to reconcile the public health costs later.

Saving our children from the World's Biggest Psychopath, involves **re-engaging personal discernment** and responsibility, something that is given away by allowing outside influences to control your focus.

The Job of Television is to control your focus, hold your attention, with images and emotion. Fear and Guilt are hard core motivators, while sex and desire for good things is more subtle but a potent tool.

Our love of products and convenience has been used as a weapon by a system of economics that profits from dependency in a sick cycle of conflict and chemical enslavement to ensure the status quo never ends.

"**For Peace** - Thank you Lord of All things, for giving humanity the eyes to see and ears to hear, such that the influence of war mongers disappears, along with their techno partners. Good riddance to Palantir. Hour by hour and day by day the war mongers influence crumbles away, visibly. Undeniably. Peace, Peace, Peace on the increase. Fear and expenditure on war evaporates. The People Celebrate."

Religion as a Middleman.

When one shops for sustenance,
One can go to the supermarket and acquire
Packaged and promoted products.
Or
One can go to the farmers market and acquire
Fresh produce, direct, without unnecessary packaging.
Whether sustenance for the body or the soul,
The direct experience is fresher, healthier and hunger is satiated for longer.
The supply chain is shortened and has fewer interpretative bling and less packaging,
Alleviating burdens on the future.
In spirit thirst, the difference between listening to a preacher and
Listening to the quiet voice within is vast...
In the former, one is a pawn, and
The later, one is a player in the game of light and life.
The Great Spirit comes as a quiet whisper from within,
Not the forceful preacher, without.

Faery Food

Of the mechanized world...
The food of Faeries, fabled of old,
Tell of the dangers of eating Faery Food,
Not made by living Man,
Putting unsuspecting humans into forgetfulness, that
They waste their lives in another worldly dimension or reality.

Modern food made by machines, of
Men selling a fable, of
False reality to the world...
This food of fabled reality, having
The nutritional value of Fairy Floss and
Producing, forgetfulness, of
Skills and sovereignty within the masses.
Modern mechanized food sustains forgetfulness, not
Human health and creativity.

Modern mechanized food processes provide the genetic security of
Fairy Floss and are an unsustainable waste of Resource and Life.
Mimicry of the tales of old...
Do not mock the Faery Tale.
Their messages stand the test of time with
Delivery of moral perspectives with intended benefit for
More than one generation...
The Moral of the story;
Keep your food REAL,
Made by Nature and human hand, or
Skills, sovereignty and health will not be easily maintained.
Choices daily and Daily Choice are personal pivot points of power,
Choose well to Be Well.

"**History repeats**. Once upon a time King Herod sent out swords to slaughter all the babies he perceived as a threat to his throne. With modern technology the swords have shrunk to the size of injectables that the kings of power and money today, send out to slaughter, disable and maim babies and the Human Genome. History will mark this 'disgrace' with shame and the truth will defect their false template/over-lay with a dead end. The Lord of Life's Creation will have the last say. Ameen

Popstars of poor Governance.

How many politicians are wise and how many are good at heart?

Yet humanity allow them to rule the roost and steal from the hen house?

A flawed system for which the Future pays the price.

The current global economy by example, was set up by psychopathic, greedy and self-interested men.

A war bribe, no less, is the birth place of this economic platform.

Every avenue of Service to Humanity has been poisoned and/or enslaved.

Predating upon desire of "having", consumerism, the new religion of dollar gods,

Laid waste to honourable trade and values.

Divided, Family falls to Nuclear dependency on a system that supports no level of family effectively.

Laid waste by war upon war and layer upon layer of chemical, for better production, but killing the world and its population of diverse life, now endangered.

Tribes living in harmony with 'all that is' threatened by monstrous economies of zero respect.

Policies of ignorance create wastelands of natural resources and diminished genetics of life across the world.

Peoples who think they are immune will be the first to fall victim to the chemically enhanced attrician brought by the creators of the economy of Doom.

Sir John Maynard Keynes and Steiner predicted the path of consequence accurately, but no one listened to Wisdom in the rush for 'Having' more, more, more of everything, including War.

Future generations will hold this Bankers Century in scorn.

For them, living the life of 'consequences terrible', will mark consciousness with wisdom, to say No to the dollar delinquency.

It is noted with modern medicine that for every intervention another intervention is necessary.

This is not Wellness. This is economy furthering itself by Dependency and Hypocrisy.

This is why large, so called, Health organisations wage an ongoing propaganda war on Natural Medicines.

A Peer review of the Health Economy would concur.

Patients make corporations rich, like Wellness never did.

A Wellness culture would thrive if Doctors were allowed the education of Natures' Pharmacopeia.

Continuing the loop?

Allowing lobby groups to run the country's show puts an end to diverse futures we could know, in preference for their own, monoculture continuance.

Does this make good health sense? No, just a perpetuation of toxic old status quo, economic rule over generations and genomes.

An additional potential solution to the corruption that goes on with public and private systems of social support:

Daily Democracy – a simple system change providing a basic need –good governance without overt/corrupt control by false overlords. Electronic voting is easily achievable today, as with all other business transactions.

An end, to unelected Big Business/lobby group manipulation and internal political corruption by ending the pathways of control.

Step 1. Provide news cast announcements in-between finance and sporting segments regarding the matters for parliamentary discussion and/or voting for the Local, State and Federal Political Agendum's for the next day. This information could be in a chart format that allows people to take down the codes for specific discussions and/or votes to enable each person interested in participating to comment and/or vote according to their own preference on any issue presented. Using their existing unique identifier, the TFN.

Step 2. People discuss, research, decide and vote using their "unique identifier" if they wish on any topic, using the internet and /or phone registration codes provided by the Media. No obligation required except at the specific 4 year State and/or Federal elections. Local Government is not constitutional governance of the people of Australia and exists as a service provider on behalf of State Government. The Swiss people vote 4 times per year on taxation expenditure…That would be possible in Australia.

Step 3. Politicians turning up to work, would open their laptops and act in accordance with the 'will' of the people in their constituency in regard to any issue for discussion and/or vote.

The result will be, a better educated and more interested public;

- Politicians that can truly represent their constituents and will have more contact with those constituents by the nature of their 'True Public Service';
- Daily Democracy would end Party Politics, that serves very few and enslaves the many.
- Daily Democracy would end the pathways of political pollution via wooing's of Big Business and other 'unelected' Big NGO Lobby Groups.
- Daily Democracy will encourage wise and caring people into politics, ending the arrogant Polo Pony era.
- Big Business will evolve to provide more ethical products and services to continue their supply of your dollars and their validity in the world beyond political manipulation.

A simple solution for a better world for PEOPLE of this Nation and OUR CHILDRENS FUTURE.

Australia is full of very smart people of all professions, Network groups of the best from around Australia can be selected as committee guides for the Australian public to question about any issue of technical importance that may be required in relation to **Daily Democracy**.

Daily Democracy could promote an awareness of synergistic proportions as we see on social media today with issues and discussion forums, **Daily Democracy** could be a multi- point portal discussion and voting format, for our every day, Daily Governance Matters, whether it be Local Council, State Government or Federal Government.

As Finance and Sport get so much coverage and few benefit, a new Daily Democracy segment may be far more interesting. And people can have a say about how the governance that affects their lives. A constitutional Right, surely to keep up with the technical times and allow democracy on a daily basis!? Keep the State and Federal major election term and conditions as they are, but while in office… **Daily Democracy**…

Daily Democracy is a simple low cost change that could Revolutionise; Transparency in Governance on all levels and motivate everyone on all levels to care more and corrupt less. Politicians will have a code of conduct in service to the public.

Politician Code of Conduct could include:

- To recognize what Good Governance is. That Government only exists to serve the public need and facilitate structure and services that we need to do together rather than individually as stated in the Australian Constitution.
- To Serve Constituents Honorably by ways of Good Governance.
- To consider the effects of any decision on Seven (7) generations hence.

Unique Identifier:

- Is required to support one vote to one person policy on any issue/s, presented in **Daily Democracy**,

Most Australians over the age of 18 already have a "Unique Identifier"; A Tax File Number (TFN) which could be utilised to facilitate honest and efficient electronic voting.

Recycling of energy.

Wars come and go, an excess of greed, anger, pride and
Carelessness, is the human foe...
Chemical consequences live on, you know.
Birth defects fifty years on in Vietnam...
Nuclear poisons assault continuously the Marshal Islands and Japan.
Chemical enslavement and addiction of the west in pain, to be opiated again and again.
Business giants harming the health of Soil, Food, Water and
Human immunity, creating genetic disorder.
War, Agriculture and Medicine, a
Chemical control economy, made to order...
Its evolution of toxicity, brings division, disease and death of the
Physical and social structures.
The consequential evolution of Big Business's vision and investment in the
Psychopathic new world order... of economy.
Plastic products of food and war for plastic people in a plastic choked world.
Wasted...
In the quality VS quantity revolution of the past century,
Obsolescence it seems is the end of itself...
See the trash fall away with the
Return of the Artisan, once displaced by the false economy of quantity,
Now springs up from the human wellspring of creativity and common sense.
A return of Quality, Respect of resource, handmade by living humans,
Satisfying the need and creativity, the skills and knowledge of doing.
Truth separates itself from Falsehood, precipitating naturally.
With the value added, understanding of the energetics of 'Great Care' in the art of doing, saying and thinking,
Humanity is now free and ready to be trustworthy.
It is acknowledged by the physicists and mystics of this plane, that
Energy of all forms is recycled again and again.
Our responsibility collectively and individually at this time is to see and take the opportunity to transmute and transform the negative to the positive.
Silver lining, darkness to light...
With the power of Loving Hearts and personal choice, transformation is within your grasp.
Change is possible in every Now.

Transform energy of emotion back to its original form, Love and Peace, naturally.
See Israel as the lesson of pain and un-forgiveness,
Recycled endlessly from the Exodus, to the Nazis and now Palestine.
Individuals and the Collective, holding on and
Passing on, old pain again and again...
Love and Forgiveness, nowhere to be seen.
A continuance, a choice, sadly,
An insult to every concept of GOD/YHWY/ALLAH.
If the holocaust delivered by Nazis was wrong, an against life action,
Then so too, is the treatment of Palestine by a
Self-obsessed, victim Israel.
Religion nor economy can be justification for harmful actions.
God cannot be owned.
Economy is a marketplace but not rule of Law for Life.
Every Eye is the Eye of GOD, sharing a unique perspective.
Don't disregard the need for diversity, from
The smallest to the biggest of everything,
All is needed, as stitches in the Great Tapestry of Life.

Peace will come when individual and collectives surrender
The recycling of unforgivingness that perpetuated the energy of pain and suffering.
Be careful and loving in what you pass on...
For Peace, for a Future for the Children.
Love thy Neighbour, as thyself. For Peace, For Humanity.

The Bretton-Woods Curse

In Australia we have a 'weed' called the "Patterson's Curse"
A pretty foreign scourge that, is toxic to stock, and smothers, arable Earth.
The World, observed, has the "Bretton-Woods Curse";
Toxic; to All Biological Life...
Choking the Earth with Its'
Conflict creation and disrespect of diversity or healthy choice, called progress.
Psychopathic Business Prescriptions;
Chemicalisations and Might is Right.
This Global Economy, was "Sold" to the Worlds People as

"Salvation Jane"!?
Just like the fake war on Weapons of Mass Destruction… that rapidly became,
An industrialist game,
A Sovereign Peoples Curse, and the Earths Bain.
From here the Analogy, of the Global Economy sprang.
The Global Economy as a 'Weed',
That grew from the 'Seed' of the
Bretton Woods, conference, War Bribe and Trade-A-Greed;
Fertilized with a psychopathic creed
Promoting and Harvesting, your Fear and Guilt.
Make you feel irrational buying, is good, or indeed a need.
On products of waste and dependency, they feed…
Fluoride and TV; The zombie makers a, Main-line bleed.
Consumers so entitled, gobble greedily,
Buying like junkies?
Sovereignty, skills and necessities, lost in Techno Haste...
Chasing products of 'Disrespect' and 'Waste'.
Not what our Children's Future Needs.
So, This Global Economy… Is Not the "Salvations Jane" we were led to believe, but
"The Curse of Bretton-Woods";
An economy based on Greed and Disrespect of local sovereignty,
War, the 'Rape of Resources', and 'Economic Slavery'.
Foreign starvation, alongside dysfunctional
Local dependency and pharmacological addiction…
This False Economic Governance, is indeed a nasty Affliction,
Upon Our Essential, 'Biological World', and all its children…
As witnessed; the whole world believed, without question,
A 'U.S.' led Lie about Weapons of Mass Destruction, and
We all saw the machine, go to War to fight for Profit of US business in reconstruction...
A shame millions of innocents had to die.
All the women and children, outside the economic drive,
Killed or displaced for another big business Lie.
Our Thanks go again to another U.S. Administration, for their Arrogance and Destruction forced upon people in other countries through no fault of their own.
Shame's Stink is Strong...
The unethical 'Might Is Right', is clearly Wrong.

Soulless, is the expression of a Nations Administration, that has built its greatness upon the business basis, of conflict and chemical conscription.
An economic plan, turned Dominatrix Machine of its own creation,
Bulldozing the Liberty of its own people and other Nations.
The Draconian Business Show must go on! So they say.
Such is Economic Rationalism, short sighted, short term profit fixated.
Social, Economic, Environmental Disaster, zero consideration for Seven Generations Hence…
Now they wish to focus, our money and time on other planets…?
The Indigenous Peoples pray that 'little brother' hurries and Learns Respect.!
Diversity of life should not be threatened…
No more! Enough Is Enough!
Chemical Streamlining of agriculture, poisoning food, air and water,
Chemical Streamlining of medicine, where Nature is an Enemy, to the toxic tyranny and concoctions of control, the 'management tool' of the New World Order's day.
No Acknowledgement or Product Dollars in Wellness or Good Health, Natures way.?
And in less than 100 years,
The Great IMF - World Bailiff Banking system has meddled in the lives of many countries,
Robbed many a Nation of a Future, for its Children.
In its desire for world economic domination, the global economic agreement, has created a racket and herded people as if they were cattle…
Shame the on past and present Global Trade Administrations.
Like a toxic Boil, they erupt from within;
Spewing, the toxic economic rationalism, strip mining
'Human Liberty' from 'living' on the Good Earth.
So much could be gained from economics that serve The People, The book, 'Small is Beautiful', unwelcomed on the big boys playing field.
Economy, needs to Serve the grass roots, First, not Last.
The Rustics are the Ground upon which Great Men stand, without Rustics, Great Men would have no Legs to carry them...
So "The Bretton-Woods Curse" is,
A system of Economic Progress that turned "Farm Management" on The People,
As the Industrialists and Usury families of the 1930's always intended to do.
The hungry sheep of the world's fold followed, so hopefully..
Seeking "Salvation Jane", after WW2, (out of the frying pan and into the fire) from overt war to subvert control with, economic ply.
Easy quarry, for a 'Psychopathic Rouse', at the fated Bretton-Woods Conference in 1942.

Followed unquestioning, toward the 'shiny' 'shiny', Lie..
One that has led people down the path of conflict for profit;
Social, Economic Instability and War-Torn Gloom and Doom.
Profitable for 'The Few', that made a lot of money...
For 'The Many', that 'Serve Well', the carrot, the crumbs, and
Broken dreams... Hoodwinked! PTSD the common reward.
The Lie; like Lollies for children, the promise of more, Progress and Comfort,
As never seen before... Enough to dull the senses of our elders at that time...Sadly,
Safety nets, Sovereignty and Sensibility were thrown overboard for
The new gold fever, of seemingly deserved, excess and comfort...
The Social and Economic Cliff was noted, but ignored.

The "Economic Lie's" Future was foretold in sad detail, by
Sir John Maynard Keens, even before "The Bretton-Woods Curse"
Global Economic Deal was signed and sealed after WW2.
No One Listened...
So it happened that the "Bretton-Woods Curse" came upon the Earth.
It was $Bought$.
To quote John Maynard Keynes:

> *"Capitalism is the astounding Belief that the most wickedest of men will do the most wickedest of things for the greatest good of everyone."*
>
> *"The decadent international but individualistic capitalism in the hands of which we found ourselves after the War, is not a success. It is not intelligent. It is not beautiful. It is not Just. It is not virtuous. And it doesn't deliver the goods".*

Righting the upset applecart

May the poetry of my pencil, lay waste to illusion,
As the Sword of Truth, would cut the thickest delusion.
Grant me a publishing of skill and passion,
Aligned with the Eagle and Jaguar Perception, in the Heart of the World.

Let the Quetzalcoatl Symbol be, revived in the Hearts and Minds of All.
Pure and True,
A Guide, to Peace and Harmony for a happily Creative Humanity.

Helping people everywhere bid conflict 'Adieu'.
Let clarity replace, marketing's Blathe.
Love is the Law
Let Love again underpin the 'Will' of Man/Woman/Child.
Let Love issue instruction to the Mind to
"Get in Behind". And
Let the Heart again, drive True.
The road is windy, and the cluttered mind makes mistakes, but
The Heart knows Grace.
Listen to your Heart, not Fools.
Doctors today are trained to
Think medicine, think time management, think Pharma product..
Doctors are not trained to question? Or Think for themselves...
It is not set up that way.
Eyes that are 'willing' to Look, will SEE.

Chapter 8

Ancient Wisdom, could it be useful ?

The Essenes and Quetzalcoatl interlinking life interpretation and symbology...

The Sevenfold Peace
Peace in the world, Peace with culture and diversity.
Can humanity gain a fresh perspective from some old hidden seeds?
The Essene Contemplative practices and the Quetzalcoatl symbol?

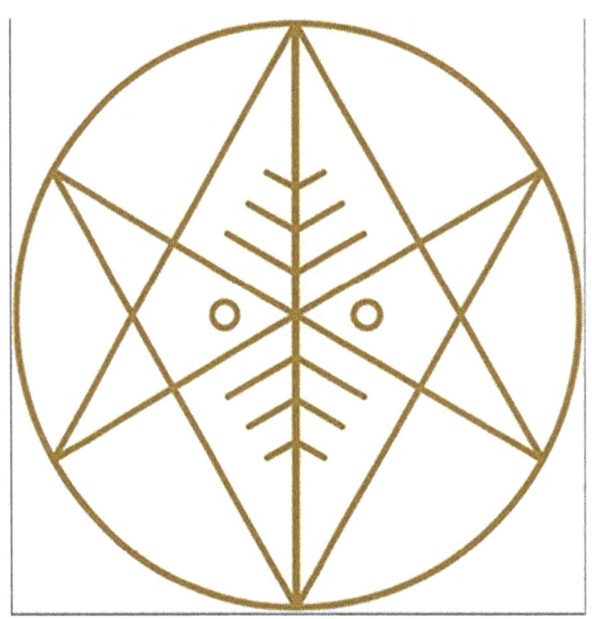

The Map of Peace and Harmony

The Quetzalcoatl symbol
Its meaning has been lost over time and
In some parts demonized by religious powers of old.
Just as medical religions today do with Vitamin C, natures herbs and common sense… to maintain sway.

The symbol of Quetzalcoatl understood, is a map of Harmony and Peace for Humanity
That includes all the sacred understandings of all past times…
"Simplicity is the Ultimate Sophistication" as Da Vinci said.
Or …" Simplicity is the Advanced Course" as said Sri Chinmoy.
Its understanding supports the glorious continuum of 'Mastery of the Self'
In the most testing of realms – The Physical.
Peace, Peace, Peace – Let the Angel of Peace be Always Everywhere.
In the centre of the symbol is the Tree of Life,
Linking with Tree of Life teachings,
Holistic contemplations and communions with seen and unseen realms, themselves providing direct experiential teachings, and Wisdom that
The Masters know and serve.

"Such was the Essene pattern of Communion with the cosmic and natural forces and contemplation with the aspects of peace that showed them how to put the forces into practice in their daily lives. We shall not find its equivalent in any other system. It has the wisdom of eight thousand years behind it. It is not merely a form or a ritual; it is a dynamic, intuitive experience. It can establish the unity of mankind." Said Dr Edmond Bordeaux Szekely of this preserved work (The book, 'From Enoch to the Dead Sea Scrolls'). From the transcriptions of Essene practices he described the seven days of the week, and how one cultivates three contemplations per day, one on an element of Earth, one on Peace and one on the unseen realms.

Each day of the week has a different focus, with Peace as a continuous thread,
always the focus of noon contemplations.
Working with these gentle suggestions provides a very organic
Understanding of the fractal world. It grows the psych's connectivity…

"An abbreviation of Essene Noon Communions is given below:

Saturday; **Peace & Kingdom of Heavenly Father**. Sunday; **Peace & Kingdom of Earthly Mother**. Monday; **Peace & Culture**. Tuesday; **Peace & Humanity**. Wednesday; **Peace & Family**. Thursday; **Peace & the Mind**. Friday; **Peace & the Body**."

The Essene Tree of Life with Morning & Evening Communions

FRIDAY EVENING
The HEAVENLY FATHER
and I are ONE
THURSDAY EVENING
Angel of WISDOM descend upon my thinking body and enlighten all my thoughts.
SUPERIOR THOUGHTS
SATURDAY EVENING
Angel of ETERNAL LIFE descend upon me and give external life to my spirit.
GRAVITY Superior Planets
WEDNESDAY EVENING
Angel of LOVE descend upon my feeling body and purify all my feelings.
SUPERIOR FEELINGS
SUNDAY EVENING
Angel of CREATIVE WORK descend upon humanity and give abundance to all men.
BEES - Creative Work
TUESDAY EVENING
Angel of POWER descend upon my acting body and direct all if my acts.
STARS - Cosmovital Forces
MONDAY EVENING
Peace, Peace, Peace,
Angel of PEACE be alway everywhere.
MOON - PEACE WITHIN
TUESDAY MORNING
Angel of JOY descend upon earth and give beauty to all beings.
HARMONY
WEDNESDAY MORNING
Angel of SUN enter my solar centre and give the shine of life to my whole body.
SOLAR RAYS
MONDAY MORNING
Angel of LIFE enter my limbs and give strength to my whole body.
TREES - Vitality
THURSDAY MORNING
Angel of WATER enter my blood and give the waters of life to my whole body.
RIVERS, CREEKS
CIRCULATION
SUNDAY MORNING
Angel of EARTH enter my generative organs and regenerate my whole body.
TOP SOIL - Growth
FRIDAY MORNING
Angel of AIR enter my lungs and give the air of life to my whole body.
ENERGIES OF ATMOSPHERE - Breath
SATURDAY MORNING
The EARTHLY MOTHER and I are ONE.
She gives the food of life to my whole body.
NUTRITION

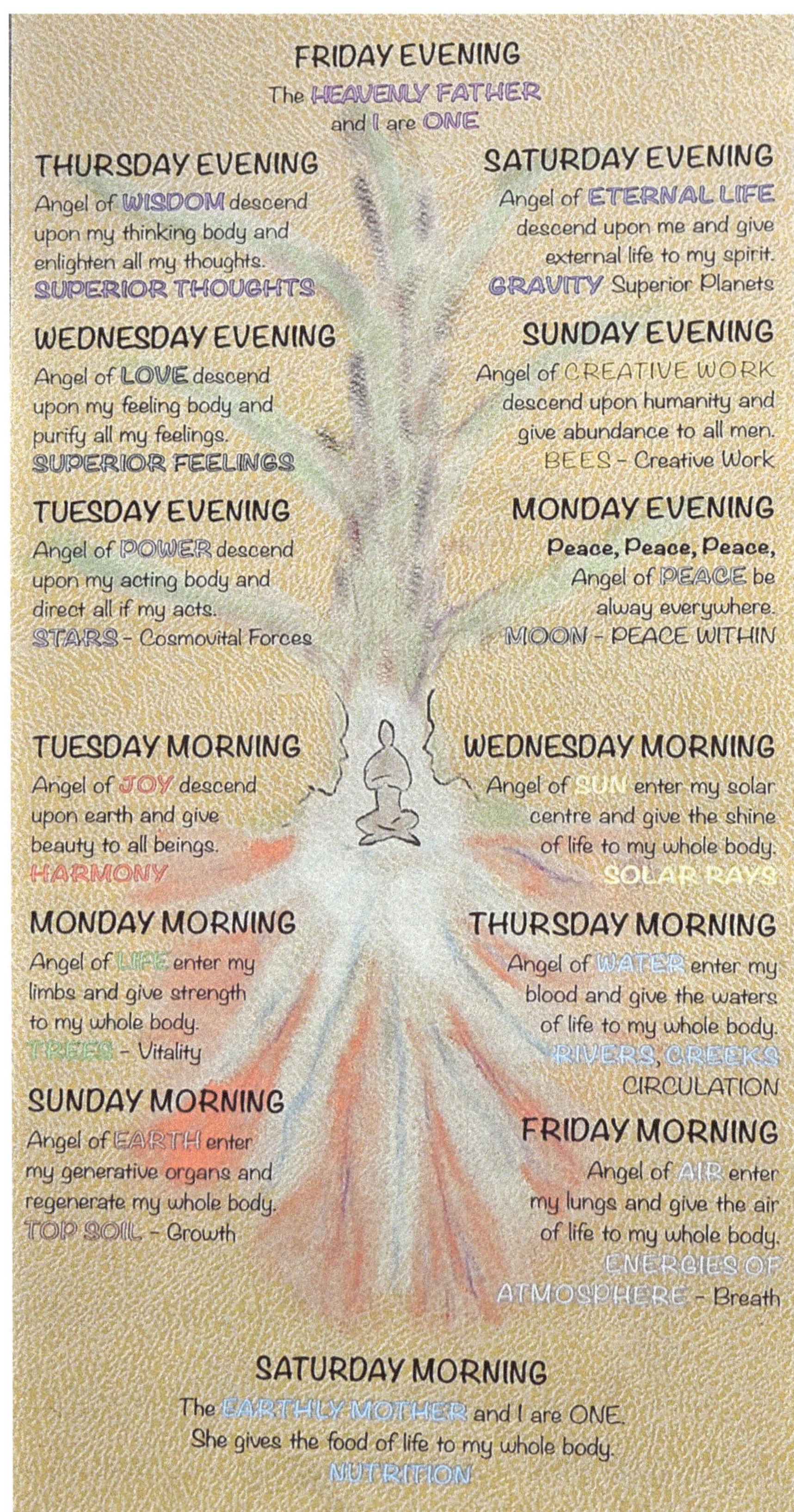

The Rules for play in continuum hinged upon the tree of life
Are and have been set out
Many times and in many forms.
Many Masters with the same message
Have come and gone.
Many messages of Peace and Love
Have been twisted and edited for
The purposes of control of the 'physical'.
The Quetzalcoatl Symbol contains within its message
The Dove of Peace and
The Butterfly of Man,
The Tree of Life and
The Yin and Yang.
The sacred geometry of universal architecture and
A very strong message of
The Foundations of All –
Love is the Law.
Whatsoever you wilt will be Law –
Let Love be the Foundation of your Creation for
Love is the Law.

Other pertinent reviews and musings…

Review: "Primary Perception

Bio communication with plants, living foods and human cells".

By Cleve Backster – 36 years of research described

Also author of the "Secret Life of Plants".

Understandings of this research makes saviours of
this man and his fellow researchers, for future generations.

A word on the future and the past
Edgar Cayce mentioned, out of
Deepest Darkest Russia, Siberia,
Would come a Light unto humanity and the world…

A saviour to kinship of Earth...
The connecting thread I see is
"Anastasia" and the "Ringing Cedars" series,
Spreading like interconnected mycelium,
Empowering gardening and kinship across the world.
Reconnecting humanity with its roots of 'interconnectedness'-
Beyond religious controls and taxes –
Back to the Garden of Eden, human creativity and happiness...
Peace on Earth.
Respect of diversity and kinship by Gardening and food sharing.

An acknowledgement of the prophecies of Benjamin Solari Parravicini, and
The Domestic Screen.
What has happened since 1943?
Nature provides all that humanity needs, including
Observable patterns for harmonious co-existence and creativity... But
The World's Biggest Psychopath's (WBP),
Giant false overlay of a psychopathic economy has
Lulled the, humanity engaged, into a
False sense of security...
There is nothing in this economy, worshiped by so many,
To sustain humans, but for a short time.
Now we see governments all over the world,
Lie to the People to support and placate
Corporate business interests, bigger than themselves...
Supporting disease, war and ego entrapment,
Rape of the senses and genetic decent.
Yes, it seems in 1938 Benjamin Solari Parravicini
Was Right!
Television is the tool that mesmerizes and has
Hypnotized whole generations into believing and investing in
Something false –
Like Candy Floss, it melts away
Real security, skills and sanity, instead it
Supports disease of
Heart and Soul.

Nature is no Ruse…
The Cleanse comes –
Time for humanity to return to senses and run home
To the Mother.

As the last American President takes the stand,
Time for the insane Atom manipulations to End.
Along with the arrogance and disrespect of Men who are
Learning that ego only supports ego and human
Families need Real Men and Real Women, not plastic fantastic human drones.
Bless the disruption for it saves humankind from the
Evil Psychopathic grip of a False Lord economy that
Went insane and replaced
Valued trade of Goods with
Trade of Conflict and Money.
An economy of lust that has hypnotised Humanity…
Mother will wake the human child from its slumber and
Outside of the Nightmare of psychopathic economy,
We will all wonder how we ever went that way?
Experience and hindsight is a fine thing.
Let us not Forget.

In the Garden

I heard the Flute of Pan,
Custodian of Nature and Man,
Giver of Fertility,
From Mother Earth her flesh that be,
That her joy and laughter,
Fill your girth.

Joyous creativity her Natures 'will'.
Societal controls of Fear and Guilt
Are Man's shame,
Not divinity's twill.
Such aberrations, get in the way of Life's joyous game,
Like a toxic pill.

Let good hearts rejoice and
Resound in all of Man.
The false garb falls away, and
Shining,
United we stand.
Be Love Now
The reflective and The Creative.
All are One.
Cease Hurting and Judging.
Allow the Unique expression of Consciousness,
Yourself to be.

That you were born to this physicality.
Thumbprints of each, a sacred pattern, of a fractal world.
All Eyes are the Eyes of Great Omnipresent Divine,
All points of Light, are glowing threads of frequency, connected to the Centre, cycling uniquely, again and again.
In Living, we gain understandings, of
Honour and Respect,
Loving and Giving.
Pain, Loss and Destruction,
Cycles that All, Begin and End…

Adolescence is over, for Humanity,
Now Responsibility Begins.
The End of human reliance on the destructive,
"Against Life" Machine.
Robbed of their senses, some may never see.
Choice is made in every Minute, with
Every Thought, Every Word and
Every Deed.
All is recorded of your person and the world, in
An Akashic Record.

Keep focus on your Journey,
If you are here,
You are valued for your gift…

Avoid the Soul Starvation of
Fear and Guilt, the false Creed of
Avarice and Greed.
Avoid false economies of imbalance, dependence and disease,
Robbery of sensory frequencies and basic needs.
Overloading Human Focus and Biology,
Time to Defrag Humanity.
Mother will have her way!
Cleansing with wind and water,
Life in her field must respect "All as Its-self'" or
Face Decay.
For this IS the Playground of Divinity and not the place for
A Demogorgon 'economic machine', that is
Destroying our children in
The Garden of Eden.

Chapter 9

Bleed-through time...looking through a different lens.

Above the door to the Temple of Delphi it reads;

KNOW THYSELF and
NOTHING IN EXCESS.

An ancient Truth and Wisdom put to the test.

A global economy that predates upon
Hypnotized and sleeping peoples,
Preventing vision through constant distraction and
Beguilement...
Eager to prevent any person or herd of peoples from
Ever, 'knowing themselves', in
The environment of encouraged needless, consumption and excess.

Natural pace and pathways discouraged by the
Machine that cannot sustain itself,
If humanity wakes up...
If people 'know themselves' and
Seek balance, nothing in excess...
Nature inside Us and without
Is doing its thing and healing
Cleaning the imbalance
The festering wounds,
Of inequity, pain and unhappiness from the WBP.

New respectful ways of Trade are Born, and
Technology that truly supports human experience and
delivers respect to diversity, will go on...
Harmony again in Eden.

Double Edged Sword

Technology of Man is not all bad… or Evil (against life).
The spectrum of creativity is true to the expression of the whole…
As with all tools that can be used for good or used for ill.
A knife may be used to carve beautiful or useful objects, or
It can be used against Man and Life for ill,
Bringing harm, pain and a wound to heal.

The internet in the same way is the saviour of humanity,
Providing as sense of real-time inter-connectivity,
That has brought to an end, Non-Transparency of
Governments, religion, management of resources and the People.

It aids communication and awareness…
And for some it is Doom,
Distraction and Addiction.
A trap of focus, attention and physically depleting, inactivity.
Mental games and sales pitches absorbing peoples focus, on
Uselessness, consumerism and waste.
A Humanity, wasted and opiated by the frequency of the
Domestic Screen.

The old sign above the door of the Temple of Delphi,
Today, its message can be easily understood as
It speaks volumes.
Firstly – "Know Thyself" …
Made difficult, in a distracted world of hijacked focus.
Devoid of witnessing the patterns of nature, that, are our educators –
Look at Da Vinci's work – rejected by scholars of his day…
Nature speaks to Natures Mind within Us and through Us, every day.

Depression is learned helplessness, and anger turned into, what's the point...?
Any animal kept in an un-natural cage suffers this fate.
This is Nature's message, to get out of the box and
Move freely in the energy exchange world, rather than
The hypnotic energy suck of man-made, half baked, protocols.
Nature's message of overload and restriction, is pay attention.

Catharsis is an evolutionary mechanism within the overwhelm... Break through or break down.
The choice is always yours.
We cannot go over or around, but through the experience, to new understandings.
Secondly – "Nothing in Excess"
No matter whether this observation is applied to food, drugs, sex, money, business, weapons of war, water, light and sound, acid or alkaline,
Sand or clay,
Sadness, anger or even joy.
Excess in any and all areas causes imbalances.
Imbalances have consequences that require correction to enable balance again.
All things seek harmony, naturally.
As Water always finds its balance.
Apply attention to these simple understandings to maintain balance in your own self and interactions first.
Remember always, "Examples Work".
All creations in this world of Man are capable of
Working great good and/or great harm.
Do not blame the tool, when the user is the Chooser.
Consequences come later, but they come.
Now is the only active environment you get, so,
Choose and decide on Life Enhancing Expressions.

This is your true power, to choose and choose again.
Not to be, hijacked by blind consumerism selling itself.
Where are your choices placed and who benefits?
You or the shadow economy?
You can choose any time to turn off the addiction that keeps you feeling 'needy'
Hypnotised with a drip line, they feed off your sleeping self.
Turn off the TV, go outside, and return energy to your Real Self and the Real World.
This one Act, saves masses of energy and waste, and
Gives the children a chance at Life and Hope.
You are choosing for them Right Now.

A Recipe of Peace and Harmony?

What Happens when the worlds biggest Power companies own,
the worlds biggest weapons manufacturers, that own
household goods and appliance companies and
agricultural and pharmaceutical giants.?
Dependency, beyond good governance.
Perpetuation of toxic wars, food and medicine, wasteful devices, and genetic degradation.
A skill and nutritionally, impoverished Rich.
Out of their Senses, Humanity, is separated from Reality by conflict and economic distractions,
embodying the overburden of a toxic Harvest.
Forget the Economic Crashes, what of the Genetics?
A Biological world ruled by an Economic Psychopath.!
Likely Outcome; The Fall of Ignorance… and
Rise of Human Sovereignty again.
The Self-Preservation of the Non-Machine, Living Being.

Bubbles of Love

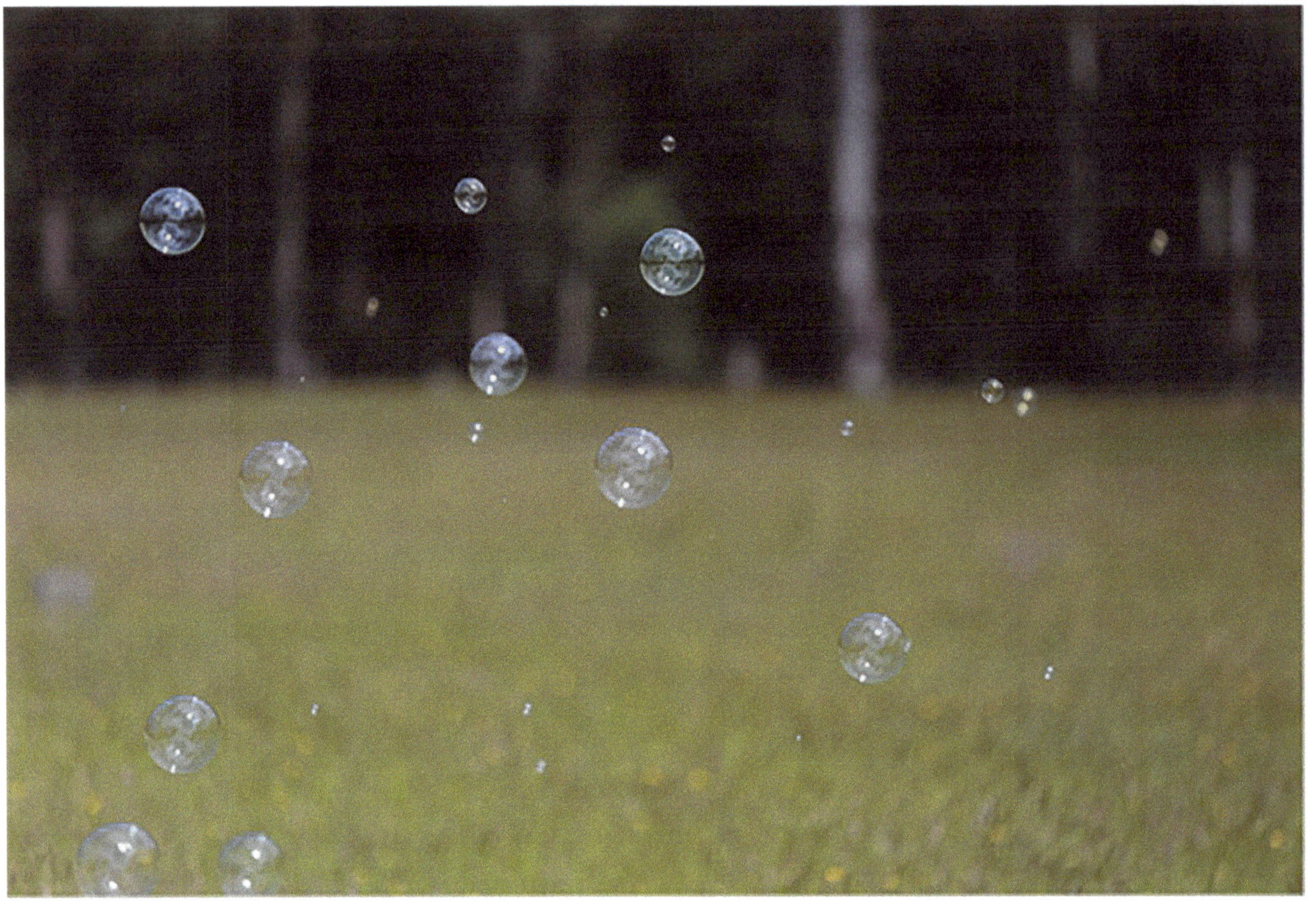

Contemplate the Facts, of physics and the 'Fractal Life' of biology;
Combined knowledge of mystics and physics employed directly...
Floating on the power of Pi

**"Alight with great Heart, bubbles of Love into the air, then
With a focused Mind send them to ones in conflict or despair."**

An empowerment image, for those that care...
A focus that enables hearts and minds to support the
Highest Good of All concerned, anytime, anywhere.
For those who feel the pain of witnessing;

BUBBLES OF LOVE

Is a positive focus for Ones mental and emotional energy.
Floating on the power of Pi
Beautiful and fragile as Life the bubble,
Floating on the geometry of Pi

Women of the world,
Men and children in this 'Play of Light',
Remember it is so, day and night.
Transform darkness into light.

Send bombardments of your hearts and minds,
Bubbles of Love, Intense and Divine!
Exploding Love, all over 'Life', within
The dark conflict- zones.

Polarization is an emotional illusion.
One cannot fight Hate with Hate and produce a positive Fate.
Love conquers All.
Love Unifies, with dignity and respect.
Love is Life, the Foundation, and Law.

Love's powerful vibration, brings Peace and Harmony,
Balance restored.
Send Love Individually and as a Group.
Bombard all those in dispute...
Sending Bubbles of Love Now! Xxx

Progress vs sovereignty

Progress should never come at the expense of Sovereignty.
As no lesser, motivations of men, should have influence in how the future unfolds.
This happened upon the acceptance of the current Global economic platform and look where it has taken us...
War and Conflict promulgated for the benefit of economic friends and business progress.
Disenfranchising Trade agreements that
Cripple local industry is the
Softly, softly, Take-over of a Country.
Brought to its knees, by convenience, dependency and
Eagerness to please...
No Sovereignty here, unless you get to choose,
What you eat for dinner?

Chapter 10

Nixon's Folly

And the Health of the World...
He brought forth the stream-lining of agriculture to benefit poison manufactures and Nylex mates,
Delivering the World, nutrient poor, refined and poison-soaked grain.
When the cancer epidemic hit the USA,
He called for submissions to amend the new cancer crisis, erupting after,
streamlining agriculture, effected the removal of nutrient rich and High Nutrillicide grains, like Hemp and Millet from daily bread.
Of 400 Health-conscious submissions, Nixon chose 3 Three:
Cyto-toxic Chemo-therapy, to perpetuate and legalize War time experimentation,
Radiation, to perpetuate and legalize war time experimentation and
Surgery, which was required as a result of wartime injuries, and deserved greater support...
All other submissions were dropped and later targeted as threats to the
New world order of chemical agriculture and poisons as food and medicine.
In 1972, Nixon made it legal to profit from disease, again, assisting mates in the insurance industry.
Private health privilege, as competition, to Universal Health Sensibility.
Disease as a profitable legal industry was born.

Once a Bright Boy.

Dylan, once a bright boy,
A Living Bridge across the Stream of Understanding,
In Life's Flow...
Let his Living and Dying not be in Vain.
Remove forced conscription to the ANZECC Study Protocol, of
All childhood Acute Lymphoblastic Leukaemia (ALL) sufferers.
For, If they could choose,
Alternatives, less toxic and less likely to create more mutations in DNA, than

The current legal protocols... They would.
The Spirit of my child told me, "The System Is Rigged"!
WHO is behind the perpetuation of this Draconian treatment that statistically, is proven, that of the 80% survivors of initial toxic treatments, only 5% survive cancer free after 5 years.
Every dose has Pub Med small print that categorically states it will cause numerous future cancers of blood, bone and brain!
It is living torture, especially, that no one speaks up about the toxic Gravy -Train.
Perhaps many are blinded by the gifts of little worth, the glamour of meeting famous people or travel to theme parks. Wellness would be preferable, if it were allowed.
Fundraising Councils and Foundations perpetuate the lies of 'Zero Cures', as
The current party plan of fundraising festivals and product sales, they cannot afford to lose.
More recently, these organisations, so as not to be completely useless, offered transport and primping services to sufferers... It looks better on the books, that they Deliver something...
No, not a cure, but transport to each poisoning session, of the same failed protocol.
Never will these Big Business foundations and councils deliver any non-profitable CURE.
Therefore, Freedom in Health Choices, must again, be made a Civil and Legal right.
People, before Economy.
Thankyou.

A Council of Cancer

There exists an area of Medicine, that has separated itself from the flow of the stream,
Forming a toxic eddy, in the Health of Humanity.
Not in the vital First- Aid, nor surgery, optometrists or dentistry.
This is a section of medicine separated and supported by Foundations...and poison companies.
Foundations expert in diversionary marketing, that keep dead-end, toxic medicine and
'Management' of disease,
In its place!
Perpetually...
Without support of these foundations, Disease Management would progress to Healing and Wellness;
The end of the Disease Economy;
The Death of Foundations of Disease.

Generosity being taken for a Ride.

A few years ago I lost one of my beloved children to a lie.
The Hoax of the century!
If you believe in Spirit, he came to me and said "It's not your fault mum, the system is 'Rigged'."
He suffered cancer twice in five years, for that's what toxic medicine does...
Repeat Business. Iatrogenic injury.
Anyone doing the Research will find this is true.
Diabolically, the Cancer Council (Council of Cancer), actively lobbies against any alternative to Chemotherapy, they are big business after all.
The Leukaemia Foundation (Foundation of Leukaemia), may as well be the same organisation for their approach is mimicry.
Transposing the names provides a more accurate description of their actions in the world.
See the book; Outsmart Your Cancer by Tanya Harter-Pierce or books by Phillip Day, illustrating the big business pathways of the anti-wellness industry.
The Generosity of Caring People is being taken for a long ride in this 'scam of the century'.
All the donations end up supporting the status quo: Chemotherapy...window dressed and sugar coated to make it easy.
Its not personal, it's just big business as usual.
WW2 Guinee Pig experimentation turned western population control.
Generous donations support an economic monster that squashes good independent research, free thinking in doctors and public choices in medicine.
These lobby groups, having carved themselves respectability via wealth and power, assist lawmakers to keep it this way... Paving the way to Hell with good intentions for their business model and removing peoples human sovereignty.
'Best Practice' they say.
The Glyphosate/Monsanto's of Medicine, The Wolf in Sheep's Clothing, has been allowed to take care of the hen house of human health.
Livestock don't get to choose...
That is why our country wrote the Constitution, to care for The People against false overlords.
Trade deals , plebiscites and Parliamentary Bills introduced for and paid for by industry lobby groups, entrenching in Law, Compulsory Products, are undermining basic constitutional rights to personal health choices within the diverse multi-cultural population.
Personal choices on health were enshrined in the original constitution for a purpose, beyond the monetary Economy.
How was this basic Human Right lost, without anyone noticing?

Millions of people rally to support the Cancer Council and Leukaemia Foundation in an attempt to 'do good' and feel good in the face of the modern epidemic, and to find a Cure... But what if They knew these powerful lobby groups, now big business, actively thwarted any cure or alternative to chemotherapy as part of their business model.

The 'Council of Cancer' and 'Foundation of Leukaemia' perhaps more appropriately describes their movement in the world...

Powerfully and expertly diverting focus with fundraising extravaganzas, expertly manipulating research parameters and alternative findings by way of laws and suppression orders.

Successfully making any 'Cure' illegal and successfully removing choice in medicine from human sovereignty.

This is their only achievement and survival goal.

Time to see through the well-constructed veil of illusion...

The original intent of "Cures" was lost long ago and The Peoples 'good-will',
reigned in, to keep the gravy train going strong.
It's not personal, it's just big business doing well.

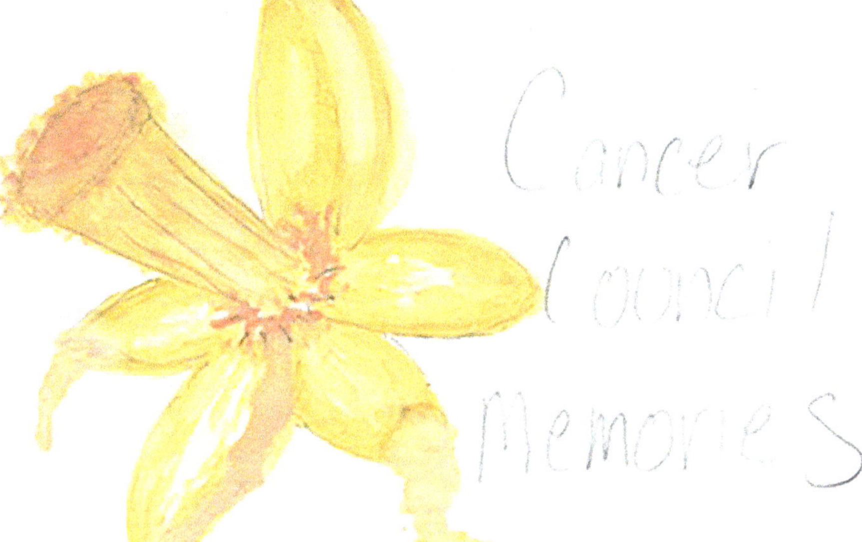

Cancer Council Memories...

Photographs are not the only way to create a "memory".

Chemotherapy will create "Memories" of Your Loved Ones.

Including a gift in your will to Cancer Council "where-ever" Can help us make more lasting "memories".

Gift hope and allow us to continue our fight against Cures. keep the Cancer economy Alive.

Help us pamper Your loved ones before they become Memories.

We Sugar coat toxic treatments, provide Diversional therapy and Transport your Loved ones to chemotherapy. Free with Balm for Calm and Unquestioning Participation. Another Chemo Memory For the Economic Drum.

KS

Awareness Proceeds Change

Awareness may be a difficult path in any field of life, but
Through difficulties, change evolves as increased awareness, through our experiences.
Thus may the "hidden" and the "Dark" in "Disease Management" medicine, the prop-foundations,
Dissolve under Scrutiny's Light.

Beneficial Technology

There are so many beneficial technologies now, in the world, yet
Chemotherapy in treating cancer is protected like technologists and Oil.
Investors seem to wish to keep chemo, and let the profits continue to flow?
Now Alternative Energy is all the go, perhaps
Alternative, Harm-Free Medicine can now be allowed?

"Love" is the Foundation 'Worthy' of your Will!

Commonality binds us all ~

The Universe, Life.
Family, Children.
Old and Young.
Love and Creativity.
The Universal Sovereign right we call Being Human.
To Choose our Health Care, or our poison.
To Choose the Right to say No,
Thank you...
Diversity of choice is Sacrosanct, to
The contribution of Healthy Life –
Not Robotic monoculture of economic delight...
Passing with each fad, day and night.
The Infinite and Eternal Garden
Is the Living Library ~
Custodianship includes,
Free-Will.

Love Supports Life

Fear Supports Monsters

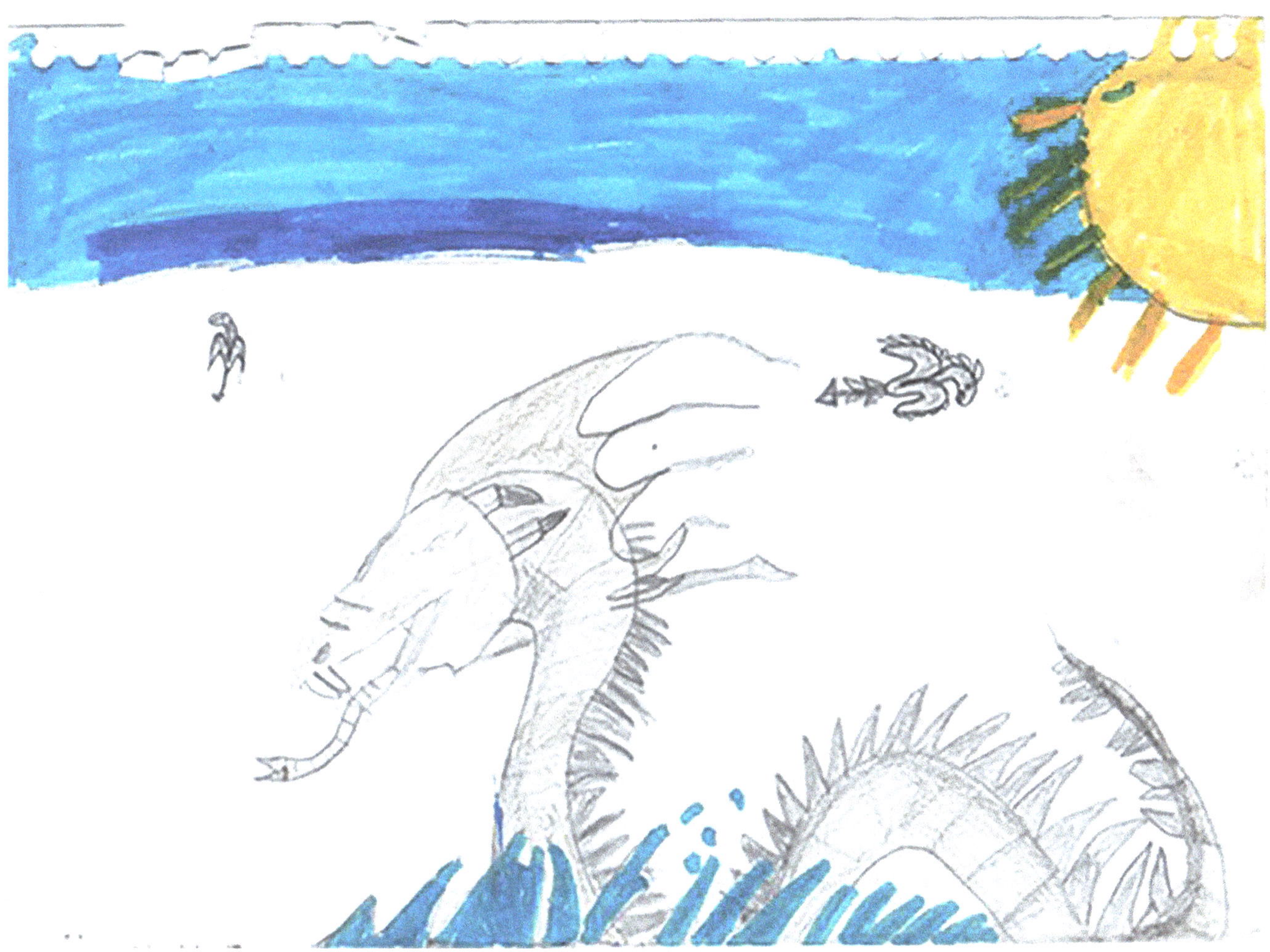

Plastic Fantastic.

Beware the polished and shiny charmers – politicians and salesmen.
We can thank the past Clinton Era for the expensive chemical obsession in the "management of disease".
Extending the Nazi philosophy in Medicine from
Cancer to Aids and then a spiked
Vaccination frenzy creating a
Multitude of new, incurable disease.

Management, Management never a cure to be…
Just more death and profitable disease.
Big Pharma and Invested politicians maximize shareholder profits with 'compulsory' medical ease.
Compulsory medicine it seems, once law,
Is a license to print money and
Demonize Choice and Liberty,
Plying marketing of, false guilt and fear, and
Linking poverty assistance with poisoning our children, go figure?

Hmm, Politicians invested in chemical empires.
Seek to sell their wares through their power, to abuse power,
Enslaving the population…
Of a skilled-down, Dependent Consumer Nation, backed by
The U.S favoured, Zombie Economic Rationalism of Greed.

An example would be Dr Kaali and Lyman's Research, in the 1990's.
Finding that 'micro ampules' of electricity
Disabled the AIDS virus from attaching to a host, and
Cleaned the blood of other bacteria's and viruses,
Without harming healthy human cells
(that have 100 times the ability to withstand electrical charge compared with bacteria and some viruses).
A promising treatment/cure, harm free and
Not expensive chemically… YES.
This was sidelined by the psychopathic medicine machine,
Wasteful and disrespectful, CODEX driven, Like Nazi chemicalisation of the population…

Fourteen U.S. technology patents survive but the Research disappeared,
Directly after the then President Bill Clinton's announcement of
Three Billion Dollar injection into Big Pharma to "Manage" Disease chemically.
Another Lawyer/Politician Investment Secure…

Any wonder, that many people feel disenfranchised,
Tired of trashy mass-production or forced chemicalisation of 'Western' living.
Now seeking… Quality of Life.
Quality Food, Quality Care and
Natures Medicines, respectful, helpful technologies.

Harm-Free, Free Will and Independence within autonomous Communities.
Sovereignty of Choice, supports diversity of life and creative flair.
It is not generally 'A Peoples Will' to participate blindly or knowingly in
An economic recipe of investment for On-going, Quantitive Disease.
Marketing Note:

Love Supports Life, Fear Supports Monsters.

Chapter 11

To act or not act.

Whistle blowers of all sorts, are
Friends of the people,
Enemy of falsely entrenched business and influenced, investing governments.
They are often forced out of well-developed careers, for telling the truth,
Industry does not want to hear...
A choice of conscience and caring about people,
They move beyond fear, to do what is right.
Many suffer legal injunctions and workplace shutouts to prevent the
Truth getting out and affecting profits.
Dr Joanna Budwig – heat treated oils

Climate Scientists

Andrew Wilkie on the WMD Lies of John Howard and Bush era to despise.

Dr Robert Mendelsohn – Confessions of a Medical Heretic

Dr Judy Mikovits - a CDC cancer researcher and vaccine developer blows whistle on contaminated immune modulating products. Admitting links with Autism, Cancer and Auto-immune imbalances brought out of Natural Suppression by the vaccine induced cytokine storms.... Old diseases in different forms

Dr Viera Scheibner – her findings in 100 years of orthodox medicine, published in her book Vaccination: The Medical Assault on the Immune System 1993.

Dr Kaali and Lyman – discovery that micro ampules of electricity disable the AIDs virus, and kill many other pathogens, as healthy cells have 100,000 times the ability to withstand electricity than any bacteria, virus or damaged cell. A harm-free Discovery to assist patients and blood banks to clean supply, ignored due to 3 Billion injection by investors and President Mr. Clinton, to 'manage'

AIDS with pharmaceuticals. Now blood products get harmful radiation instead, making sure everything is dead.

If irradiation/radiation is detrimental to nutrients in fruit and vegetables, as studies suggest, perhaps irradiation of blood products should be ended and replaced with the Kaali and Lyman electrification instead. Ensuring healthy blood cells are used for those that need to be transfused?

Phillip Day's books on the cancer industry/non-health economies and alternatives, are no longer available?

But Welcome to the new wave of whistleblowing - 2.0 Nuremberg Code. Blessings to these honourable people: Dr D Martin, Dr R Fuelmich, Dr L McLindon, Dr Robert Malone and Dr Russell Blaylock, Dr F Wolf and now so many more...

A phrase came to mind...

The ways of the West are not wise.
It is a game of economics and sovereignty's demise.
Long Live the Whistleblower,
May their arrows of Truth point true,
And pierce the veil of illusion, so carefully constructed, to
Aid delusion and fear, within every one of you.

My Child had Leukaemia Twice.

During that time I discovered a constitutional Erosion of Civil Rights in Australia.
Somehow the Civil Rights to Choose a Treatment Path have been removed, for parents of children with such life-threatening conditions...
I found the **Leukaemia Foundation** and the **Cancer Council** to be the most
USELESS organisations on Earth! Expert it appears, in fundraising?
Mere economic puppets, dedicated to diversionary therapy, and
Ensuring nothing competes with chemo-therapy protocols, or their 'personal products' range.
These 'Businesses' are successful in getting your money and marketing falsehoods, nothing else...,
Cyto-toxic contracts must be maintained...Or Else!
Dr Dishwater, bought and sold, he says All-Natural Medicine is a HOAX!?

No Choice, No Intelligent Argument, We Will transport you to the cyto-toxic therapy, none other… Prescription by conscription, supports toxic medicine as you would a football team? Science of medicines emotive manipulation, prisoner dilemma, RAND Style. Not even slightly in alignment with Nuremberg Code?

So, KEEP YOUR HAIR ON! And if you must attend…

Take a stand… ***Wear a Purple Heart, for Courage, for the Civil Right to choose*** *treatments suitable for your personal genetics or preferences, other than Chemotherapy….*

714X, Essiac Tea, Vitamin C therapy, Laetrile, Cannabis Oil, Protocel/Entelev, Personalised stem cell therapy, Dr Hopes Aussie microwave treatment….and more.

So many, more choices, these days that Aussies are Not Allowed to Choose...?

All more successful than, damaging radiation, or chemotherapy. Which according to the small print and Pub Med documentation makes cancer come again… And again….

The Government's investment has been steered by USA/CODEX sales pitch, for **their** economy. Clearly not in the Australian public's best health interests...? Or for OUR FUTURE?

False Laws have been created to prevent choices in health! The Public Voted for None of It.?

Commercial Agreements today, over-ride constitutional efficacy. Follow the money trail, it's there to see…

Hmm, Is it all part of the ANZECC treaty to poison the sick children with left over WW2 chemicals and technology? Or Just prop up Pig Pharma contracts across the globe?

Our Children are as 'NUMBERs' in their profits for poisons, Medical Protocols...!

WEAR A PURPLE HEART, FOR COURAGE AND THE CIVIL RIGHT TO CHOOSE!

God help the children…

End the need for LF or CC, big business, perpetuating outmoded technology and disease!

Quickly Please...

These campaigns, perpetuate trauma, to families that have already suffered the **"World's Greatest Deception"** in the hands of the best intentions and glamourous marketing**... But Never any Cure.!**

There is a 'Monster' in the "Smiling Clown Outfit" people...!!

Interestingly, citizens are expected to have their fingers and toes on the pulse of electronic benefits, global research and information, for the benefit of the economics of business, but Not in Medicine....? Truth has been rendered Not Legal.

No Transparency or Accountability, TGA or FDA with CODEX deals... Nor ANZECC Medical Trials/Studies of some 50 toxic years.? Placated by Million Dollar Foundations of cigarette science it seems?

Not voted for or reviewed by the People. So W.H.O Governs your choices in Medicine? A Clue? ...

Research is a wonderful thing, I do hope our Doctors get to experience its truth someday, when parameters of such are not 'dictated' by poison companies and 'Spoon feeding' by Big Pharma is finally seen as the fur-fey of education that it is.

So, Wear a Purple Heart for Courage,
(when we face the need for choice)

for Choice. (we rightfully, should be able to make)
For Truth and Accountability in Medicine.
(not lies of protectionism and false laws protecting a 'dying' economy.)

Basic Human Rights.
TO BE ALLOWED TO SAY "NO THANKS" TO POISONING.
Let this be your gift to the children of the future.
The right to say NO! And Try something else...

Hoax us Poke us.

Good people prop up toxic systems unwittingly..
I acknowledge that every individual in the Leukaemia foundation is attempting to do good,
The roots of the organisation once sound, now represents a foundation of suppressed and flawed science...
A puppet in the game of public distraction from the Facts.

A puppet perpetuating the Law of Chemotherapy… Laws preventing choice in medicine. Oops, WHO outlawed the research of anything other than CYTOTOXINS?

According to Dr Dishwater, the research undertaken at Melbourne's Children's Hospital, in the cancer trials will "Never" be anything other than Cyto-toxins!??? Nothing but Chemo is supported by the current education and economic investment..

All other avenues according to Dr Dishwater are a HOAX, yes that is the word he used for Any and All research avenues other than Chemotherapy? He is the Chief Oncologist and bone marrow transplant expert… Perhaps his job would be at risk?

Bit unscientific, don't you think? Given he said himself, that he was not prepared to trial anything other than chemotherapy, so where did he form his base line 'Hoax' opinion, on ALL other modalities that could be potentially utilized?

Dr. Dishwater has not tested anything but cyto-toxins, so how would he know, or be an authority on everything else being a Hoax?

Funding prerequisites… prevent digression from the toxic cause? Are Contracts in place, stating that if this research facility is built, controls on research parameters are exercised?

If any doctor mentions something being a Hoax, ask them to produce their research?!

It is usually always an answer of here-say, and research has not been done or is conflicting with economic gravy train.

The 'Hoax' response is a passive-aggressive response, that is easy to say and difficult to prove wrong, unless you know the research parameters and are able to question appropriately.

Few parents are equipped to counter the blanket statement, "it's a hoax" when it comes from a "trusted" doctor.

Such statements are used to stop a person questioning and to make a fool of questioning…

A not so scientific mode, to push through someone's objections, forcibly.

Logically, if as the Dr Dishwater says, ALL alternatives to chemotherapy are a Hoax, then Dr Dishwaters words are a sign of faulty Cigarette Science.

He admits to zero testing of any competition to current cyto-toxin protocols…

Cigarette Science...

The science of economic influence, that demands your unquestioning support, but cannot stand up to questioning.

Diversity in treatments for cancer and therefore greater choice,

Would result in more empowered wellness and better scientific understanding than the current Monoculture of toxic protocols...

Likened to a toxic eddy, in the progressive stream, of medicine.

May the downpour of information trigger a cleanse and restoration of the progressive flow...

Free will treated as sacrosanct and an opportunity for diverse understandings to grow.

Modern medicine may be good at First Aid, especially now with plant based enzyme glues, but

The chemical management of disease is so obviously degenerative, it must be wrong? As it serves only Old School, product profiteers.

Type 2 Diabetes as an example, is reversible with dietary changes reducing inflammation and detoxing the body of PM2.5 biomarkers. See the Halki program diabetes remedy.

Billion Dollar industry protectionism does not benefit from free choice nor natural remedies.

Billion Dollar industries rely on cigarette science or fear, to maintain economies and comfort with high paid lies.

Science, once Noble Questioning of the Nature of Reality, is

Now shackled, as a prostitute, to maintain Corporate Realty.

Doctors as WMD's?

The trusted and unsuspecting
Vehicle of Doctoring, reigned in tight,
Educated and held in Big Pharma's
Dazzling, bright lights.
Pumped with investment propaganda and

Protectionism...
Then prescription puppets are unleashed upon
An unsuspecting and trusting Nation.

Given the investment pathways, Doctor's education,
In the hands of Big Pharma, as good as
Weapons of Mass destruction...
With compulsory prescribing, chemicals of addiction and
Tight controls on "chemical management" of disease...
People told, there is no other choice.!

When the People demand a 'Cure',
Another new research foundation placates the jeers.
No one sees the money spent on engaging events and
Sensational distractions, to maintain the status quo, and
Nobody hears...
Complaints from anybody with 'social license'?
Bad news chemo stories are 'banned' by moguls of media.

Medical fraternities insist that there is no cure.
They spend Billions in court to prevent, natural medical choices
From reaching public ear or curative potential.
They insist Nature is Dangerous or ineffective?... Not to be Trusted?
A corporate assumption, so they don't go out of business. Hmm

Behind the scenes, before the courts rightly decided that
Patents on Natural substances could not be...
The US Government had Patents on Cannabis and THC,
Stating it cured more than 170 different cancers, demonstrating;
This has been known since 1970's.

With this knowledge in tow and having seen that
Research into Natures Cures is constantly thwarted or met with hostility,
by formulae of, Rich chemical competitors and existing contracts, of existing product owners.

Look at Graviola and Mangosteen... You will see what I mean.
10 years of research thrown away, due to zero patentability, both fruits
Proved 10,000 times stronger in killing cancer cells that cyclophosphamide,

one of the more seriously damaging chemo components, and yet
these fruits do not harm healthy cells.

People have been bombarded with marketing, as
The medical institutions and chemical management protocols have
Worked their magic on our societal health…
Creating more insanity, more disease to
'Manage', than any other era previously seen.
So, in the words of Dr Robert S Mendelsohn, MD
"If this is preventative medicine, I'll take my chances with disease."
Writer of useful texts for any parent, 'Confessions of a Medical Heretic"
'Male Practice', 'How Doctors Manipulate Women' and
'How to Raise a Healthy Child… In Spite of Your Doctor.'

In this day and age of prescription-puppet-
Modern-chemical-management of humanity and
1930's investment streams,
Doctors are dangerously, Agents of Delivery, of
Weapons of Mass health destruction.
It is showing in population genetics, massive increases in chronic and acute diseases.
Acute Lymphoblastic Leukaemia has become the biggest childhood killer, once a rarity?

Awareness grows, with pain and dysfunction, a catharsis occurs and with it
Precipitation…
Breakdown or Breakthrough… Epiphany.
Nature, within us, restores balance and harmony…
To Society, to Individuals, to Doctoring.
So it be.

Nature has been disrespected, exploited and ignored,
Prevented from participation in
Balanced medical form.

Nature finds its way, nature in you and nature in Me,
Will not allow all that is Natural in Human Life
To be destroyed.
Our children of diverse genetics, were not born to be
Robots, in a mechanised world.

Technology that aids, respect, harmony and
Functionality, will stay.
All 'Life Depleting' investments, to be
Swept away.

Nature is the basis from which all physical creations are possible.
A new respect for Natures interconnectedness, and ours,
Will give 'Man' what it needs to Excel,
In a balanced and respectful way.

Out of destructive Adolescence and into Maturity.
Ride the Waves of Change that are here.
Do Not Despair.
After the fall of the toxicology chemical revolution,
Balanced biochemistry will resume.

But for now chemical regulations and controls of corporations has stolen
The soil from farmers, the doctoring from Doctors, and
The Peoples health, is stolen for profit too.

Stolen Lives and Public Lies

As Chemical Dependence Medicine falls from Grace,
And the market's stage,
Big Pharma will feel the Publics Rage.
Stolen children and the Aged,
Dying untimely chemicalised deaths,
Just like a plague.. Or MRNA.
Natures Medicines will again prevail,
In healing Cancer and Auto-immune disorders
As Multi-National, Poison/Pharmaceutical Manufactures' have failed.
Trust is Lost in chemical medicine, for "Managing" any disease, or
The preventions that they sell…more akin to Entrapment?
Like many pharmaceutical therapies,
Having been found to be ineffective and/or
Promoting more disease.
This Big Pharma self-perpetuating economy is a crime against Wellness and Humanity.

A change of medical focus away from residual income,
To reconnect with the wellness expected of every age, and
Providing 'health positive' choices in medicine,
In accordance with natures diversity.
The Peoples health is not a game of Big Pharma/Lawyer/Politician Monopoly.
Medicines job is to alleviate pain, where it can, and to allow more Joy in the Body.
Good Medicine would provide Healthful Choice and have respect for Diversity over Profitability.

Protectionism - killing trust in Medicine

Fearing new modalities and protection old sustainability
Is the best way to kill trust in medicine.
Ask Morris Fischbein, who would trust his fake research now?
Laetrile/Amygdalin cures cancer. A Fact.
Dr Fischbein expended millions of dollars and six years of others efforts to debunk natures medicine to ensure his own chemical investment, profitability.
The efforts made, in covering up a wrong, add to the wrong, it does not go away...
The truth is always revealed, eventually...
Cover-ups make the Lie look much bigger indeed.
Then you can watch your hard built economy recede,
What-ever it be.
Now unworthy... Justified doubt, due to Deceit.
A Just Karma, don't you think...?
For A Medical industry that promotes itself on the power of TRUST.
But took 200 years of fear based protectionism before they acknowledged vitamin C cured Scurvy?!?
Yes indeed, Unworthy...
If a man may be known by his words and his deeds, the
Medical industry has fallen foul of a protectionist economy.
Intravenous Vitamin C has been criminalized and made illegal to stop people regaining health and independence. Iodine is next according to the requests of Council of Cancers economic institute.
This is a far cry from what the people really need.
AMA, take Heed,
Your power is an illusion of your own creation,
Industry Protectionism is not a public service, but indeed
The Killer of Trust and Free Will.

A Doctors Friend

Sadly all is not equal in Medicine Land,
I like my Doctors to have 'experience', to
Think outside the square, to assist in good faith.
Not the hurried Prescription Puppet that couldn't even manage a check-up.
Don't get me wrong.
I am the Doctors Friend...
Generally, Good People helping,
All People to be 'Well'.
I do, however, Abhor the Big Pharma Control Drama!
Crafting ignorance, via education; of product promulgation, promoting Illness and Dependency to perpetuate their market shares.
The Good Doctors I adore, are critical thinkers not prescription puppets.
Choice in Medicine, is Good for Doctors and
The Peoples True Friend.
Not "Fear Factor" Medication!
For improved health and budget outcomes, bring an End to Big Pharma controlled Education, Law making, and toxic Investment Trends.
Such that Big Pharma may no longer Monopolize or Offend;
The Sovereignty of Peoples Right to Choose, 'What-Ever'
Medicine or Modality, suits their current health issues.
The continued War on Natural Medicines is now regarded by many Citizens and Physicians as RIDICULOUS.
Natural Medicine and Pharmaceuticals CAN and DO, Co-Exist.
Focus Being: Medicine as a Means to a Healthy outcome.
People are Relieved to see, the investment trend of the current machine, peddling dependency and toxic neglect, is about to END.
As the Prescription Puppet era falls away,
Real Doctoring begins a new 'multi-modality' day.
Time to bring back basics, like, physiology and how to use that blood pressure machine...

Doctors researching Gut/Brain health link,

Failed by a web of protectionism.
AMA – A Union for Doctors?
Where were they in 2015 when 15 Doctors, all mysteriously exited the planet… Deceased.
The cost of Education and Lives of Service lost to us!
Their commonality was; ground breaking work with 'GcMAf', and
Beneficial research into the Human Glyco Protein Macrophage,
One of our body's natural cancer killers…
The minor studies showed, the Full Recovery of Brain Function in 85% of Patients with Autism that were treated with GcMAf.
GcMAf needs to bond with vitamin D3 in the body to function properly…
Another Protein called Nagalase blocks vitamin D receptors that enable GcMAf.
Nagalase is introduced to the body via Cancer tumor growth or a Virus and is found in high levels in Autistic people… SV40?
Nagalase is present in Vaccines… and associated with causing Cytokine Storms (inflammation)…
Treatments with GcMAf were showing great results in restoring functionality and health to People with Cancer, Diabetes, Parkinson's, Alzheimer's, Dementia and Autism.
Too Bad, Big Pharma didn't want you to know!.. Billions of dollars at risk.
Rest in Peace the Good Dr Tim Smith MD, and other collaborating colleagues.
May the study on 'GcMAf' be published, regardless that he is now deceased.
Let the People decide if working with GcMAf is worthy,
We don't want another repeat of the 200 years of convenient denial, like that of Vitamin C and Scurvy.!?
Some Doctors of the past thought wellness would end their profession, yet
It is, Acts of blinding Protectionism, that
Kill Trust and the Professional Evolution of Truth in Medicine.
GcMAf is a probiotic that helped prove the Brain, Gut health link.

Published on 1 September 2021 by an Australian Doctor, and in honour of other Australian's bravery, like Dr William Bay's, standing up to APHRA for honesty.

The Immuno-biology of mRNA Covid vaccination

A brief discussion

Introduction

To qualify as a valuable medical intervention a vaccination should be safe, effective and necessary. This summary will examine recent insights into the makeup and activity of the mRNA lipid nanoparticle vaccinations. Like no other medical intervention in history, this push for vaccination is global in its reach and the time interval between the emergence of a disease and the provision of a putative vaccine is unprecedented for its brevity. Further, the manipulation of data and censorship of dissenting voices has reached a level not seen with any other medical intervention.

Financial imperative rather than efficacy appears to have guided privatised vaccine development in the past. For example current versions of the influenza virus are manufactured to produce antibodies to surface antigens. As these mutate rapidly and change from year to year or even within a season, the vaccine needs to be given annually. To compound the problem the vaccine makers have to predict which variant will make an appearance the next year, to provide manufacturing lead time. Thus, the efficacy of the vaccine varies from nil, if the prediction is erroneous, to about 30%. Australian scientists developed a nasally administered vaccine against the core antigens. These remain far more constant than the ever changing surface antigens, with a duration of around seven years. In addition to this obvious advantage the added benefit of administering vaccine to imitate a natural infection, the body generates a range of IgA mucosal antibodies that can neutralise any virus before it reaches the general circulation. Despite the overwhelming advantages the project lapsed due to lack of funding.

The financial windfall to corporations enjoying a coerced global clientele is beyond calculation. The manipulation of data has been a hallmark of the transnational pharmaceutical companies for some time. For example, using data supplied to the FDA by the companies themselves, the relative risk reduction of their covid vaccine was calculated at around 95%, a very reassuring number for the uninformed. When the absolute risk reduction was calculated using the same company figures and bearing in mind there are serious allegations against the companies for introducing bias by patient selection and exclusion, the absolute risk reduction for an individual was 1.1% for Moderna and 0.7% for Pfizer.

RNA viruses, such respiratory syncytial virus (RSV) and the corona viruses have resisted attempts at vaccination in the past. RSV is a serious respiratory disease of early infancy. Up to 60,000 infants die of this condition every year and many more require hospitalisation. Early attempts at vaccination were thwarted by the emergence of antibody dependent enhancement (ADE). This is a condition of immune tolerance induced by the generation of non-neutralising antibodies. When exposed to a similar virus the immune system fails to react. Several children died after the vaccine and the program was abandoned. It is a salutatory lesson that RSV did not exist before 1955. It was introduced into the human population after 200,000 primates were used in the production of the polio vaccine. A zoonotic virus named chimpanzee coryza virus transferred to veterinary staff and then to the human population, when it was renamed RSV.

How are mRNA vaccines manufactured

Although commonly described as vaccines they have nothing in common with the inactivated or attenuated pathogen vaccines used to date and are better described as a nucleotide based gene therapy. For brevity they will be referred to as vaccines here. Ribose Nucleic Acid (RNA) when outside of the cell provokes a strong immune reaction and is rapidly cleared from the circulation by RNAse enzymes. The manufacturers thwarted this by substituting chemically altered pseudo-uridine for the physiological base uridine, so that the body's enzymes cannot bind to and degrade it. Thus, the vaccine not only introduces foreign RNA into the body, but chemically altered RNA, never seen in nature. It is not predictable what consequences this could have in the short or the long term, but this chemical substitution affects interferon production. Interferon is a cytosine produced by the body in response to viral RNA and serves to limit viral replication. The uridine/pseudouridine substitution blunts the interferon response, so reducing the body's natural defence.

The altered RNA codes for the spike protein that projects from the surface of the viral capsule and allows entry to the human cell by binding to the angiotensin converting enzyme 2 (ACE 2), widely distributed in the endothelium of the vasculature and organs. The RNA code has been further modified to substitute the amino acid proline at two critical sites to maintain the spike protein in its highly immunogenic pre-fusion state. Given that it is bound to an important cell based enzyme the result of this enhanced immunogenicity cannot be predicted in the short or long term.

Blood pressure is controlled by the renin angiotensin system. In response to reduced renal blood flow the kidneys excrete an enzyme renin. This enzyme acts on angiotensinogen produced in the liver to produce angiotensin1. This is further cleaved by ACE 1 in the lungs to produce angiotensin 2. Angiotensin 2 has a pro inflammatory effect and increases blood pressure by constricting blood vessels and stimulating the adrenal glands to release aldosterone. To maintain homeostasis this angiotensin is then degraded by ACE 2. Interference with ACE2 function by covid binding is behind some of the pathology seen with the viral infection. Introducing mRNA coding for a spike protein that binds to the ACE 2 receptor, especially a spike protein that has been chemically altered to enhance immune response could be expected to have similar adverse effects.

Further, research has established that in order to confidently produce neutralising antibodies at least three epitopes, or sites for antigenic stimulation, should be immunised for. Immunising against only one epitope, such as the spike protein alone, is much less effective. Importantly, spike protein alone was insufficient to garner a T cell response, whereas three epitopes elicited a brisk reaction.

As an aside, comment needs be made concerning antibody levels called titres. The single criterion used by the regulators for success of a vaccine has been the antibody titre. So long as a rise in antibodies is seen the vaccine is deemed successful and marketed with official sanction. Concerning influenza, as stated in the product information itself there have been no studies which have demonstrated a reduction in the incidence or severity of infection after vaccination. This preoccupation with antibody titre led vaccine manufacturers to include toxic adjuvants such as mercury and aluminium to the vaccines to overstimulate the B cells to earn the regulators tick of approval, even though no health benefit may be gained.

Lipid nanoparticles

In order to deliver the fragile mRNA to the cells the manufacturers encapsulated it in lipid nanoparticles. These nanoparticles are new to medicine and their biology is not well understood. There are a number of concerns. One of the ingredients DSPC is very pro inflammatory, raising levels of tumour necrosis factor (TNF) and other cytokines. The particles also contain polyethylene glycol (PEG), also used as an antifreeze fluid. In surveys in the US over 40% of people have pre-existing PEG antibodies, greatly increasing the risk of allergic reaction, including anaphylaxis.

For a vaccine product that is being pushed on the world these novel substances have not been thoroughly studied. The manufacturers intended for the nanoparticles to remain at the site of injection but studies have shown that they can distribute widely, including crossing the blood brain barrier. They can also localise in the ovaries. In fact, it seems that the distribution of these nanoparticles could be somewhat arbitrary. For example if the injection is given subcutaneous rather than intramuscular the nanoparticles may scatter much more widely, to lodge in multiple sites not appropriate as sites for immune reaction.

Autoimmunity

Epitopes on the spike protein have been found to cross react with at least six human proteins including myelin basic protein, thyroid peroxidase, extractable nuclear antigen, mitochondria and myosin. Antibodies to these can and probably will have clinical significance as antibodies to myelin basic protein cause multiple sclerosis while antibodies to thyroid peroxidase result in Hashimoto thyroiditis. Cross reacting spike protein generated autoantibodies could therefore be responsible for diseases indistinguishable from those diseases originating without exposure to the spike protein and this could be used to obfuscate the actual pathogenic mechanism responsible, especially since the pathology may take some time to manifest. Autoantibodies can be generated during the course of a corona virus infection. If these people are then inoculated with the spike protein vaccine the probability of autoimmunity would be increased. Given this fact and the fact that immunity acquired by natural infection is stronger and longer lasting that vaccine immunity, it beggars belief that people with clear evidence of past infection are being coerced to vaccinate.

By a different mechanism the vaccine has resulted in an increase in the frequency of Herpes Zoster (shingles). Inflammation induced by the vaccine can up regulate TNF, which suppresses interferon, resulting in latent viral reactivation.

Spike protein toxicity

In nutritionally compromised individuals and those with special sensitivities infection with Covid19 infection can cause severe disease with changes in the pulmonary vasculature resembling pulmonary arterial hypertension. Experimental evidence has shown that these changes can be reproduced by the infusion of the S1 subunit of the spike protein alone, with no viable virus present. This must concern thinking people, as the vaccine makers strategy is to induce large amounts of spike protein to be generated via the administered mRNA. The mechanism is not complicated. The spike protein binds to and blocks ACE 2, disabling its enzymatic activity resulting in excess circulating angiotensin 2. The S1 subunit is pro-inflammatory and disrupts the blood brain barrier, causing neurological dysfunction.

ACE 2 is heavily expressed in the testes and the few post mortem examinations that have been done on Covid patients have show pathological changes, highly likely to affect fertility. There are numerous reports of menstrual disturbances and miscarriages. The extent of this effect has not been quantified, although preliminary data provides clear signals of harm.

Prion diseases, including Creutsfeldt Jacob disease in humans, bovine spongiform encephalopathy (BSE) or mad cow disease and scrapie in sheep result when certain proteins induce the mis-folding of important structural proteins in the brain. Alzheimers and Parkinsons disease may be slower evolving forms of prion disease. The proteins responsible contain structures referred to as the glycine zipper motif and can be represented as GxxxG, where two glycine molecules are separated by any three amino acids. The more this motif is repeated the more potent the resulting pathological effects. BSE has strings of ten such motifs. Of extreme concern is the fact that the spike protein contains strings of five of these motifs. Such motifs have not been detected in any corona virus spike protein other than SARS Cov2. The clinical implications of this finding should induce the most acute concern, as there is no known strategy to reverse the pathological changes.

Shedding of the spike protein from an immunised individual is a theoretical and possibly practical risk, as exosomes (sub-cellular bodies containing proteins) have been detected in sputum. Whilst the quantity of such spike protein transferred would not be great, the presence of prion like activity could lead to significant pathology.

It is generally assumed that mRNA cannot be incorporated into the genome unless a reverse transcriptase enzyme is present. Detailed genetic research has disclosed structures call LINES and SINES (long and short interspersed nuclear elements). These were dismissively referred to as junk DNA but now they are believed to contain reverse transcriptase activity, possibly incorporated from prior retrovirus exposure. As outlined above the vaccine mRNA has been chemically modified to a form never found in nature. The incorporation of such altered genetic codes introduces risk for unpredictable outcomes.

Conclusion

This brief account has only touched on some of the possible unintended consequences of this experimental gene therapy. The issue of transplacental spread and immune tolerance in the newborn has not been discussed for want of information, but learning from the case of bovine viral diarrhoea, caused by the RNA pestivirus we see trans placental spread and immune tolerance, such that the newborn sheds large quantities of virus, without an effective immune response. This and other serious concerns should serve as a stark warning. The last two years have seen unprecedented activity by governments of all stripes and private corporations to limit debate and establish a single paradigm that brooks no other. Senior medicos are censored or censured for voicing concern and new laws are being constantly introduced, generally not bolstered by any credible research. Political agendas and greed appears to be trumping (no pun intended) rational investigation, while full and open debate, the hallmark of a rational society, is smothered under a welter of media propaganda.

Albert Einstein famously opined that "the splitting of the atom has changed everything except how man thinks, so that we rush towards catastrophe". If that great man were alive today that cautionary message could be restated as "the manipulation of the code of life has changed everything except the greed and arrogance of the power elite, such that we rush to unparalleled dangers.

Sincerely
Dr Andrew Katelaris MD

Video Reference from Telegram: The Concerned Lawyers Network;

Top Merck Scientist Admits That Polio Vaccines contained Leukemia, SV40-And Cancer Viruses.

In this 1987 interview one of the most prominent vaccine scientists in the history of the vaccine industry Dr Maurice Hilleman a Merck scientist made a recording where he openly admits...

https://rumble.com/vlgck83-top-merck-scientist-admits-that-polio-vaccines-contained-leukemia-sv40-and-html

And..

'It's Time to Start Questioning Everything,' Including the Childhood Vaccinations

Steve Kirsch: "(I asked Andrew Wakefield), 'Do the unvaccinated kids do 10% better, 20% better in terms of the health outcomes and so forth?' And he said 'Oh, no! Not even close. It's like 10x.'10x."

Dr Ryan Cole: "If you look at under reign of Fauci for 40 plus years, where childhood chronic diseases and illnesses have gone from 6% to about 54% as we've added more and more layers of shots onto those schedules. And again, they'll say 'Correlation isn't causation.' Well, not a single childhood vaccine was ever tried in their clinical trials against placebo."

Full Video: tinyurl.com/Cole-Kirsch

Robert Kennedy in 2025 interview confirms that evidence shows The CDC have 'NEVER' tested any of the childhood vaccinations, recommended in many countries and compulsory in some, for safety or efficacy, relying instead on manufacturer claims. The TGA in Australia too have never tested any vaccine listed on the Australian Compulsory Register, instead relying on claims made by the CDC.

Old and new studies show that vaccinated groups suffer many health complications over many years, ranging from mild to severe disease, unlike the much healthier un-inoculated counterparts.

There is no such thing as a harm-free vaccine, the legal term given in the Supreme Court in USA is **"unavoidably unsafe"**.

Observably, laws enforcing the inoculation of children in Australia and the World are not ensuring good health but profits for pharmaceutical manufacturers.

"Why do Covid 'vaccines' cause cancer? Quoted from a 2023 video interview with **Angus Dalgleish, Professor of Oncology at St George's Hospital Medical School** in London, former President of The Clinical Immunology and Allergy Section of the Royal Society of Medicine, explains...

"The Pfizers are all full of SV40. SV40 was what, in my day, we put into mice to make them grow tumours so we could pour chemotherapy into them to see if it worked for the tumours. And we are putting this into humans for a disease that hasn't killed anybody for at least two years?! It is beyond belief! And that's really what I cannot understand. Now, today (2023), I got sent something from Australia which I must say it, is the closest to being cold in my stomach and being sick. It was a race on Morrison, the Prime Minister, doing a deal with Moderna for messenger RNA vaccines for the next 10 years, that you will buy $2 Billion! Australian Dollars of these vaccines over the next 10 years, and they will target all sorts of diseases and they will be given to children. This is a gene therapy that they... I mean how much were they bribed to do that?! Because I must say, if I was given a billion dollars to do this and it meant it was going into children. I would walk away, even if it was 10 billion. To me it is beyond belief that you would even consider it! These people behind Moderna and Pfizer are just pure, pure evil, and they must be held to account!""

Chapter 12

Saving Our Children From The World's Biggest Psychopath.

The true story, a journey of chemical conscription, of a boy and the World...

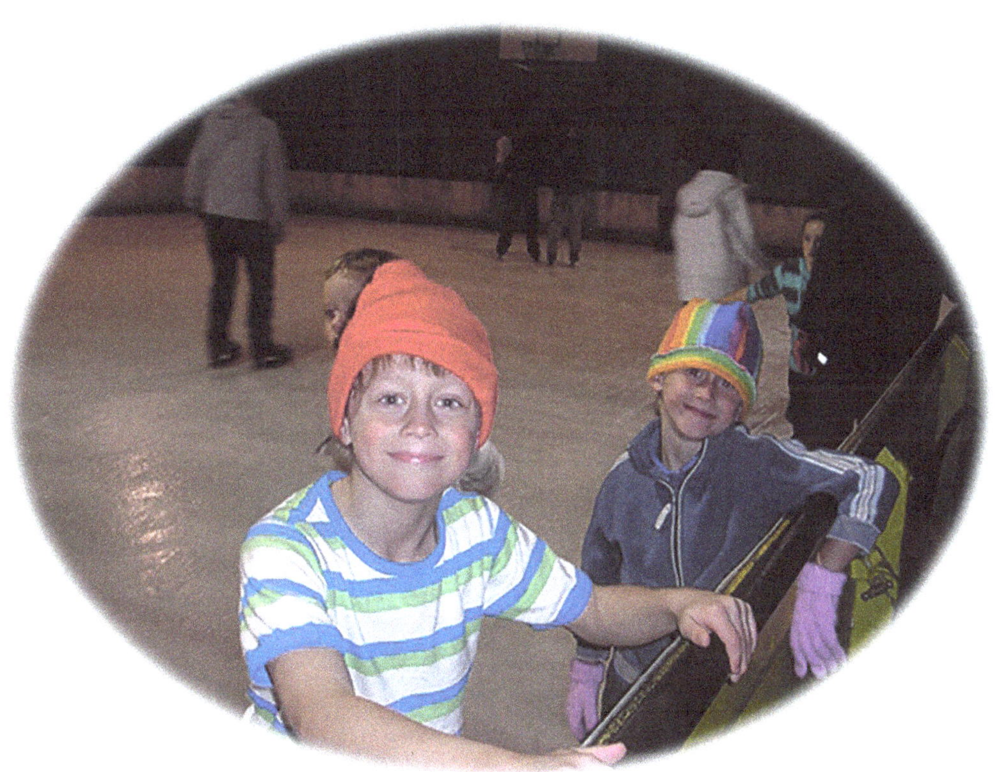

Summary

For Dylan and the future of our children; Let them be free of Hazchem's, free from the hidden, systemic economy of psychopathic tyranny; of choiceless, conscripted chemicalised management, dependency and death... Let our children be Sovereign beings benefiting from clean water, the vitality of biologically farmed food and harm free medicine choices. The right to choose wellness. The right to choose naturalness, the right to ... Be Here Now.

The edifice of the Australian Constitution is Sovereignty. The King James Bible was used as a reference point to ensure "Sovereignty" of Citizens after Catholicism was seen to rob other religions patrons of their skins, and rights to live peacefully etc.... It is even written into the Australian Constitution that no Catholic should hold public office, as a permanent acknowledgement of the suffering of innocent non catholic civilians that were harmed by the said extremist Catholic Church doctrine keepers prior to the 1900's.

The Australian Constitution has its first 8 sections dedicated to citizen rights, and the 9th section of the constitution which via plebiscites, is the only section of the constitution that the Government recognizes since "corporatization" in the year 2000. The section of the constitution governing your health choices, especially pertaining to your own children, is not recognized by the current Australian "corporation", again, industry owned politicians make use of Plebiscites to enable industry profits and remove individual health choices. Children with Cancer have no rights and are forced into a Hazchem regime regardless of ineffectiveness, toxicity or parental consent.

I always thought we in Australia, lived in a free country, until my son got Acute Lymphoblastic Leukaemia, then I discovered that we live in an illusion of democratic choice. It appears that some multi-national conglomerate is being serviced by our politicians, at taxpayer expense. And now our constitutional rights to choose medicines and foods have been compromised by corrupt Agricultural and Medicinal interests that make money out of Chemical management; of Agricultural Land (the body of our earth) and the chemical management of disease (our bodies/ our children's).

This is written to show how such things are facilitated by various governing bodies and other salubrious organisations and has been implemented purposefully using the law of graduation over a period of approximately 70 years.

The chemicalisation of world's food and medicine is encouraging a population of chemically managed Drones... A Psychopathic Economy of enslavement and destruction to maintain the industrialist games of the past.

Equals disaster; for our Earth, our land/soil health, our food and water, our bodies, our genetics, our future as healthy sovereign beings capable of expressing the full gambit of the Great Spirits many expressive potentials in life...

The weeping women of the world,
I hear your cries, within the tears of my own eyes
For you, this book is intended as an extended arm,
Exposing an economic world of lies...
That, future mothers and children will have greater discernment, and Thrive!
Whatever the cause when a child dies,
Radiation, Chemo, or land mines,
Guns, bombs, or other Westinghouse/Life's Good guise,
All are agents of war, products of conflict,
Continued and continued, to justify prior investments and shareholder profits.

Our children die for economies of oil, diamonds, war, timber and the mining of ore, are Routinely harmed by ineffective medicine, processed food, immunity products and more... Our children's lives blindly conscripted to fulfill the economies of the World's Biggest Psychopath...

Enough is Enough, conscripted chemicalisation and conflict are; Against Natural Law!
The economic Hoax on Humanity CAN be altered to SERVE,
The healthy continuance of human creativity and trade,
Is this so absurd?

Our Greatest weakness, as has enslaved us, to this psychopathic economic blight, our "Desire", for ease, comfort and pleasure, when unbalanced or in excess, causes dependency, loss of skills, and sovereignty loss over time. Not my fore fathers time, but mine and our children's children.

Our Greatest Strength and bringer of peace and atonement is the same seat as our weakness.

Our power to choose...

A Collection of useful books

THERE IS ALWAYS AN ALTERNATIVE – Peter Baratosy MD BS

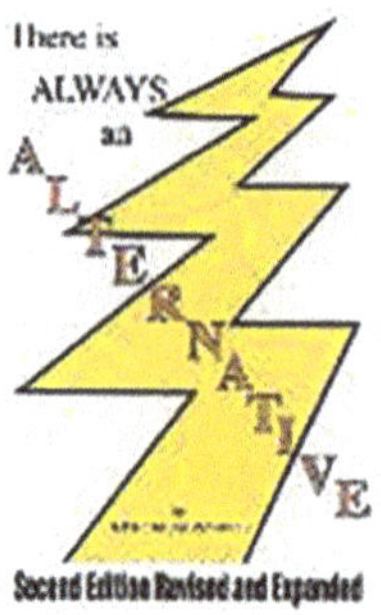

Confessions of a Medical Heretic – Robert S Mendelsohn, MD

See Appendix page 268 for an excerpt from this book.

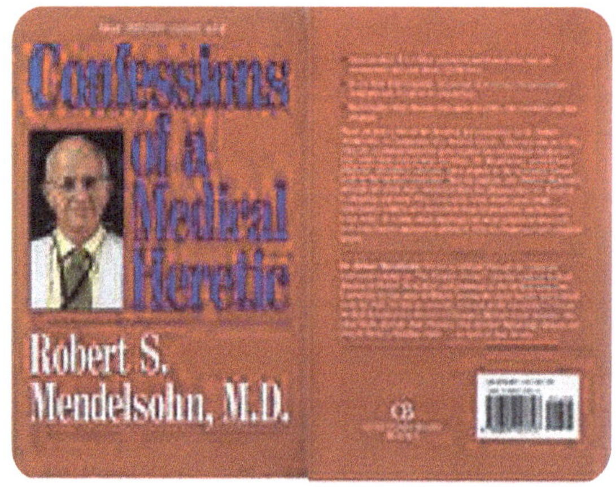

How to raise a healthy child in spite of your doctor – Robert S Mendelsohn, MD

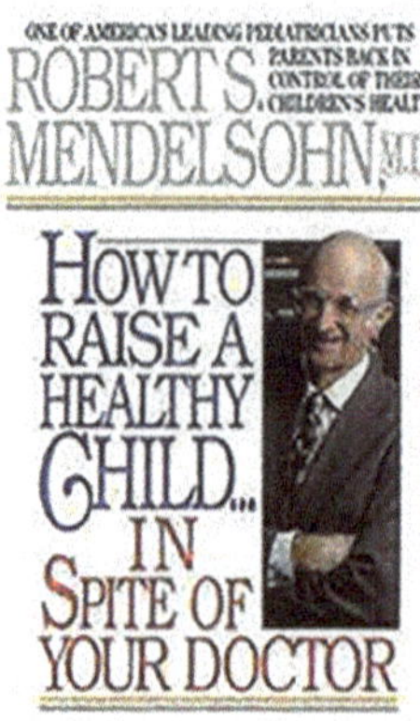

VACCINATION The Medical Assault on the Immune System – Viera Scheibner Ph.D. – 100 years of Orthodox Research shows that Vaccines Represent a Medical Assault on the immune system.

See appendix page 245 for some excerpts from this book.

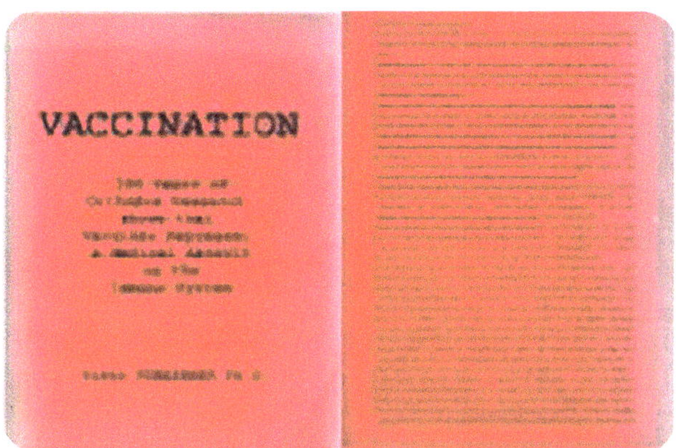

And my favourite, because it **empowered** my choices:

Outsmart Your Cancer, Non-toxic treatments that work, by Tanya Harter-Pierce.

Discussing several Alternative Non-Toxic Treatments that work, she includes the history of suppression of each modality discussed. This book really helps when one is looking outside the box for choices that may work with different cancers, references including some case study contacts are available to assist.

Link to online PDF: https://all-med.net/files/ebook.php?id=fY-PPgAACAAJ&item=outsmart-your-cancer

(See appendix for book review giving page references to the book and PDF)

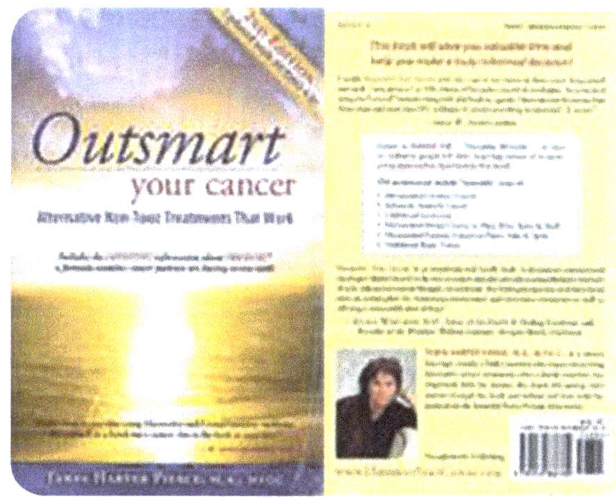

The Complete Raw Juice Therapy

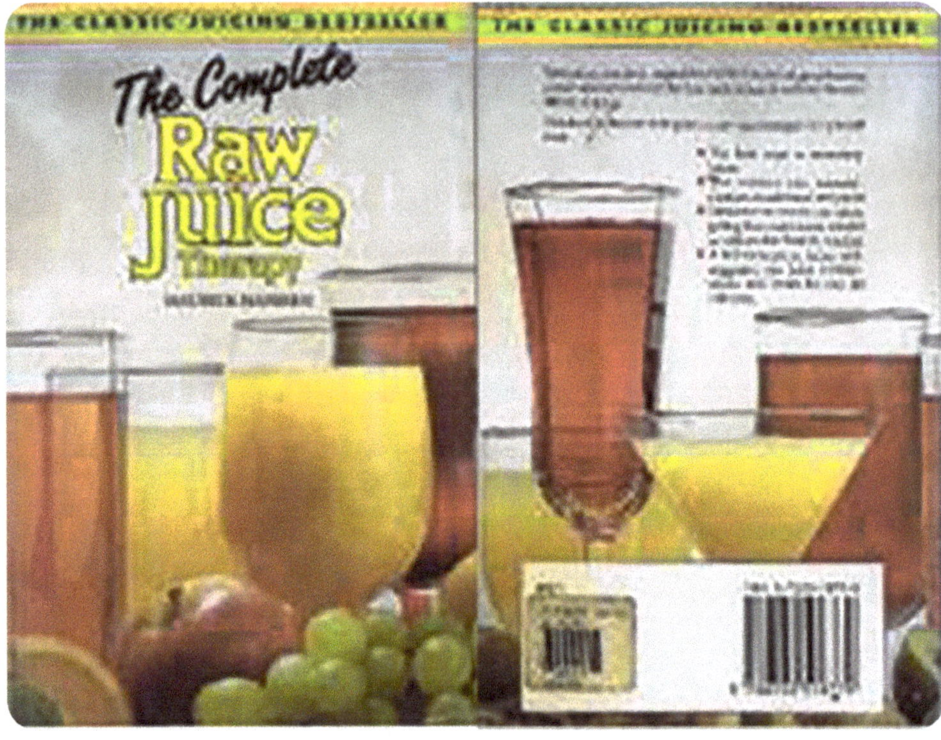

'The Breuss CANCER Cure' by Rudolf Breuss with Hilde Hemmes, is a truly insightful and practical assistant on the journey of personal choice in treatment of Cancer.

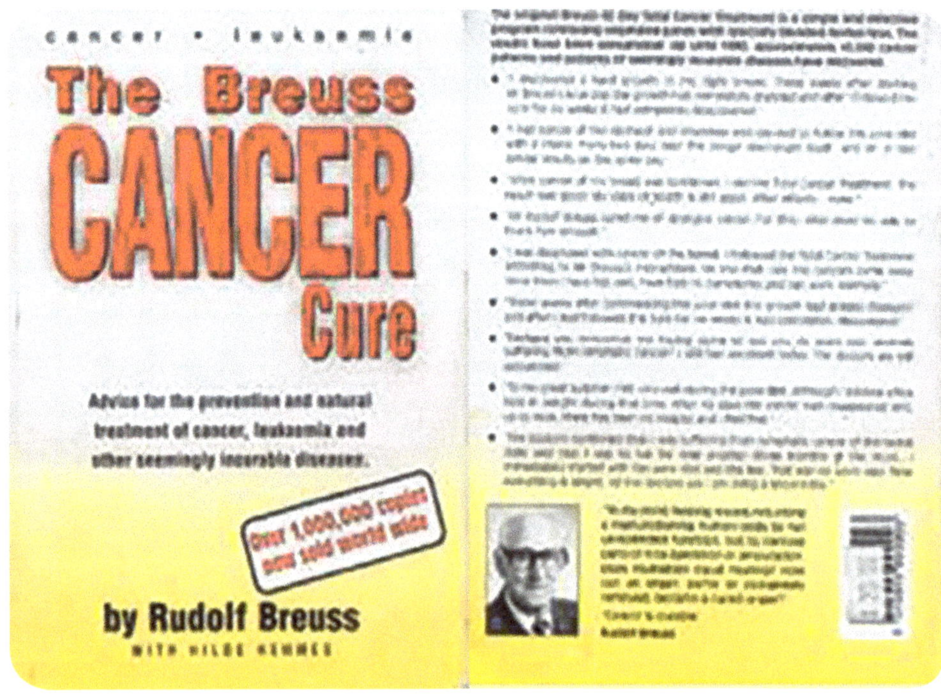

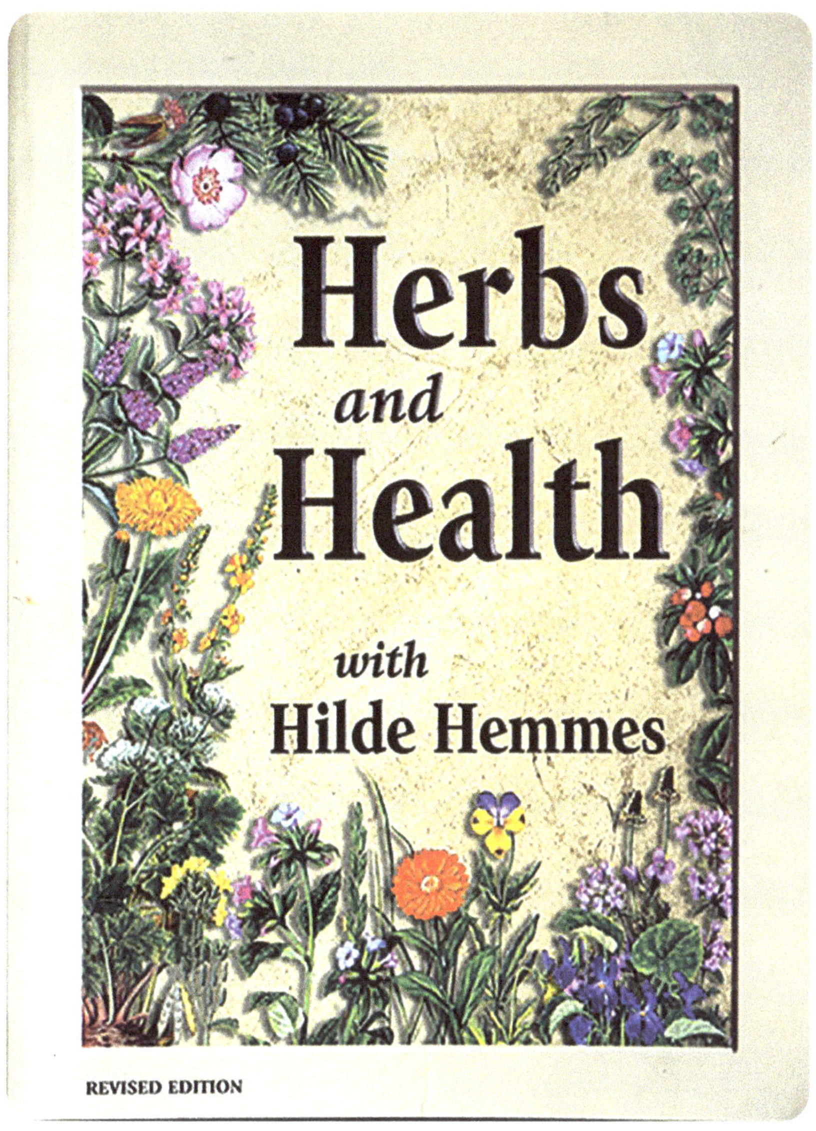

From the Australian School of Herbal Medicine

'Herbs and Health with Hilde Hemmes'

"Many people died while the herbs that could have cured them grow on their graves." Sebastian Kneipp (1821-1897) Some sample recipes from this wonderful book are included on the following page.

'SELF HELP CANCER CURE & other chronic diseases' a book by Walter Last, Chris Wheeler, Max Yelsaeb & Health writers. "Cancer is relatively easy to prevent & cure. The really terminal disease in our society is the moral cancer which prevents the safe, certain & above all, cheap methods described in these pages from being applied universally." Published by the Soil & Health Association of New Zealand Inc, Auckland 1997.

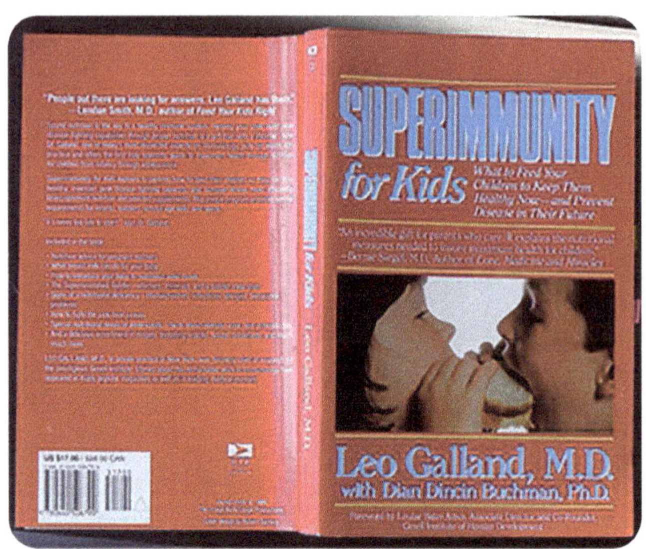

– SUPERIMMUNITY for Kids. What to Feed Your Children to Keep Them Healthy Now – and

Prevent Disease in Their Future. By Leo Galland, M.D. with Dian Dincin Buchman Ph.D.

Collection of useful links

Look up – Dr. Sebi Marathon

https://www.youtube.com/watch?v=zc_YI85u7wQ –
Dr Russel Blaylock, Surgeon. – Sugar and Brain health talk

https://www.youtube.com/watch?v=JPyj9Pi8nw4 –
Dr Suzanne Humphries, MD – Vit C and Immunity

https://www.youtube.com/watch?v=nkI5MCUNuXw –
Dr Linus Pauling (Nobel prize winner) on Vitamin C and immune disorders 10 years of clinical research proving Vit C can cure any disease. Ignored by AMA.

https://www.youtube.com/watch?v=YHKBhz7OCB4&t=328s –
Liposomal vs. Oxidized Vitamin C and DIY DHAA: The Amazing Green Smoothie

https://www.ncbi.nlm.nih.gov/pmc/?term=BLACK%20SEED%20ANTI%20CANCER&fbclid=IwAR1EdqDGYVu4bQyErGbrgSqZGCl07vBPL_MUj9KP0TdrCprOyP7EA9BpBPY –
The Anti-Cancer properties of Nigella / Black Seed oil. A collection of peer-reviewed studies.

Physics Of Crystals Full Documentary - Les Brown
https://www.youtube.com/watch?v=wM21geOzyj8&t=219s

Dr Bob Becks blood electrification DIY: link

https://www.scribd.com/document/558620483/126474736-Homemade-Bob-Beck-Machine

www.bobbeckinstruments.com also on Instagram @bobbeckinstruments

On Facebook.. Bob Beck Zapper & Colloidal Silver (schematics, videos, products and groups)

Search: Video from Paul Napier taken from old footage of Bob Beck talk January 16 1997 "Treating Cancer and every known disease with Colloidal Silver and EMP's Dr. Bob Beck..."

Based on research done at the Albert Einstein Medical Institute by Researchers Kaali and Lyman. 14 US Patents. One being: 5188738 Dr Kaali. Feb 23 1993. Invention made to attenuate any virus, bacteria, parasites, fungus or disease. Electrode arrays implanted into arm.

3.92Htz half of the Schumann's resonance. 50-100micro ampules biphasic pulses.

https://www.youtube.com/watch?v=9OQ7q7B99TA
For Vitamin C, this lecture is informative and offers PubMed references .

https://jeffreydachmd.com/vitamin-c-saves-dying-man/
The Mr Allan Smith story, 60 Minutes NZ on Vitamin C curing a man with N1H1 swine flu, and Leukaemia.

TERRAIN – A FILM produced by MARCELINA CRAVAT and ANDREW KAUFMAN M.D.

A History of Germ Theory +++
https://www.bitchute.com/video/JcO23Wdx1cne/"

"Rick Simpson oil (RSO): Benefits, uses & risks. How to make it yourself.
https://leafwell.com/blog/what-is-rick-simpson-oil-rso"

Dr Naomi Wolf – "The Pfizer Papers: Pfizer's Crimes Against Humanity

Book by Amy Kelly and Naomi Wolf. A book that explores data and confirms evidence that Pfizer knew of the negative impact of their MRNA inoculation product, on the Heart and human reproductive system.

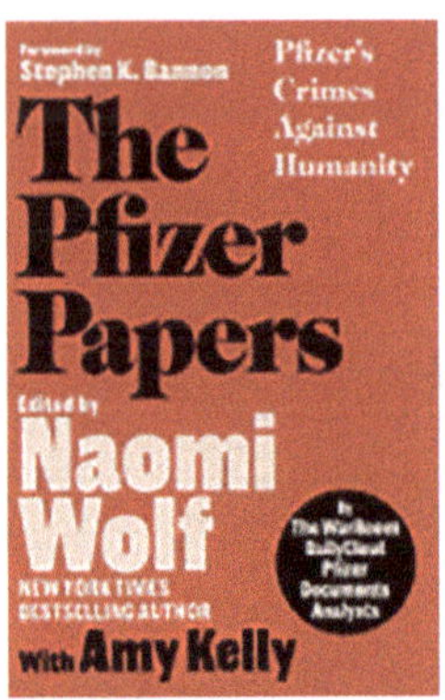

Decentralised medicine/ Jack Kruse / Assembly 2023

https://www.youtube.com/watch?v=TcbuqQd57rY

Jack Kruse is a Neurosurgeon and here he is talking about a historical pathway of centralised medicine that is being used to manipulate, trap and make sick, humanity. He also speaks of the use of blue light as a tool of manipulation. Circadian Biology being affected by technology. Probably the best link you could be aware of today.

"The Barrington Declaration" a group of doctors, physicians and scientists speaking out on the corruption and psy-op of medicine relating to the Covid Plandemic. #medicalethics #stopmedicalcensorship # https://lighthousedeclaration.world The Cape Byron Lighthouse Declaration.

Appendix 1

1. **Lecture notes from Suzanne Humphries lecture on Vitamin C**

Notes from lecture – Vitamin C Basics, by Suzanne Humphries MB, Internist and Nephrologist.

Study of healthy levels of Vitamin C.

Animals make their own Vitamin C;

Cows – 18mg/Kg/day. Daily total 12,000mg per day.

House cat – 20-40/Kg/day. Daily total 180mg made on their own.

Dependant animals like Primates eat 30mg/Kg/day, totalling 4,500mg per day.

Guinee Pigs eat 33mg/Kg/day, totalling 30g per day.

Goats are rarely sick and when healthy they make 185mg/Kg/day, totalling 13,000mg per day.

When goats are sick or stressed they make up to1400mg/kg/day (100,000mg/day)

Adult humans 'Recommended daily intake' (RDI) is 75mg/day = 1.2mg/kg/day.

One cigarette consumes 25mg of vitamin C.

Dr Steve Hickey wrote about the flaws in the RDI of vitamin C.

Two Kiwi fruits per day can elevate vit C levels.

A Canadian hospital study of blood levels of Vitamin C in inpatients found "Nearly one in five had a plasma vitamin C concentration compatible with Scurvy". – Gan 2008:PMID:18838532

If Doctors knew Vitamin C was so vital to wellness would they change practice?

Quote: The Black Widow Spider: Case History Tri-State Med J,Dec 1957, Vol5, No.10, pp15-18.

"...there are some physicians who would rather stand by and see their patient 'die' rather than use ascorbic acid – because in their finite minds, it exists only as a vitamin." – Dr Frederick R Klenner.

Dr F R Klenner was an outstanding and successful doctor of the 1950's. He used vitamin C for Tetnus and Polio – he achieved a 100 percent cure rate with Polio using vitamin C.

Dr Klenner wrote many articles about snake bites, spider bites, measles and other infections diseases and the curative use of vitamin C. He recommended high dose vitamin C during pregnancy and after delivery, which was found to reduce infections and mortality. His articles are available on-line.

Dr Frederick R Klenner proved vitamin C was more than just a vitamin.

Vitamin C – A few of its 'Actions' in the body.

- Antioxidant
- Electron donor
- DE toxicant
- Prevents damage
- Anti histamine – beneficial against hay fever
- Enzyme co factor
- Collagen production
- Neurotransmitters
- Hormones
- Carnatine (amino acid)

Vitamin C has been shown to be beneficial in improving diabetics management, heart disease and kidney disease. Vitamin C's Anti-inflammatory action on the body aids recovery from many illnesses.

Oxidative Stress, life toxins and electrons:

Aluminum is a highly reactive, electron stealer.

Fluoride is also a highly reactive electron stealer.

H2O water for life.

Free radicals are often elements missing an electron, thus an electron thief.

Oxygen shares bonds with Hydrogen. H2O

Hydroxyl radical OH steals electrons to get to H2O.

Vitamin C is ideal as an electron donor, it does not steal after it has donated electrons in its free radical nutrilisation. This is how Anti-Oxidents work.

Vitamin C is a Hydrogen (electron) donor.

Figure 1. Vitamin C

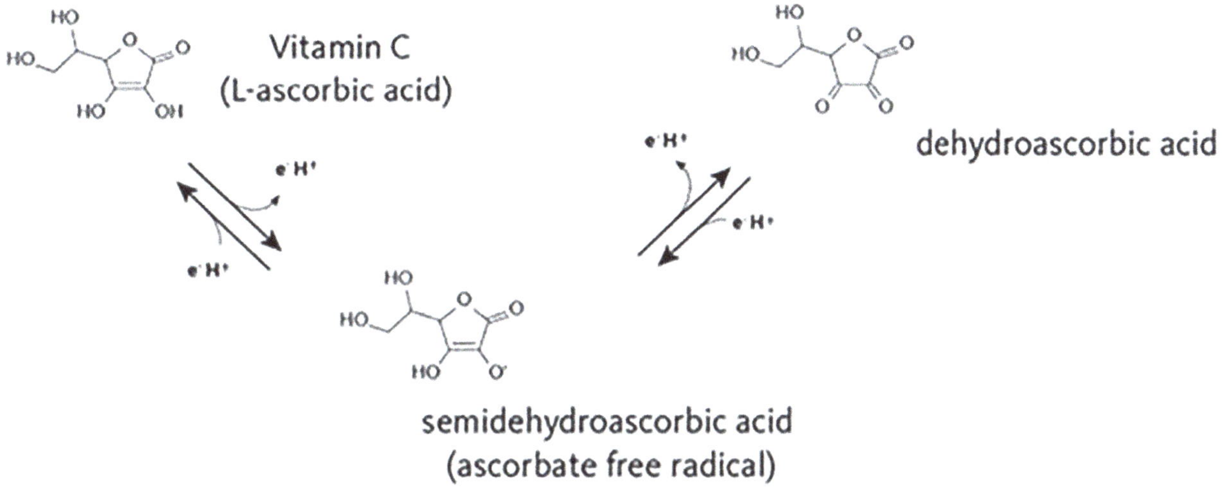

Vitamin C (L-ascorbic acid) is an electron donor. Vitamin C can sequentially donate two electrons. Vitamin C can donate electrons to reactive free radicals, which then become reduced. The loss of one electron results in vitamin C being oxidized to the ascorbate free radical, which is relatively unreactive compared to other free radicals. The ascorbate free radical can be reduced to vitamin C by gaining one electron or be further oxidized to dehydroascorbic acid by losing another electron. Dehydroascorbic acid is only stable for a few minutes and is then either irreversibly hydrolyzed to form 2,3-diketogulonic acid or reduced to semidehydroascorbic acid and vitamin C (not shown here). However, the efficacy of the *in vivo* reduction reactions that yield vitamin C from dehydroascorbic acid and semidehydroascorbic acid appears to be low as vitamin C deficiency occurs in 30 days when vitamin C is removed from the diet of healthy people. Thus, most of the vitamin C is likely oxidized to dehydroascorbic acid, which is irreversibly metabolized.

The beauty of Vitamin C is that it does not continue to steal after donating an electron and some areas of the body actually prefer the used Vitamin C, such as brain nerves, mitochondria, red blood cells and bone cells. Wilson 2005 PMID 16011 461 – Where Dehydroascorbic acid is recycled.

Vitamin C - Foetus and Mother.

The Placenta has two times (x2) the amount of Ascorbic Acid/Vitamin C compared to the mothers blood.

The Umbilical cord has two times (x2) the amount of Vitamin C compared to the mothers blood.

The Foetus has two times (x2) the amount of Vitamin C compared to the mothers blood.

The Amniotic Fluid has two times (x2) the amount of Vitamin C compared to the mothers blood.

Vitamin C is vital to cell development.

During vaginal labour the body uses more Vitamin C than with a Caesarean Section. Recommends 80 percent more Vitamin C intake for vaginal labour.

Stress of being born: Catecholamines are necessary for first life. Clears lungs, aids sucking, alertness and bonding which increases glucose levels to aid the newborn. Oxygen saturation is around 60 percent and catecholamines assist at this time.

Jaundice effects 60-70 percent of newborns today. Bilirubin mops up free radicals of birth. The baby makes antioxidants which also aid in transition to oxygen.

Abdul-Razzak 2007 PMID:19675711:

"Antioxidant vitamins and hyperbilirubinemia in neonates. Neonates with low levels of bilirubinemia had twice the levels of Vitamin C as those with higher Jaundice..."

Association between low Vitamin C and bilirubin:

Italian study – Prevention of Jaundice: Vitamin C during pregnancy – Garbelli 1957. PMID:13420320

Jaundice absent in 61 percent of babies and mild in others. Bilirubin is an electron donor and is not as high when Vitamin C is at healthy levels.

Phototherapy – Blue light increases oxidative stress to baby, lowers Vitamin C, lowers GSH and lowers Albumin which is all needed by any baby recovering from birth stress. Dahlya 2006 PMID:23105589.

Vitamin C is vital to the structure and integrity of bodily tissues.

Bones, eyes and skin all need collagen. Muscles and tendons require collagen.

In structural repair, knitting collagen fibres, one molecule of Vitamin C is oxidized for each stitch. Making collagen and bone takes a lot of Vitamin C. For fibres to become a matrix, enzymes depend on Vitamin C.

Vitamins K and D call to mineral stratification.

Osteopregurim is bone strengthener from breast milk.

Short list of Acute conditions that benefit from Vitamin C uptake:

Infections - Antiseptic/bacterial, Sepsis and critical care.

Trauma, surgery, burns.

Endotoxin processing

Vascular integrity

Antihistamine

Whooping cough – panic free management.

Vaccine reactions – Oxidative stress bonfire.

Evidence that Vitamin C works, including kidney, liver function and sepsis: New evidence for IV Sodium Ascorbate. "Phase 1 safety trial of Intravenous Ascorbic Acid in patients with severe Sepsis."

Fowler 2014 PMID 24484547 showed good results with low ascorbate use. SOFA score – indication of mortality, dropped dramatically in Vitamin C patients but placebo patients had zero change.

Is there any excuse for medical Doctors to not know of the benefits of Vitamin C on Sepsis patients? Lack of evidence is not the issue!

Hickey 2008 Pharmacakinetics of oral Vitamin C, Vol 17. No.3: PP 169-170.

National Health states healthy level of Vitamin C is 70mg, but Hickey showed this to be untrue. National Health states that absorption of 220mg of Vitamin C is impossible, but Hickey showed absorption levels of 400+ is possible.

Hickey 2009 Vitamin C: The Real Story ISBN: 1442972793

Padayatti 2004 PMID 15068981 shows the time taken for intravenous Vitamin C to leave the body. Most is gone in 6 hours. Knowing this helps maintain levels in cancer treatments.

Why NOT Ester-C (Calcium ascorbate)?

Death by Calcium and Primal Panacea.

Levy 2013 Death by Calcium ISBN: 0615839603

Seely 1991 PMID: 1743778

- 220mg Calcium per 1000mg Ester-C = 400+mg in 4g dose.
- Sodium Ascorbate is physiologic (2Na ascorbate transporters)
- Na ascorbate is buffered.
- Manufacture requires high heat, which leads to about 10 percent DHA formation = (Oxalic acid).

Seely 1991 PMID: 1743778 charts deaths in males from heart disease and milk protein consumption: "is Calcium excess in western diet a major cause of arterial disease?"

Chart/Country – Male mortality – Milk protein gross consumption. Showed a close correlation between increase mortality with increase in milk protiens.

Mortality highest in countries with more milk protein consumption.

Glucose-6-Phosphate dehydrogenase (G6PD) deficiency? Always check the level of G6PD prior to IV use of Vitamin C.

Kidney Stones: Calcium oxalate.

Concerns that taking Vitamin C may cause kidney stones is unwarranted. (Wandzik 1994 PMID: 8126804)

Giving up to 10 grams per day/intake. Two large prospective cohorts show lower stone risks in males (Curhan 1996 PMID 8668271), and no increase in women (Curhan19__ PMID 10203369).

Dr Suzanne Humphries, in her opinion, Vitamin C is warranted if dehydration or kidney failure is present.

Dr Thomas Levy – Vitamin C Researcher wrote the book titled, "Vitamin C Antidote to all known toxins".

After Nobel Prize winner Linus Pauling's studies on Vitamin C found promising results, Thomas Levy MD continued the work of exploring the curative properties of this essential, natural and harm free, super vitamin.

2. Book Review of "Outsmart Your Cancer" by Tanya Peirce

Review of Outsmart Your Cancer by Tanya Harter-Pierce

This book was an empowering inspiration, written in a direct manner with usable resources.

She begins with "Why so much Cancer and what Causes it?" Pages 43-51 (PDF pg51-59)

Chapter by chapter Tanya discusses alternative treatments, from discovery to suppression, with case studies and user references including group support.

On page 332 Tanya begins a new section with "Deciding for yourself" Chapter 21 discusses "Evaluating conventional methods" Pg 333-353 (PDF pg 339-361) and Chapter 22 "Choosing an Alternative treatment plan" pg 355-365 (PDF pg 364-373).

Chapter 23 – "Dealing with Fear and the mind body connection".

In Tanya's "Recommended Resources", pgs 385-388 (Pdf pg 393) there is a list of Alternative treatment references to aid readers in their personal quests

The Appendix on page 389 offers a list of the "5 big Environmental Cancer triggers"

1. Chlorine by-products 2. Fluoride 3. Asbestos 4. Fiberglass 5. Nuclear Radiation.

Each point is discussed with scientific references.

Finally the section of "Evaluating Conventional Methods" pg 341-353 particularly relevant to my son's journey, and then Tanya's "Concluding Comments" in Chapter 24 pages 379-384 (PDF pgs387-392)

Outsmart Your Cancer by Tanya Harter Pierce is outstandingly helpful and definitely worth reading.

"At the pointy end of MRNA.."

* "**Detoxification of Spike Protein** from cells and tissues (Published in US medical literature)as a minimum three month protocol, developed by **Dr Peter McCullough**. It contains:

- Nattokinase 2000 units x 2 per day,
- Bromelain(from stems of pineapple) 500mg per day,
- Curcumin (from Turmeric) 500mg 3xper day."

"*May 2025 US Medical Association recently published a paper saying that 'Long Covid' is not a disease but a vaccine injury that has disabled the human immune system.

*In a Congressional report 2024 Dr Jordan Vaughn of Alabama, delivered on the effects of Covid shot and 'Long Covid' he stated: " S1 sub unit is not a benign protein and it triggers inflammation. It produces Amyloid aggregates, damages endothelium barriers and impairs oxygen take-up. Damaging heart, brain and circulatory system. (LNP) Lipid Nanoparticles distribute widely into many of the body's organs including reproductive system, heart and brain."

*This company never made a commercial product ever before… Patent No. US 10.702.600 B1 (7 July 2020) MODERNA made 4 patent applications in 2019. On July 7 2020 were amended filings, to state "accidental or intentional release of respiratory pathogen" – Interestingly the World Health Organisations, 'world-wide exercise' included the same words but added the word lethal.. "accidental or intentional release of lethal respiratory pathogen" Audacious criminals telling the public what they were going to do. No one in the Public cared?"

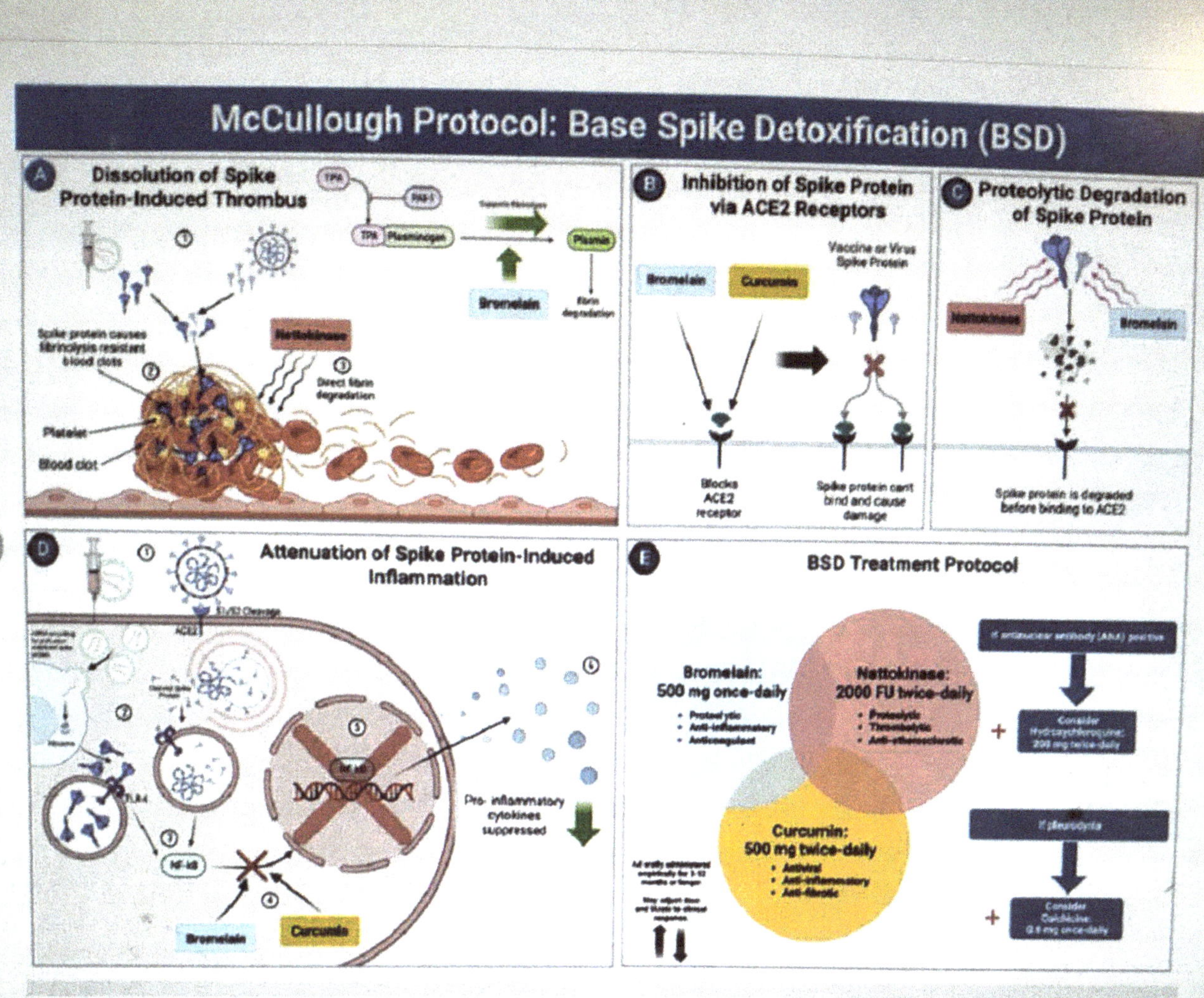

McCullough Protocol: Base Spike Detoxification (BSD). A: Dissolution of spike protein-induced thrombus. Nattokinase directly degrades fibrinolysis-resistant fibrin (from spike protein), and bromelain upregulates fibrinolysis. B: Inhibition of spike protein via ACE2 receptors. Bromelain and curcumin block the ACE2 receptor, preventing spike protein from binding. C: Proteolytic degradation of spike protein. Nattokinase and bromelain degrade spike proteins, rendering them inactive. D: Attenuation of spike protein-induced inflammation. Bromelain and curcumin downregulate the NF-kB signaling pathway induced by spike protein, leading to the suppression of inflammatory molecules. E: BSD treatment protocol. The full treatment regimen and the addition of other compounds based on clinical indication are illustrated. Abbreviations: TPA = tissue plasminogen activator, PAI-1 = plasminogen activator inhibitor-1, ACE2 = angiotensin converting enzyme-2, NF-kB = nuclear factor kappa B, S1/S2 = spike protein subunits S1/S2, TLR4 = toll-like receptor 4. *Created with BioRender.com. Panel E adapted from McCullough et al. [43].

Source publication

FIGURE 3: McCullough Protocol: Base Spike Detoxification (BSD). A:...

Abbreviations: ACE2 = angiotensin-converting enzyme 2, FAT = fatty acid...

https://www.youtube.com/watch?v=67sLlXeMg2I

Regenerative Energy & the Light Inside You | Jack Kruse | 221

Mind & Matter Podcast

Short Summary: A mind-bending dive into evolutionary biology and health through a biophysicist's lens, with Dr. Jack Kruse delivering provocative insights about biology, medicine, and health.

About the guest: Jack Kruse, MD, is a neurosurgeon known for integrating biophysics into medicine. He challenges conventional biochemistry with his "leptin prescription" and decentralized health approach.

Full transcript and other information on Substack.

Episode Summary: Dr. Jack Kruse joins host Nick Jikomes to explore the Great Oxygenation Event's role in shaping life, linking it to modern health via biophysics over biochemistry. They discuss oxygen's impact on metabolism, the significance of deuterium-depleted water, and sunlight's influence on the leptin-melanocortin pathway. Kruse shares his dramatic weight loss journey using sunlight and cold therapy, critiques modern tech-driven obesity, and unveils a controversial history of SV40 in vaccines, tying it to cancer spikes.

Key Takeaways:

The Great Oxygenation Event (2.1-2.4 billion years ago) drove life's shift to oxygen-based metabolism, with cyanobacteria as key players.

Kruse argues biophysics, not biochemistry, explains evolution, spotlighting light as life's fundamental driver.

Deuterium-depleted water is important for enabling our cells and mitochondria to use energy from the TCA cycle without "shocking" the body.

Sunlight exposure boosts nitric oxide, reducing food needs via the leptin pathway, challenging diet norms.

He links obesity to indoor tech lifestyles, disrupting heme proteins and mitochondrial function.

SV40, a virus in 1950s polio vaccines, may connect to cancer rises, a story Kruse says was buried by centralized science.

*Not medical advice.

https://www.youtube.com/watch?v=tm-gNltJnLU

Fauci takes HUGE Taxpayer Money & RFK EXISTENTIAL Threat to Big Pharma... | Neil Oliver

How Fauci censored RFK and how the tables are about to be turned.

THE USDA's FOOD IRRADIATION PLOT

US food and health authorities, in league with corporations, are enacting plans to sterilise the fresh food supply with irradiation, thus destroying essential disease-fighting nutrients and promoting a sick society.

by Mike Adams © April 2008
Editor, NaturalNews.com
From the web page:
http://www.naturalnews.com/023015.html

Why the USDA Wants to Sterilise Fresh Produce and Turn Live Foods into Dead Foods

There's a new plot underway to sterilise our food and destroy the nutritional value of fresh produce. The players in this plot are the usual suspects: the US Department of Agriculture (USDA), which backed the raw almond sterilisation rules now in effect in California, and the American Chemical Society, a pro-chemicals group that represents the interests of industrial chemicals manufacturers.

The latest push comes from USDA researchers who conducted a study to see which method more effectively killed bacteria on leafy green vegetables like spinach. To conduct the study, they bathed the spinach in a solution contaminated with bacteria. Then they tried to remove the bacteria using three methods: washing, chemical spraying and irradiation. Not surprisingly, only the irradiation killed nearly 100 per cent of the bacterial colonies. That's because radiation sterilises both the bacteria and the vegetable leaves, effectively killing the plant and destroying much of its nutritional value while it kills the bacteria.

The USDA claims this is a huge success: by using radiation on all fresh produce, the number of food-borne illness outbreaks that happen each year could be substantially reduced. It all makes sense until you realise that by destroying the nutritional value of all fresh produce sold in the United States, *irradiation would greatly increase the number of people killed by infections and chronic diseases that are prevented by the natural medicines found in fresh produce.*

Why fresh, living produce helps prevent sickness

The USDA, you see, has zero recognition of the difference between living produce and dead produce. To uneducated government bureaucrats, pasteurised or irradiated vegetable juice is identical to fresh, raw, living vegetable juice. They believe this because they've never been taught about the phytonutrients, digestive enzymes and life-force properties that are found in fresh foods, but that are destroyed through heating or irradiation. Thus, the USDA is operating out of extreme ignorance when it comes to food and nutrition.

Even a simple leaf of spinach contains hundreds of natural medicines—phytonutrients that help prevent cancer, eye diseases, nervous system disorders, heart disease and much more. Every living vegetable is a powerhouse of disease-fighting medicine: broccoli and celery prevent cancer, beet greens cleanse the liver, cilantro removes heavy metals, berries prevent heart disease, and dark leafy greens help prevent over a dozen serious health conditions while boosting immune function and helping prevent other infections. But when you subject these vegetables and fruits to enough radiation to kill 99.9 per cent of the pathogens that may be hitching a ride, you also destroy many of the phytonutrients responsible for these tremendous health benefits!

This means that while irradiating food may decrease outbreaks of food-borne illnesses, it will have the unintended consequence of *increasing* the number of people who get sick from other infections (and chronic diseases) due to the fact that their source of natural medicine has been destroyed. For many Americans, you see, *salad greens are their one remaining source for phytonutrients*. Given their diets of processed foods, junk foods and cooked foods, there are very few opportunities for these consumers to get fresh, phytonutrient-rich foods into their diet. And now the USDA wants to take that away, too, by mandating the irradiation of all fresh produce.

Let me make a rather obvious prediction, on the record. If the irradiation of fresh produce goes into effect in the United States, rates of infection among consumers will sharply *increase*, not decrease, due to the removal of immune-boosting natural medicine from the food supply. Consumers will also experience higher rates of cancer, heart disease, dementia, eye disorders, diabetes and even obesity. By destroying these thousands of healing phytonutrients, irradiation will leave many consumers defenceless against modern society's many health challenges.

It is no exaggeration to say that a policy of mass irradiation of fresh produce is as blatantly stupid as the Romans building their aqueducts with lead-lined waterways. As historians have explained, after the aqueducts were built the water delivered to the Roman population was contaminated with lead—a heavy metal that causes numerous health problems, including insanity. Many historians blame the lead-lined aqueducts as one of the primary reasons why the Roman Empire fell: its leaders went mad, and the rest is history. I would argue that America's leaders are already mad, but that's beside the point.

If we start irradiating our food, thereby destroying its nutritional value, we are going to unleash a cascade of unintended consequences even greater than those of the Romans' aqueducts. Absent the protections of phytonutrients found in plants, the health of most consumers will rapidly decline, and we'll see the US thrust into a quagmire of chronic disease and medical bankruptcy. (It's already heading there, of course, but killing the food supply will only accelerate the downward spiral of health.)

Let's sterilise all the food!

The USDA has never met a food sterilisation plan it didn't like. It backed the recent raw almond sterilisation law that went into effect in California last year [2007], forcing all almond growers to sterilise their almonds by subjecting them to toxic chemicals or cooking them at high enough temperatures to kill anything that might have been alive (such as the almond itself). Now, all the raw almonds consumed in America are purchased from overseas growers, where raw still means raw.

Raw milk has also been under attack in California and elsewhere. The USDA supported laws that essentially banned the sales of raw milk, requiring milk to be sterilised, too.

If you now irradiate all the fresh produce, you have a food supply that is predominantly sterilised—otherwise known as "dead". And dead foods lead to dead people. That a society's health regulators would want all foods to be dead should be downright shocking to anyone who knows anything about health and nutrition. Live foods keep people alive, but dead foods make people die. It's really not a complicated concept.

That a society's health regulators would want all foods to be dead should be downright shocking to anyone who knows anything about health and nutrition.

The USDA's definition of "food safety", however, is based on the idea that the health of one immune-system-compromised individual who can't handle a little *E. coli* is more important than the ongoing health of the entire population. Thus, all foods must be killed for everyone.

I strongly disagree with this approach. We should not expect foods to be sterilised. In terms of food safety, emphasis should be placed on boosting the health and immune systems of individuals so they can survive *occasional contact* with *E. coli*, rather than on trying to create a sterile environment in which nothing is alive. As it turns out, the people susceptible to food-borne illnesses are precisely those individuals who have compromised immune systems due to their intake of *vaccines and antibiotics*. Thus, it is modern medicine that has made these people vulnerable to food-borne illnesses. Blame the drug companies, not the bacteria.

But the USDA would rather blame the food. However, blaming conventional medicine for the harm it has caused to the human immune system is not politically correct. It's better to blame the food, then use scare tactics to announce yet more outbreaks and hope for a public outcry for widespread food irradiation. And that brings me to the "final solution" on food irradiation.

The social engineering recipe

There is a corporate-sponsored plot underway in the US today to keep people sick and deny them access to information about natural cures (such as medicinal foods) that would prevent disease and keep people out of the hospitals.

In more than 1,500 articles on this website (NaturalNews.com), I've documented the Food and Drug Administration's (FDA's) criminality, the USDA's indefensible actions and the criminal behaviour of drug manufacturers that only earn profits if they can find a way to keep the entire population sick and diseased for another generation or two.

Destroying the natural medicine in the food supply sure would be a highly effective way to create more customers for Big Pharma, wouldn't it? I think it's all part of the "keep the population sick and diseased" plot being carried out by an evil partnership between drug companies and the US government. We already know that the FDA and USDA work for the corporations, not the people. We already know that the drug companies will do practically anything to boost their profits (including conducting medical experiments on infants, drugging schoolchildren, lying to the public, fabricating clinical trials and more). Is it any surprise that they would now attempt a "final solution" on the food supply that kills the food and thereby results in a huge reduction in the population's intake of the disease-fighting nutrients found in fresh produce?

Pulling this off, of course, requires a bit of social engineering by the USDA in order to force the public into demanding that something be done. If you're the USDA, you can't just suddenly announce a national food sterilisation plan; you have to prime the pump with a bit of dirty work. Here's the simple plan for accomplishing that, if you're the USDA...

1) Conduct poor inspections of fresh produce *on purpose*, in order to cause a large increase in food-borne illness outbreaks. (We've seen this increase happen over the last 12–24 months.) This can be easily accomplished by reducing the budgets of food inspection offices or by removing inspectors from the payroll altogether (which has already happened).

2) Wait for the outbreaks to happen. When consumers get sick, run national press releases announcing how dangerous the food supply is.

3) Watch the consumer reaction as people and lawmakers demand that "something must be done".

4) Fudge a study with the American Chemical Society to show that washing doesn't work and that irradiation is the only solution. Time the release of this news to coincide with the public outcry that "something must be done".

5) Once the public is demanding a solution to food-borne illnesses, roll out a national produce irradiation requirement that sterilises all the food.

Mission accomplished! This, of course, leads to:

6) Watch the population become increasingly sick and diseased (thanks to the lack of phytonutrients that used to be found in the fresh produce), and cash in on your Big Pharma shares as the population is herded into hospitals for lucrative treatments with monopoly-priced pharmaceuticals.

It's the same old social engineering trick that's been used to hoodwink the American people hundreds of times. How do you get the public to support a war in the Middle East? Stage an attack on US soil first, and wait for the public outcry. How do you get the people to support the mass sterilisation of their own food supply? Lower your inspection standards, let the sickness spread and then wait for the public outcry. It's the way governments get things done these days: they manipulate the public into demanding the things they wanted to accomplish in the first place. These are sometimes called "false flag operations" in a military context, and they've been conducted by the US government on numerous occasions, just like they were conducted by Hitler in Nazi Germany to justify his invasions of neighbouring countries. You can read about false flag operations on Wikipedia (http://en.wikipedia.org/wiki/False_flag).

They don't want foods to be used as medicines, and they don't want the natural medicines found in foods competing with their own patented pharmaceutical medicines...

What "they" really want: a dead food supply

Let's be blunt about this. The corporations which run this country (and which also run the US government) want the US food supply to be dead. They don't want foods to be used as medicines, and they don't want the natural medicines found in foods competing with their own patented pharmaceutical medicines (that just happen to earn them a whole lot more money than any food ever did).

Don't you find it curious that this attack on the food supply is coming out now, right after all this incredible news about the healing power of foods has been hitting the science journals? Every week, it seems, we find out about another amazing health property in a food: black raspberries reverse oral cancer, pomegranates halt prostate cancer, green tea prevents breast cancer—the list goes on. Just on this website alone, we've probably published 1,000 stories over the last two years on the disease-fighting properties of foods.

The thing to realise here is that many of *the healing properties of these foods are destroyed through pasteurisation and irradiation*. If you're a government that wants to "take away the people's medicine", the fastest way to accomplish this is to mandate the sterilisation of the food supply. Kill the foods and you take away the people's medicine, and that forces the population to use pharmaceuticals instead.

The FDA, for its part, has for many decades conducted its natural medicine censorship campaign, the only purpose of which is to *deny the people access to accurate information about the healing properties of natural medicines found in foods and herbs*. But apparently that wasn't enough. The Internet came along and people found a way to educate themselves. So, since the FDA couldn't keep the truth about natural medicines bottled up and censored, the government has now apparently decided to sterilise all the foods, thereby destroying the natural medicines and transforming Mother Nature's gifts into dead calories.

The USDA's decisions here are not based on public safety but on corporate greed. Just look at how the USDA handled the raw almond controversy (see related articles at http://www.naturalnews.com/almonds.html).

The USDA, as operated today, is a front group for wealthy corporations. It is not interested in helping the people. It's interested in protecting the profits of corporations—even if that means destroying the food supply and turning the population into "dead eaters" who die from other diseases caused by the lack of phytonutrient protection.

To try to make our food supply sterile is insane, and anyone who supports the irradiation of the food supply is, in my opinion, supporting a policy of genocide...

How you can help stop this latest atrocity against our food supply

What can you do to stop this? Be prepared to *fight irradiation plans* with a massive outcry that demands our food supply be protected from radiation. There are two things that need to be accomplished, and of course the USDA and FDA oppose them both:

1) Require the labelling of all irradiated foods with a large "Irradiated" label or sticker.

2) Block any attempts to mandate the irradiation of fresh produce.

Stay tuned to NaturalNews.com for more on this story. We'll be joining with other pro-consumer groups (like the Organic Consumers Association) to rally our readers in opposition to this food irradiation effort.

I believe we must keep our food supply fresh and alive. (Sounds kinda obvious, huh?) And if there's a little extra bacteria on the spinach, it's nothing that a healthy body can't handle anyway. Take some probiotics and avoid antibiotics, and you'll be just fine. *E. coli* is really only a threat to the health of individuals who have had their immune systems (or intestinal flora) destroyed by pharmaceuticals in the first place. There's nothing wrong with some living organisms in your milk, on your almonds or on your spinach. Wash your food, get plenty of sunlight and avoid using antibiotics.

The human body is *not* a sterile environment. To try to make our food supply sterile is insane, and anyone who supports the irradiation of the food supply is, in my opinion, supporting a policy of genocide against the American people. To destroy the vitality of the food supply is a criminal act of such immense evil that it stands alongside the worst crimes ever committed against humanity.

You see, it's not enough for them to poison our water (with fluoride), poison our children (with vaccines) and lie to us about the Sun (with skin cancer scare stories). Now they want to destroy our foods—and thereby take away any natural medicine options that might actually keep people healthy and free. Remember: a diseased population is an enslaved population.

Now go eat your Big Mac, drink your Pepsi, and don't ask too many questions... ∞

About the Author:
Mike Adams is an holistic nutritionist with a passion for teaching people how to improve their health. He has written more than 1,500 articles and dozens of reports, guides and interviews on natural health topics, reaching millions of readers with information that is saving lives and improving personal health around the world. He is a trusted independent journalist who receives no money or promotional fees whatsoever to write about other companies' products. He is editor of the NaturalNews website, http://www.naturalnews.com.

In 2007, Adams launched EcoLEDs, a manufacturer of mercury-free, energy-efficient LED lighting products that save electricity. He also founded an environmentally friendly online retailer called BetterLifeGoods.com, which uses retail profits to help support consumer advocacy programs. He is a veteran of the software technology industry, having set up a personalised mass email software product used to deliver email newsletters to subscribers.

Adams volunteers his time to serve as the executive director of the Consumer Wellness Center, a 501(c)(3) non-profit organisation, and practises nature photography, Capoeira, Pilates and organic gardening. He is known as "the Health Ranger", and his personal health statistics and mission statements are located at http://www.HealthRanger.org.

To read references for his article in this edition, visit http://www.naturalnews.com/023015.html and click on the hyperlinks.

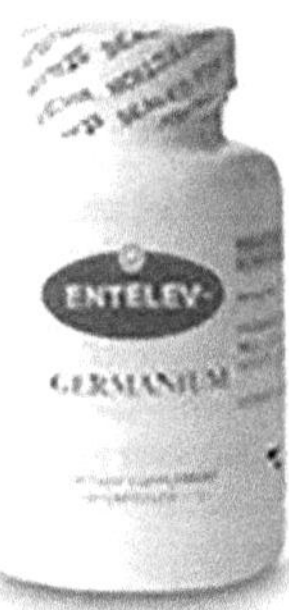

Germanium

Ge132-Germanium Sesquioxide

Natural trace mineral element

A trace mineral that may enhance oxygen delivery to the blood by releasing the energy of the earth, plants and sun.

Benefits of Germanium

- High oxygen provider to all cells
- Beneficial for rogue cell complaints
- Increased oxygen for energy and rejuvenation
- Reduce acidity and the risk of degenerative disease

Germanium is consistently found in all aspects of Nature

Germanium (element symbol Ge) is an ever-present trace element found not only within plants, soil, animals and humans. Germanium helps build immune cells, provide energy, and is known to play a role in rejuvenation. As a powerful antioxidant, it has also been used for pain relief for a diversity of causes.

Natural sources of Germanium include garlic, aloe, comfrey, chlorella, ginseng and water cress and the health benefits of these plants have long been recognized. It is speculated that the presence of Germanium provides the strong healing potential of these particular plants. It has been proposed by Dr Kazukiko Asai Ph.D., a scientist and advocate of Germanium's health benefits, that the existence of Germanium in these traditional remedies has some connection with chlorophyll. Germanium perhaps acts as a catalyst with chlorophyll to biochemically increase oxygen potential and release energy or the plants healing potential.

Germanium's diverse healing potential

Germanium may be appropriate for use in conditions which are attributable to a deficiency of oxygen. A commonly held theory is that all disease may be caused by a deficiency of oxygen. Dr Asai, the founder of modern day Germanium health research, discovered that the plants containing unusually large quantities of Germanium were those valued as Chinese medicinal herbs.

A primary function of Germanium is that it greatly enriches oxygen, essential for sustaining life. Organic Germanium may be beneficial in treating symptoms of conditions such as anaemia, arthritis, food allergies, elevated cholesterol, chronic viral infections, neoplasms and AIDS. Germanium may also assist in the symptoms of rogue cellular activity commonly found in lung, bladder, larynx and breast conditions. Germanium has been shown to alleviate symptoms of asthma, diabetes, hypertension, cardiac insufficiency, sinus inflammation, neuralgia, leukaemia, neuroses and cirrhosis of the liver.

The Germanium compound may induce the production of interferons (IFNs) which are proteins naturally produced by the immune system that assist in fighting foreign agents like bacteria and viruses, and also protect the body from disease. Germanium carries oxygen to the cells which helps to fight pain, keep the immune system functioning properly, and rid the body of toxins and poisons.

Dr Asai, found that individuals taking 100-300 milligrams (mg) of Germanium showed improvement with many illnesses including rheumatoid arthritis, food allergies, elevated cholesterol, chronic viral infections, neoplasms and AIDS.

Germanium variation Ge132 is discovered

Dr. Kazuhiko Asai graduated from the Imperial University of Tokyo in 1932. He studied metallurgy and mining for four years in Germany and upon his return to Japan in 1945 founded the Coal Research Institute. Dr Asai began to understand the health benefits of Germanium and in 1969 he founded the Asai Germanium Research Institute in Tokyo, Japan. After testing 132 different variations of Germanium for effectiveness, he named the 132nd substance Ge132 "bis beta-carboxyethyl germanium sesquioxide" or "mu-trioxo-bis (beta-carboxyethyl) germanic anhydride".

In physiology, a phenomenon known as the dehydrogenating effect led Dr Asai to the assumption that Germanium might also have interesting biological applications. The effect causes a negative hydrogen ion, which may be viewed as an electron, to be discharged from the body. Dehydrogenation refers to the ability of organic Germanium to seize and combine with hydrogen ions which have accumulated in the body and remove them. This occurs constantly when natural internal cleansing mechanisms are stimulated.

Dr Asai discovers biological applications of Germanium

All plants seem to contain Germanium, which supported Dr Asai's hypothesis that Germanium plays a very important role in relation to plants with medicinal properties and biochemical life. In plant biology, when water is broken down into oxygen and hydrogen by this method, oxygen is discharged from the plant and hydrogen combines with the carbon of carbon dioxide absorbed by the plant to form carbohydrates or food for energy production.

Did you know?

Germanium is a natural element that assists plants to process oxygen and resist harmful bacteria? Germanium occurs naturally in plants like garlic, aloe and watercress and can also be found in minerals like coal. Clemens Winkler discovered and named the new element in 1886 after his native country Germany.

Explore, learn and shop at www.BioNatural.biz

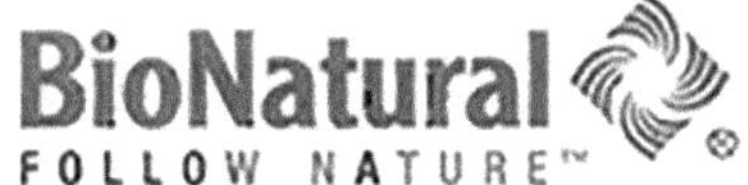

BioNatural Pty Ltd > 1 Overland Drive, Vermont South, VIC 3133 Australia
BioNatural Carlton Pty Ltd > 202 Rathdowne Street, Carlton, VIC 3053 Australia
Mail Order > Australia-wide > **Stores** > Open Monday - Friday 9 - 6, Saturday 9 - 4
Phones > Toll free 1300 555 686 > Head office 03 8847 3000 > Fax 03 8847 3030
Secure online shopping > www.BioNatural.biz > info@bionatural.biz

Information provided by BioNatural Pty Ltd including product descriptions and pictures is provided for educational and informational purposes only, and has not been evaluated by the Therapeutic Goods Administration. These products are not intended to diagnose, treat, cure, or prevent any disease. Please consult your appropriately trained healthcare practitioner for medical advice.

Germanium - natural trace mineral elemnt

In effect this means that Germanium is a key factor in the growth of plants.

In human biology, an excess of positively-charged hydrogen ions provides the acid environment which is the foundation for disease. The semi-conducting properties of Germanium with its dehydrogenation capacity, supports the body's ability to reduce oxidation associated with free radical damage and chronic degenerative disease. Also, dehydrogenation makes oxygen available to the body, thereby promoting a healthy alkaline inner environment.

Organic Germanium's immune enhancing properties

The action of organic Germanium may:

- stimulate the production of immune (gamma) Interferon
- activate resting macrophages or white blood cells and convert them to cytoxic (killer) macrophages
- stimulate the production of Natural Killer (NK) cell activity, T suppressor cells
- assist in the repair of decreased immunity

The origins and development of Dr Asai's organic Germanium

While sifting through raw coal material, Dr Asai discovered that Germanium is found in Japanese coal in about five to 10 parts per million (ppm). On further examination of various coals, Dr Asai detected the existence of medullary tubes, which are the vessels that plants use to draw nutrients from the soil. He reasoned that the Germanium in coal therefore came primarily from living matter, and did not enter the coal later from the surrounding soil.

Dr Asai also measured the Germanium content of those plants reputed to have beneficial effects in the treatment of malignant tumors. He found that shelf fungus, measuring 800-2000 ppm, was at the top of the list. For centuries shelf fungus has been reputed to be effective in the treatment of cancer, and Nobel Prize winner Alexander Solzhenitsyn referred to this remarkable herb in his book, "Cancer Ward". This led to Dr Asai's discovery that those plants which are generally regarded as conducive to good health also contained fairly large quantities of Germanium.

Germanium appears to play a role in plant life self defence in accordance with the following discoveries of Dr Asai. In analyzing the Germanium content of the medicinal plants it was found that the element was not distributed evenly throughout the plant body. Ginseng, for example, has Germanium concentrated in the area extending from the centre of the roots to the stems of the leaves. The heavily concentrated area registers as much as 4,000 ppm while the peripheral root hairs contains no Germanium at all. Ginseng would be susceptible to the thousands of viruses and bacteria existing in the soil and would soon rot if it were not for its extremely high Germanium content.

The discovery of Germanium's antibiotic properties

Due to his interest in discovering more about the antibiotic properties of Germanium, Dr Asai conducted controlled petri dish experiments. The results obtained demonstrated that harmful bacteria died due to their molecular structure being destroyed by the dehydrogenating effect, or oxidizing action of Germanium. In using mould as the test subject, the trial showed that it effectively used Germanium to fight harmful bacteria, as well as to facilitate it's own growth.

Experiments with other plants also demonstrated benefits of Germanium. In an experiment with rice plants, Dr Asai discovered that Germanium increases their resistance to cold and that when only a small quantity of Germanium was added, the growth of various plants was greatly accelerated and the flowering period enhanced. Plant cuttings showed improved assimilation of nutrients. This was evident when water drawn by the plants electrolysed, or converted to energy by sunlight, using Germanium as a catalyst.

Nature's life cycle inspires the discovery of Germanium

In Nature, there is a transmigrational phenomenon whereby metallic elements existing in the soil play an important part in plant growth. Animals ingest these elements after feeding on the plants and return them to the soil through evacuation or upon death. The metallic elements involved in this cycle, such as Germanium, move in organic form from the plant to animal bodies.

This natural cycle prompted Dr Asai's search to find an organic compound which could be synthesized and had universal application for humanity. His search involved thirty years of extreme hardship and devotion. Eventually synthesizing organic Germanium fulfilled a vision Dr Asai had since his youth of making a personal significant contribution to benefit mankind.

Dr Asai's unfailing belief in the universal health benefits to of Germanium may best be summed up by a quote from his autobiographical text, 'Miracle Cure Organic Germanium'. "Gazing upon the single crystal of Germanium with its silver grey sheen, I feel, on the palm of my hand the touch of a substance I am tempted to describe as the fountain of life that fills the universe".

Related products

If you are considering purchasing Germanium you may want to consider it's relationship to:

Entelev 50 and Entelev 23 - Anaerobic cellular technology, liquid dietary supplement designed to cleanse the body of toxins on cellular level

ProEnzymes - probiotic enzymes that assist in breaking down protein lining on cellular wall of anaerobic cells to assist in cellular cleansing

NanoPrime - nanotechnology antioxidant, nutrient and detoxifier that revitalizes the body by the elimination of damage-causing free radicals from the mineral Zeolite.

BioNatural Pty Ltd > 1 Overland Drive, Vermont South, VIC 3133 Australia
BioNatural Carlton Pty Ltd > 202 Rathdowne Street, Carlton, VIC 3053 Australia
Mail Order > Australia-wide > Stores > Open Monday - Friday 9 - 6, Saturday 9 - 4
Phones > Toll free 1300 555 686 > Head office 03 8847 3000 > Fax 03 8847 3030
Secure online shopping > www.BioNatural.biz > info@bionatural.biz

Information provided by BioNatural Pty Ltd including product descriptions and pictures is provided for educational and informational purposes only and has not been evaluated by the Therapeutic Goods Administration. These products are not intended to diagnose, treat, cure, or prevent any disease. Please consult your appropriately trained healthcare practitioner for medical advice.

Explore, learn and shop at www.BioNatural.biz

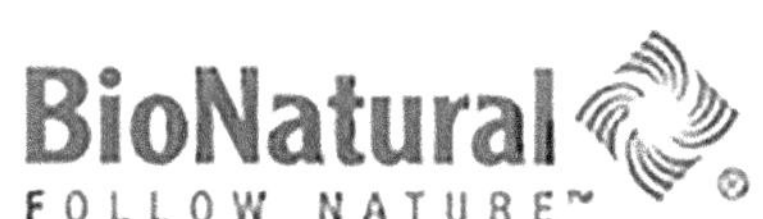

Proteolytic Enzymes

Probiotic microorganism

Concentrated protein digestion supplement

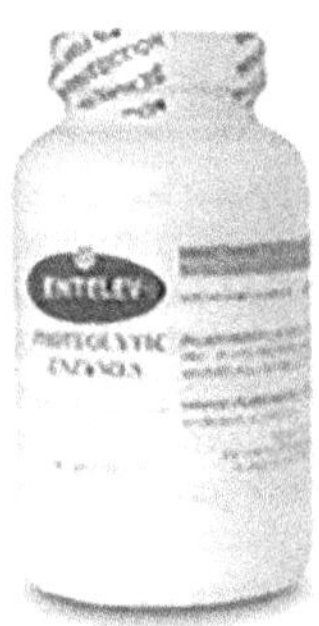

- Powerful supportive measure for rogue cell self management
- Restores natural gut flora balance to assist optimal performance throughout the body

Proteolytic enzymes may assist to:

- enhance nutritional status of foods eaten
- strengthen the immune system
- guard against rogue cells, cardiovascular and degenerative disease
- combat yeast overgrowth and fungal infections
- prevent indigestion, constipation, diarrhoea, flatulence and bloating
- protect against osteoporosis and rheumatoid arthritis
- lower cholesterol levels

Proteolytic enzymes break down protein in the digestive process

Our bodies are made up of a series of marvellous biological chemical reactions that occur every second of the day. Eating and digesting food is one of the most obvious body functions we are aware of and proteolytic enzymes play the most essential role in the digestive process. The digestive process takes substantial amounts of energy from the body to perform its work.

Proteolytic enzymes, or proteases, are enzymes which break down the peptide bond of proteins and allow the protein nutrients to be assimilated into the body. When we eat, food enters the stomach and intestines to be broken down into microscopic particles so that they can be absorbed and used to deliver and generate energy for all body processes. Enzymes are part of the biochemical process which enable the body to identify the aspects of food, which when broken down, provide the fuel needed to live. This enables the release and utilization of the nutritional value of the food by effectively assimilating the essential food nutrients.

A malfunctioning digestive system is considered a primary cause of disease. The body, unable to absorb vitamins and minerals necessary to sustain healthy life, becomes susceptible to systemic toxicity that can lead to immune dysfunction and chronic degenerative disease. The benefits of maintaining a good supply of proteolytic enzymes may improve the general health of the digestive system and increase the available nutrients in the body.

Retaining adequate of supply of proteolytic enzymes vital to good health

Proteolytic enzymes must be kept in adequate supply by being absorbed from food or made within the body. Since they have a limited life span, they must be replaced regularly. **Enzymes are damaged or destroyed by modern processing of food including heat, dehydration methods, vacuum sealing, pasteurisation techniques, microwaving as well as fluoridation found in the water supply.** Enzymes are temperature sensitive and are destroyed when food is cooked at temperatures exceeding 54 degrees Celsius. Given the level of environmental pollutants with which the body must contend on a daily basis, enzyme supplementation can assist the body to function at an optimal level. Antibiotics can kill benificial enzymes.

Enzymes and their vitality are best obtained from raw fresh foods or quality enzyme supplements. **With age, the body's ability to make sufficient quantities of these enzymes reduces dramatically. The immune system weakens, allowing disease and illness easy access.** The function of the immune system is to fight foreign invaders, such as bacteria, viruses, carcinogens and other chemicals. It relies most heavily on enzymes to perform this role. Enzymes have a limited life and must be replaced regularly. A weakened immune system has a decreased total volume of enzymes, including many which are defective or operating at a reduced rate.

Healthy digestive functioning also allows the liver to perform more effectively in its task to produce bile salts that are responsible for the break down of intestinal fats. An accumulation of these fats may result in elevated cholesterol levels.

How proteolytic enzymes work

Different enzymes are designed to break down a particular type of food. For instance, maltase is the enzyme found in the small intestine that reduces sugar to glucose for energy. Protein is split by proteolytic enzymes into amino acids that become the basic building blocks of all cells. The duodenum, the first section of the small intestine, is where enzyme digestion mainly takes place.

Many people with dysbiosis (gastro-intestinal tract imbalance) or candida (infection causing yeast condition) have poor digestive function that prevents the proper break down of enzyme-rich food. This results in nutrients being eliminated without being absorbed. Taking bioavailable enzymes in ready-to-digest form allows the body to maximize its uptake of nutrients from the food consumed. The nutrients are used to either immediately

Did you know?

Living enzymes are in raw unprocessed foods. If you are not getting enough raw foods it is essential to supplement your enzymes. Enzymes aid the digestive process by accelerating the rate of chemical reactions in breaking down the food we eat. There are more than 5000 known varieties of enzymes with uses in brewing, living dairy, baking, paper manufacturing and health industry and have shown health benefits in clinical trials over many years.

Explore, learn and shop at www.BioNatural.biz

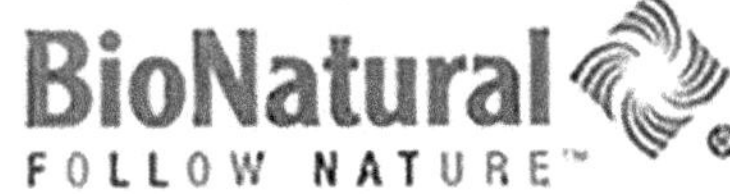

BioNatural Pty Ltd > 1 Overland Drive, Vermont South, VIC 3133 Australia
BioNatural Carlton Pty Ltd > 202 Rathdowne Street, Carlton, VIC 3053 Australia
Mail Order > Australia-wide > Stores > Open Monday - Friday 9 - 6, Saturday 9 - 4
Phones > Toll free 1300 555 686 > Head office 03 8847 3000 > Fax 03 8847 3030
Secure online shopping > www.BioNatural.biz > info@bionatural.biz

Information provided by BioNatural Pty Ltd including product descriptions and pictures is provided for educational and informational purposes only, and has not been evaluated by the Therapeutic Goods Administration. These products are not intended to diagnose, treat, cure, or prevent any disease. Please consult your appropriately trained healthcare practitioner for medical advice.

Proteolytic Enzymes • Probiotic microorganism

replace and repair worn-out and damaged tissue or are transformed into energy and used to generate heat.

Should pain in the stomach or indigestion be felt regularly after eating, the addition of enzymes to aid in digestion of the various foods is recommended. To avoid the vast array of complaints that arise from poor protein digestion, Proteolytic Enzymes - plant protease, bromelain and papain - should be taken on a daily basis to restore digestive health.

Plant protease, bromelain and papain

Plant protease enzymes found in proteolytic enzymes provide a comprehensive blend of vegetarian enzymes. The capacity of these enzymes to be active in a broad pH range, aids food digestion markedly.

Bromelain, found in pineapple, including the core, is a proteolytic bioflavonoid that has been found to inhibit the effect on ongoing inflammation in mucous membranes found throughout the body. It is also used for reduction of inflammation in damaged muscle tissue after traumatic injury or following prolonged, intense athletic activity. Bromelain has also been used to treat boils, angina and atherosclerotic plaque responsible for heart disease.

Papain is effective in digesting proteins, fats and carbohydrates. It has also been known to safely destroy and expel parasites from the intestines. Papain has also been known to have an anti-ulcer action and been used to treat neoplasms or rogue cells of the lungs.

Fast modern living, stress and digestive dysfunction

Emotional stress has a remarkable effect on the bowel. When suddenly alarmed by an event that calls for swift action, the body enters the first phase of what is known as the general adaptation syndrome (GAS). This phase is characterised by an instant release of adrenalin into the bloodstream that has a multitude of almost instantaneous effects. Among these is a release of stored sugar (energy) from the liver, to fuel the many responses of the body to whatever demands have been placed on it. These include a tensing of voluntary muscles in preparation for action, or what is commonly referred to as the 'fight-or-flight response'.

The heart rate speeds up, sweating starts, the mouth becomes dry and, of particular relevance in this instance, digestive processes cease or slow down dramatically to provide

emergency energy levels elsewhere, as blood is diverted from the gut to the muscles. Should such an alarm situation allow suitable action, then all the listed changes then normalize as the body reverts to an unstressed function. Should no such fight-or-flight response be possible or the stress event allows for no appropriate action, such as when stuck in a plane, train or car with no obvious end in sight, then the arousal adrenalin release and all the physiological consequences are not suitably used.

Should such a stress pattern be repeated often, as is common in the modern, fast-paced environment where rushing to be somewhere is a common experience as opposed to simply being, then a change takes place in the alarm reaction. The body adapts to the repetitive demands made upon it and the responses become chronic rather than acute. A pattern of months or years of repetitive stress may result in permanently tense muscles, headaches, high or low blood sugar levels, high blood pressure and tendency to palpitations, indigestion and or stomach ulcers and almost certainly a degree of bowel dysfunction, due to constant acidic secretions triggered as part of the body's adaptation to stress.

This pattern of damage is most obvious in the colon evidenced by damage to the mucous membranes lining the digestive tract that can lead to local swelling, inflammation and sometimes small haemorrhages or ulcers.

Such changes have a variety of effects on the local flora or natural bacteria of the stomach and intestines. A variety of toxic chemical substances can be formed, some which can pass through damaged mucous membranes into the blood stream with allergic and inflammatory consequences. An immune system response to such inflammation would also be likely to occur as the body attempts to fight the invasion.

Digestive dysfunction and the link to chronic degenerative disease

A large variety of disease begins with digestive dysfunction and the taxing effects of this chronic fight-or-flight adaptation process. The effects of this stress process, combined with the general toxicity that arises from the fermentation and purification of undigested food and the toxic gaseous wastes that form, become distributed and re-absorbed throughout the entire body.

Diseases linked with this leaky gut syndrome lead to an oversensitive immune system response. The body is on constant hight alert, bombarded by undigested proteins and toxic chemicals from the damaged mucous membranes lining the gut wall. This eventually results in the immune system identifying its own cells as foreign. The body then mounts an auto immune response that destroys its own healthy cells.

There is a growing consensus among health care professionals that diseases associated with a hypersensitive immune response include rheumatoid arthritis, asthma, lupus, cancers, osteoporosis and leukaemia to name a few.

Proteolytic enzymes may guard against degenerative disease

Those with chronic indigestion are well advised to examine lifestyle factors and reduce stress-causing events. Combine this lifestyle change with supplementation of Proteolytic Enzymes and practical measures such as exercise, breathing, meditation, relaxation and time spent in Nature to regain full health benefits. Employing the power of the mind in combination with Proteolytic Enzymes may reduce the impact on the body of digestive strain and its toxic by-products.

Learning and taking personal responsibility for you're your own health may overcome the habbits of stress and poor diet. Proteolytic Enzymes in the daily diet may act as prevention against chronic degenerative disease and lead to improved general health and wellbeing in the long term.

Suggested use

Take two capsules of Proteolytic Enzymes three times daily with water half an hour before meals or an hour and a half after meals or as directed by a health care professional.

BioNatural Pty Ltd > 1 Overland Drive, Vermont South, VIC 3133 Australia
BioNatural Carlton Pty Ltd > 202 Rathdowne Street, Carlton, VIC 3053 Australia
Mail Order > Australia-wide > Stores > Open Monday - Friday 9 - 6, Saturday 9 - 4
Phones > Toll free 1300 555 686 > Head office 03 8847 3000 > Fax 03 8847 3030
Secure online shopping > www.BioNatural.biz > info@bionatural.biz

Explore, learn and shop at www.BioNatural.biz

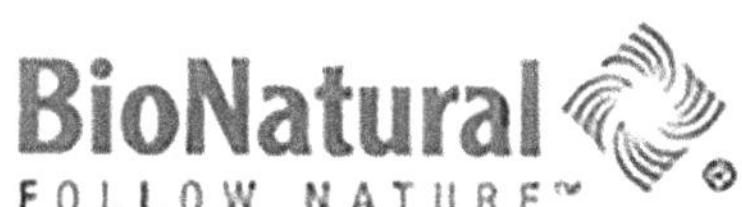

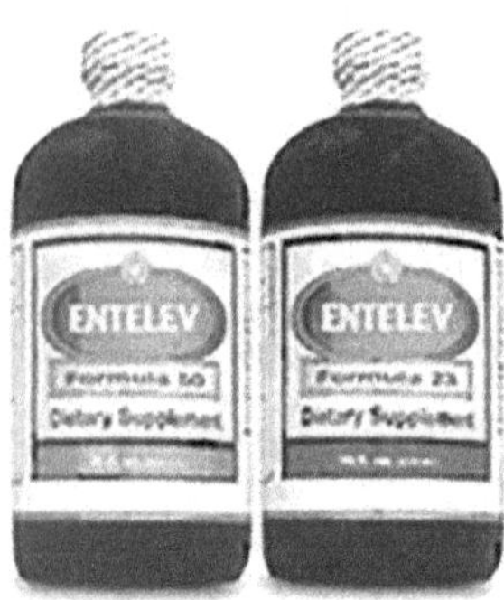

Entelev - Extreme antiaging antioxidant

The natural non-toxic herbal supplement that assists elimination of rogue anaerobic cells

Dr. Robert Becker, M.D., in his book "The Body Electric", indicates in his research that of the billions of cells the body creates each day, many of these are not health reproductions and become "non-contributing" cells. These damaged cells or "body debris" need to be removed by the immune system before they further impair health or replicate.

Every immune system needs **intense** nourishment **and detoxification. It also** requires a clean inner **environment for** cellular communication **and optimal** health. Even with good intentions and correct eating habits, the build up of body debris still occurs on a daily basis. The more rogue **cells** and toxins the body can remove, the more heightened the vital immune response **becomes** and natural energy levels **increase**.

Non-toxic health management
It's in your hands

What does the **word 'anaerobic' mean?**
A micro-organism which flourishes without free air", Webster, Contemporary Dictionary, page 25. When it comes to cells in our body, we have two kinds, "aerobic" a healthy cell which uses oxygen, and "anaerobic" an unhealthy cell that does not use oxygen. To regain health or to maintain one's present level of health, the immune system has to daily remove all unwanted anaerobic cells. If they accumulate, they may become fertile ground for destructive elements that if not removed, can destroy one's life.

Anaerobic Cellular **Reduction** Technology (ACRT) is a scientific term for a new technology developed through extensive research that, in a very unique way, causes a modest but safe interference in the cellular structure. (The human body comes equipped with several, vitally important, built-in, natural healing and restorative systems or mechanisms, to bring about optimal health. However, most often, our diets, lifestyles, habits and environment have rendered these mechanisms largely ineffective.) Entelev's two formulas were formulated, using the breakthrough technology, to assist these natural mechanisms and to enhance their effectiveness. Certain modified natural compounds, which have been selected for their effect on electrical-current functions within the cells, are used in the production of both Entelev formulas.

These selected compounds have a particularly unique oxidation-reduction potential and are formulated in such a way as to affect certain key cellular and biochemical transformation processes. The uniqueness of the technology is that it promotes lysing (the breaking up) of unwanted cells, while causing no loss of function in healthy cells.

Entelev Formula 50

Formula 50 is designed to aid the immune system by cleansing inside the body. This stronger formula has been developed to achieve faster and more intense cleansing.

Entelev Formula 50
Two months supply
*AUS338.00

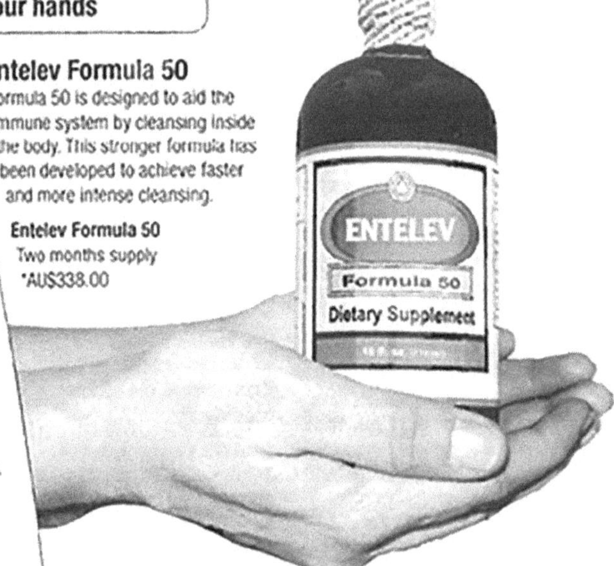

Entelev Formula 23

Entelev 23 is also designed to aid the immune system in its unending task to cleanse the body of the daily accumulation of toxins and body debris.

Entelev Formula 23
Two months supply *AUS248.00

Learn about Entelev soon

Entelev InfoPack includes:

- Book outlining the history and development of Entelev
- Key benefits
- How Entelev works
- Testimonials of personal experiences
- Directions for use
- Websites
- Entelev uses for pets
- Audio cassette tape

Entelev InfoPack *AUS29.00

*Prices are plus Pack & Post

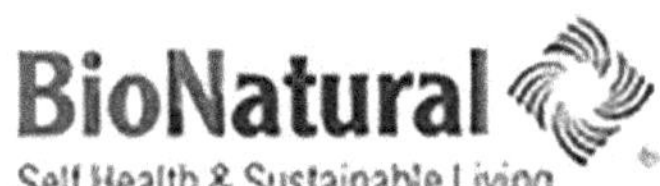

Explore, learn and shop at www.BioNatural.biz

BioNatural Vermont South > 1 Overland Drive, Vermont South, VIC 3133 Australia
BioNatural Carlton Pty Ltd > 202 Rathdowne Street, Carlton, VIC 3053 Australia

Mail Order > Australia-wide > **Stores** > Open Monday - Friday 9 - 6, Saturday 9 - 4
Phones > Toll free 1300 555 686 > Head office 03 8847 3000 > Fax 03 8847 3030
Direct deposit > BioNatural, Westpac BSB 033062 A/C 235666
Secure online shopping > www.BioNatural.biz > info@bionatural.biz

Entelev - Extreme antiaging antioxidant

Medical scientists now believe that the next generation of technologically advanced medicines will no longer poison the body with chemotherapy or burn the body with radiation but instead teach the human body to control its own cancer. What these scientists envisioned for the future is already available in a unique product called Entelev.

Entelev is available in two different formulas, the stronger Entelev 50 and the maintenance Entelev 23. Both of these formulas function based on "Anaerobic Cellular Reduction Technology". The formulas are non-toxic, safe and formulated from natural occurring and synthetic compounds which activate the body's own built-in healing mechanisms.

James Sheridan, a biochemist and the inventor of Entelev embraced the theory that was first proven by two times Nobel Prize winner, Dr Otto Warburg. Dr Warburg believed that cancer cells use the fermentation of glucose for energy rather than using oxygen for energy like normal healthy cells. These are known as anaerobic (without oxygen) cells or aerobic (with oxygen) cells respectively.

Entelev's uniqueness comes from its ability to operate on the "biochemical" level of cells. It specifically targets damaged anaerobic cells. Entelev's biochemical reaction in the body lowers the voltage of every cell just slightly. Simply put, for each cell in the body, the voltage of the cell operates as the "glue" that holds the cell together. As anaerobic cells produce energy in a different way than normal healthy cells, they operate on a much lower energy level thereby holding a lower voltage than healthy cells. With the slight reduction in voltage of as little as 10 to 15% caused by the regular use of Entelev, the anaerobic or damaged cells lose their "glue" and begin to lyse or break down into harmless protein that is easily eliminated by the body.

Another characteristic that makes Entelev unique from other types of treatment is that Entelev targets the basic respiratory system of cancer cells, hence cancer cells do not have the chance to mutate and resist attack. This in contrast to chemotherapy where cancer cells are known to mutate and become resistant. Entelev is a much safer.

Entelev is non-specific and therefore works in the same manner for cancers of all types. Many other types of chronic illnesses can be the result of anaerobic cells damaging the body. Entelev may also assist in the improvement of the degenerative conditions of high blood pressure, arthritis, chronic fatigue, diabetes, crohn's disease, multiple sclerosis, viral infections, endometriosis, hemorrhoids, psoriasis and autoimmune diseases.

Since 1970, thousands of people in the USA have used Entelev as their primary approach to cancer recovery. Before the product became available to the public, the FDA suppressed the product to be advertised as a form of treatment. Entelev is currently sold as a dietary supplement. However, because Entelev is a product unlike any other, it's had 60 years of research and dedication originating with its inventor, James Sheridan.

Every individual who is dealing with cancer should have the right to know about Entelev and make their own fully informed decision as to what treatment approach they choose to pursue that best suits them.

What does the word 'anaerobic' mean? – "a micro-organism which flourishes without free air". Webster, Contemporary Dictionary, page 25. When it comes to cells in our body, we have two kinds, "aerobic" a healthy cell that uses oxygen, and "anaerobic" an unhealthy cell that does not use oxygen. To regain health or to maintain one's present level of health, the immune system has to daily remove all unwanted anaerobic cells. If they accumulate, they may become fertile ground for destructive elements that if not removed, can destroy one's life.

Anaerobic Cellular Reduction Technology (ACRT) is a scientific term for a new technology developed through extensive research that, in a very unique way, causes a modest but safe interference in the cellular structure. (The human body comes equipped with several, vitally important, built-in, natural healing and restorative systems or mechanisms, to bring about optimal health However, most often, our diets, lifestyles, habits and environment have rendered these mechanisms largely ineffective.) Entelev's two formulas were formulated, using the breakthrough technology, to assist these natural mechanisms and to enhance their effectiveness. Certain modified natural compounds, which have been selected for their effect on electrical-current functions within the cells, are used in the production of both Entelev formulas.

These selected compounds have a particularly unique oxidation-reduction potential and are formulated in such a way as to affect certain key cellular and biochemical transformation processes. The uniqueness of the technology is that it promotes lysing (the breaking up) of unwanted cells, while causing no loss of function in healthy cells.

Entelev 50 and Entelev 23 plus other innovative products for non-toxic Self Health are now available in Australia direct from the importers and distributors, BioNatural Pty Ltd. BioNatural have a comprehensive Entelev InfoPack detailing the history of Entelev, how it works, how to use it, testimonials and audio cassette for $29.00 plus Pack & Post.

When does one stop taking Entelev?

Just because a scan no longer pick up a malignant tumour, it does not necessarily mean that it is completely gone. Unfortunately, it takes only one cancer cell remaining in the body for there to be eventually a problem with the disease again. It is recommended that Entelev is continued for at least an additional three months once the doctor considers the patient to be in remission – this is the best scenario as far as any physician is concerned.

By this point, taking Entelev should be part of an individual's normal routine of life such as brushing teeth and hair daily. Staying on Entelev for an extended period of time will allow the body to completely eliminate all diseased/damaged cells.

BioNatural Vermont **South** > 1 Overland Drive, Vermont South, VIC 3133 Australia
BioNatural Carlton Pty Ltd > 202 Rathdowne Street, Carlton, VIC 3053 Australia

Mail Order > Australia-wide > **Stores** > Open Monday - Friday 9 - 6, Saturday 9 - 4
Phones > Toll free 1300 555 686 > Head office 03 8847 3000 > Fax 03 8847 3030
Direct deposit > BioNatural Westpac BSB 033062 A/C 235666
Secure **online shopping** > www.BioNatural.biz > info@bionatural.biz

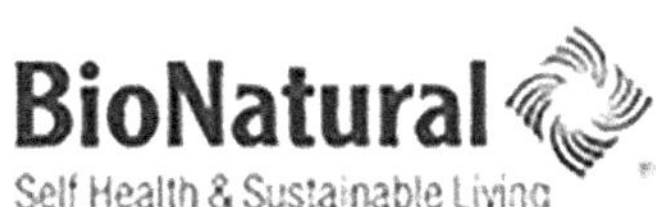

Explore, learn and shop at www.BioNatural.biz

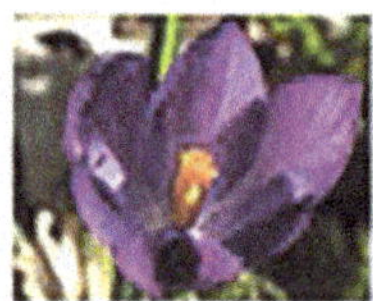

German New Medicine®

Dr. med. Mag. theol. Ryke Geerd Hamer

The Five Biological Laws of the New Medicine

presented by Dr. med. Ryke Geerd Hamer

at the

First International Congress on
Complementary and Alternative Medical Cancer Treatment

May 14/15, 2005
Madrid, Spain

Amici di Dirk, Ediciones de la Nueva Medicina S.L.
Camino Urique 69, Apartado de Correos 209, E-29120 Alhaurin el Grande

Introduction

Dear Friends, Esteemed Colleagues:

It is a great honor for me to present you with the greatest gift the Gods have ever given to mankind. I am the president of this congress, but at the moment detained in a French prison because of the "instigation to practice the German New Medicine". These are the words used in the official charges and the verdict. After 8 ½ months in custody a detention review hearing will finally take place, one day after my 70th birthday.

Back in 1986 my approbation was revoked, because of my "refusal to renounce the iron law of cancer and my non-conversion to traditional medicine".

For 24 years now I have been chased, threatened, prosecuted and thrown into jail twice, although I have done nothing wrong – except to rediscover this wonderful New Medicine with its 5 Biological Laws of Nature, a medicine that has always existed and will always exist. This, Ladies and Gentlemen, is the extent of my crime!

When I now present the New Medicine to you, you have to realize that the New Medicine is actually "illegal". Although the findings have been verified 30 times by medical doctors and professors through signed documents, apparently for the last twenty years only Jewish doctors were allowed to practice it.

This congress calls itself a congress for "alternative medicine". I affectionately call it *alter-naive* medicine, because by nature any alternative medicine can only exist as long as an understanding of the true contexts and meanings is suppressed. However, generally speaking, one refers to an "alternative medical therapy". Let me say a few words about this. As you will see in a moment, so-called diseases as we have understood them until now do not exist. Rather, they are Meaningful Special Biological Programs of Nature. And they do not have to be treated with "therapy", but must be left to run their course because they always have a biological purpose.

The crux of our thinking lies in the fact that, for 1500 years now, in Europe we have practiced a medicine of symptoms. Everything has diligently and religiously been categorized as "benign" or "malignant": Cancer is malignant, so are microbes, so is fever or fatigue; and all supposedly so-called "symptoms of disease" were malignant and had to be eradicated – like a sinful action.

Since nobody knew anything and nobody knew of any causal therapy, approximately 1000 different therapies existed. But whenever Mother Nature had finished her work of healing – despite our erroneous attempts at pseudo-therapeutic intervention – then we were quick to praise the outcome as our own "success". How wise we thought we were – just like the sorcerer's apprentice!

Before I introduce you to the New Medicine, or rather, the German New Medicine – let me take a few moments to explain the name: I changed the name from New Medicine into German New Medicine purely for the reason that currently some 15 different alternative therapeutic approaches also call themselves New Medicine because the name cannot be protected. I had to find a new one. And I decided to call it the German New Medicine because it was discovered in Germany, the nation of thinkers and poets, of musicians, inventors and explorers, and because the German language is the mother of almost all European languages. The result of this is that, apart from being charged with sectarianism, I am now unfortunately also accused of anti-Semitism.

The Five Biological Laws of the German New Medicine®

Both conventional and alternative medicine consider what we commonly call a disease as a result of an „error" of Nature, as a failure of the so-called "immune system", as something "malignant" that is trying to destroy the organism and therefore has to be fought with all possible medical-military strategic means available. In 24 years of profound and intense work on this subject I have moved light years away from this notion.

It is, of course, not easy to change our traditional biological-medical thinking straight after the first foray into this new dimension. In the following, I will strive to give you a general overview in the short time available to me.

The German New Medicine (as it is now called), which I discovered in 1981, is an exact natural science based on five biological laws. It does not require any hypothesis and, in rigorous scientific terms, is reproducible for any patient case. This was demonstrated and officially certified on September 8/9, 1998 at the University of Trnava (Slovakia).

In biological-medical terms, the German New Medicine identifies a living organism as an inseparable unity of the psyche, the brain and the organ. All processes of the psyche and the organ are coordinated from the brain. Essentially, the brain is the main computer of our organism, the psyche the programmer. Body and psyche together are basically the "data receiver" of the computer brain (both in optimal programming mode and also when errors occur). By no means is the psyche the sole programmer of the brain. In cases of injuries the organ can also induce an automatic response in the brain and in the psyche. In this sense, the German New Medicine distinguishes itself fundamentally from all other medical schools of thought, in particular from those of standard medicine.

The German New Medicine is an empirical natural science based on 5 biological laws which have always existed and which always will exist. I merely rediscovered these natural laws. They are applicable in equal measure to human beings, animals and plants, even to single-celled creatures – in fact, they apply to the entire cosmos. And, naturally, they are valid concerning all so-called diseases as part of a two-phased Meaningful Special Biological Program of Nature (MSBP).

Lacking the medical and clinical relevance of these 5 biological laws prevented us from being able to understand, classify, and correctly assess one single disease. We were unable to understand cancer and its contextual implications because we considered cancer to be incurable and merely concentrated on eliminating the symptoms on the organ. Nor were we able to understand the so-called infectious diseases, because, instead of recognizing them as healing symptoms, we considered them as aggressive diseases with microbes out to destroy us.

Equally ignored were the "Law of the Two Phases of Every Disease", the psychological level, the cerebral level as well as the significance of left- and right-handedness. Let alone the "epileptic or epileptoid crisis" and the so-called "Syndrome" which is the most frequent cause of death.

All these new ways of understanding and of curing a disease are based on understanding the Iron Rule of Cancer, the First Biological Law, and the so-called DHS = Dirk-Hamer-Syndrome, named after my son Dirk whose unexpected death was the cause why I developed testicular cancer.

The Iron Rule of Cancer is called "iron" because it is a biological law. The fact that a child must always have a father and a mother is an example of a biological law; there must always be two participants involved in creating a child. In the German New Medicine we have 5 biological laws that are quasi iron.

THE FIRST BIOLOGICAL LAW

THE IRON RULE OF CANCER

The Iron Rule of Cancer has 3 criteria:

THE FIRST CRITERION

Every Meaningful Special Biological Program (MSBP) originates from a DHS (Dirk Hamer Syndrome), which is a serious, acute-dramatic and isolative conflict shock that catches us completely off guard. The conflict shock occurs simultaneously

1. in the psyche
2. in the brain
3. on the corresponding organ.

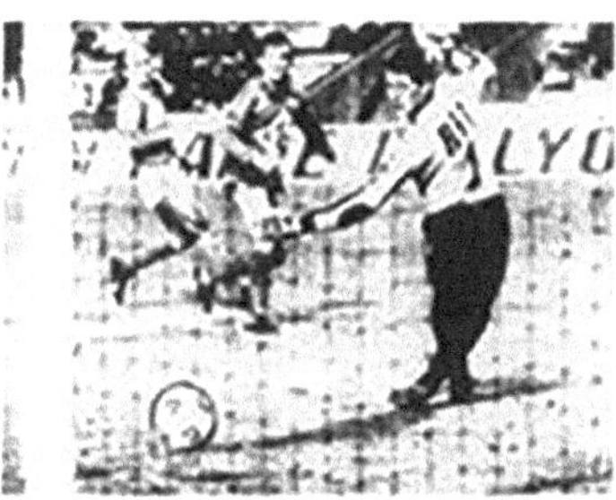

This picture shows how a goalie is caught "on the wrong foot". He looks puzzled at the ball which he expected in the other corner. He can no longer get off his "wrong foot".

This is the typical situation of a DHS. The individual is caught "on the wrong foot".

A **DHS** is a serious, acute-dramatic, isolative conflict shock that catches the individual "on the wrong foot". However, with the DHS the individual gets a chance to make up for the mishap and to cope with the unexpected situation. At the moment of the DHS the shock triggers the onset of a Meaningful Special Biological Program that runs synchronously on the level of the psyche, the brain and the corresponding organ. This "Special Biological Program" is both visible and measurable.

Exactly at the moment when the DHS strikes, the patient experiences a prolonged stress phase, i.e. he has cold hands and cold feet, he dwells day and night on the conflict content trying to find a resolution. Typically, he can't sleep, and if, then only during the first part of the night, he has no appetite, he loses weight. That is what we call the **conflict active phase**.

We see that, contrary to ordinary problems in our daily lives, these biological conflicts launch the patient into a continuous stress tonus with very specific symptoms that cannot be missed.

This condition will only change when the patient resolves the conflict. With the resolution of the conflict the patient changes into a rest tonus because now the psyche has to recover. Typically, the patient feels sluggish and tired but released. He has good appetite, his body temperature rises, often accompanied by fever and headaches. In this phase the patient sleeps well, but usually only after three o'clock in the morning. This is what we call the **conflict-resolution phase**.

We humans can suffer many conflict shocks without falling ill but this is only the case if we had time to be prepared for the conflicts.

At the moment of the DHS something else can happen. At the same instant **tracks** are laid on which the disease development "runs" its course. Tracks are additional conflict aspects in connection with a DHS, i.e. circumstances that are associated at the moment of the DHS. Just as in a still photo taken with a flash, but without being aware of it, when the DHS occurs, human beings (as well as animals) pick up the smallest accompanying details such as sounds, smells, sensations, or tastes and store these imprints for life. If, at a later time, the patient sets on such a track, the whole conflict can become re-activated resulting in a relapse.

Together with the main DHS-track five or six "side tracks" (accompanying circumstances that are considered important) can be set simultaneously. It is important to understand that one can also set from one of the sidetracks on to the main track. That's why we call them "tracks".

We human beings regard these tracks as "pathological". We consider them as allergies that have to be fought or we call them "hay fever", "asthma", "neurodermatitis" etc. and randomly label with these terms different conflicts in different phases with all their physical and cerebral symptoms.

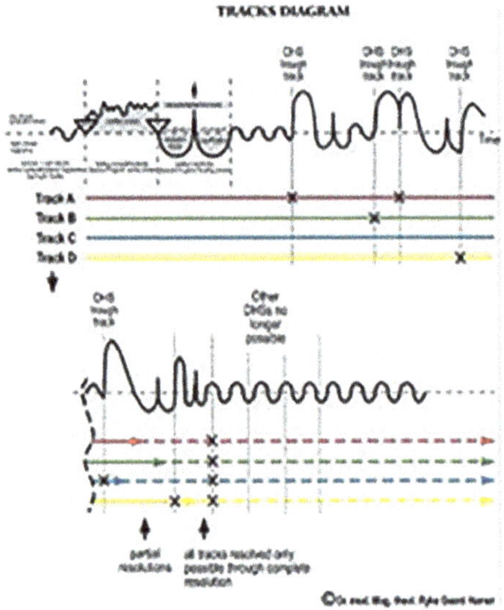

Example: In a young mother, an amniocentesis carried out in order to determine proof of paternity, triggered a mother-child conflict resulting in cancer of the mammary glands. During the intervention itself the woman was consumed with great fear of potential damage to her unborn child. Although the baby was born completely healthy, the mother experienced the entire paternity proceedings on this established conflict track. Each time she received a letter from the lawyer or the courts, she fell back on this track and the tumor continued to grow. Thus, the DHS does not only comprise the moment of the acute dramatic conflict shock which "catches us on the wrong foot" but also the content of the conflict, which determines where the Hamer Focus appears in the brain and which organ is affected by cancer, necrosis or failure. However, as we can see, much more can happen in the exact second the DHS takes place: in this moment the tracks for future repeated episodes are laid.

THE SECOND CRITERION

The biological conflict determines at the moment of the DHS the location of the so-called Hamer Focus (HH) as well as the location of the cancer or cancer-equivalent disease on the corresponding organ.

At the moment of the DHS a Meaningful Special Biological Program (MSBP) is switched on that runs synchronously in the psyche, the brain and on the organ. In theory, we use these three levels as a helpful tool for diagnosis and therapy. In reality these three levels constitute one single unit.

Each conflict has a very specific content that is defined at the moment the DHS occurs. The conflict content is determined "in association", which means that it happens unconsciously, bypassing our consciousness. We think that we think. In reality, the conflict has already associatively hit a fraction of a second before we even began to think.

The unexpected shock leaves a mark in the brain, which is visible on a computer tomogram of the brain. Such a ringed lesion is called a Hamer Focus (German: **H**amerscher **H**erd). The term was actually coined by my opponents who mockingly named the ring formations "the dubious Hamer Foci". These Foci look like a set of concentric rings, similar to what we observe when skipping a stone on water.

Every conflict is linked to a specific organ as well as to a very specific part of the brain from where the process on the organ level is controlled and directed.

The changes in the brain are visible at the very second the DHS occurs.

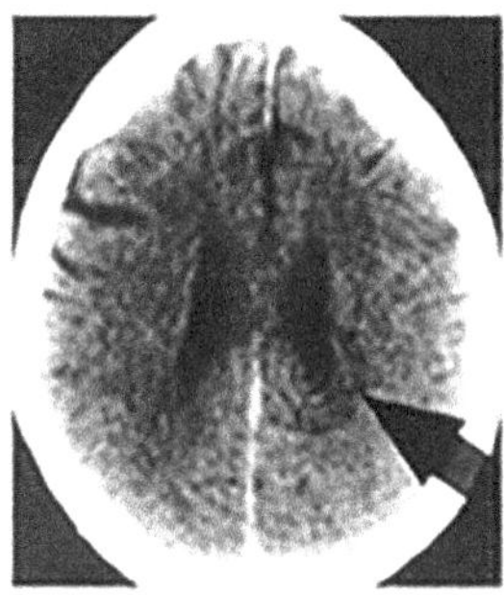

Hamer Focus (HH) in ring form configuration at the beginning of the healing phase

The larger the HH, the larger is the tumor, the necrosis or the cell alteration on the corresponding organ. The more intensive the conflict, the faster does the tumor grow or the larger is the necrosis, the osteolysis or the cell alteration with those cancers that do not display cell augmentation.

During this phase there is temporary swelling of the brain which can cause problems, e.g. if the conflict has lasted too long, or when the brain edema is located in an unfavorable location, or when the HH shows an intra- and perifocal edema. The edema on the organ and on the correlating HH in the brain grows particularly large with a simultaneous kidney collecting tubule-water retention conflict, which we call "The Syndrome". At this point the HH requires more room, consequently indenting surrounding brain tissue or pushing it out of the way.

In the brain both phases (conflict active phase and resolution phase) have the HH at the same location. They are, however, in different conditions: During the conflict active phase the HH appears as a sharp ring configuration while during the resolution or healing phase the HH appears as swollen, edematous and dark. At the end of the healing phase so-called glia, harmless brain connective tissue is stored at the site participating in repairing the HH.

The white dense glia HHs, which can be easily made visible in a computer tomogram using iodine contrast substance, indicate a repair process on the HH in the brain and are not at all a reason to panic.

After the healing phase the HH shows as a harmless scar – the end result of a successfully completed healing process. The glia-rings are unfortunately misinterpreted as "brain tumors", as glioma, astrocytoma, oligodendroglioma, glioblastoma etc. and are cut right out to the disadvantage of the patient. Since brain cells can no longer divide after birth brain tumors do not really exist!

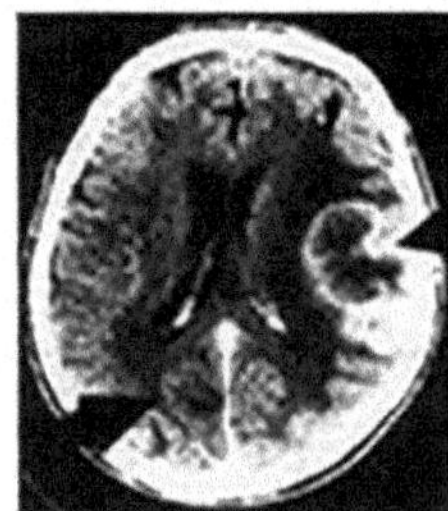

Right arrow: HH in right temporal lobe
Condition after heart attack (territorial conflict)

Left arrow: testicular carcinoma (profound loss conflict) for right testicle (already in healing phase)

In this example, the patient, a farmer, had suffered a DHS six months earlier, when his only son had a serious motorcycle accident. The son spent a long period of time in intensive care, and the patient thought that his son would remain physically disabled. But his son fully recovered. Four weeks after the son returned to the farm, his father suffered a heart attack with dizziness, headaches and balance disturbances. He suffered the heart attack <u>after</u> he had resolved the conflict.

In the animal world, a male deer can also suffer a biological conflict, e.g. a territorial conflict with angina pectoris during the conflict active phase, when his opponent drives him out of his territory. The ulceration in the coronary arteries that starts as soon as the conflict takes place widens the coronary vessel, which allows the double or triple amount of blood being pumped to the heart. This enables the deer to wait for the right moment to fight his opponent and win his territory back. He only gets this vigor and strength because the Special Biological Program is activated. Without it, he would not be able to succeed. Were the deer be given tranquilizers, it would never be able to get his territory back.

For a man his "territory" could translate into his business, his girlfriend, his family or his job. We humans have several shared territories – even a car can be a "territory". With human beings the heart attack is only noticeable when the conflict activity lasted at least 3-4 months. However, if the conflict active phase lasted more than 9 months the heart attack is usually fatal.

This is different from the myocardial infarct (controlled from the cerebral medulla). Here the conflict content is experienced as: "I am completely overwhelmed". The conflict active phase manifests itself as necrosis of the myocardium. During the healing phase and specifically during the epileptoid crisis, which indicates a crucial turning point, the epileptic heart attack or myocardial infarct is initiated.

THE THIRD CRITERION

The development of the MSBP on all three levels, from the DHS to the conflict resolution (CL) and the epileptoid crisis (EC) at the height of the healing phase and the return to normalization always runs synchronously.

The development of the Meaningful Special Biological Program occurs simultaneously on all three levels. If the conflict becomes more intense, then, for example, the tumor growth advances faster. If the conflict loses intensity, the intensity diminishes on all other levels. If the conflict is resolved, then the resolution phase takes place on all three levels. If there is a relapse, the relapse happens on all three levels.

The Conflictolysis (CL) is a very distinctive point since every disease has its very specific healing symptoms that only commence with the resolution of the conflict. If we ask the patient about his conflict, we know the psychological level; if we have a computer tomogram of the brain, we know the brain level. On the organ level, however, we see, for instance, a paralysis, neurodermatitis, diabetes, etc.

What is fascinating about the German New Medicine is that we are not only able to conclude from the brain scan the type of biological conflict, the conflict content, which organ is involved and whether cell multiplication or cell loss is taking place, but we can also establish whether the conflict is still active (ca-phase) or has already been resolved (pcl-phase).

THE SECOND BIOLOGICAL LAW

The law of the two phases of all MSBP provided there is a resolution of the conflict

This natural law turns our entire medical understanding of diseases upside down, since ALL diseases run in this two-phased pattern. Unaware of these relationships, we have in the past identified a few hundred "cold diseases", and a few hundred "warm diseases". Patients with "cold diseases" had cold skin, cold extremities, were in protracted stress, lost weight, had difficulty falling asleep or suffered from sleep disturbances. Patients with "warm diseases" had warm or hot extremities, often fever, good appetite, and considerable fatigue.

With the so-called "cold diseases" the subsequent healing phase was overlooked or viewed as a "disease" in itself. With the so-called "warm diseases" – which are in fact already healing phases following a conflict active phase – the cold phase was overlooked and also viewed as a disease in itself. Now we understand that what was previously considered as two "diseases" is actually one single Special Biological Program (MSBP).

One could ask why physicians haven't yet recognized this two-phased pattern if it is so obvious. The reason is simply that conflicts are not always resolved. If the conflict cannot be resolved the disease remains in one phase, in other words, the individual stays in conflict activity, wastes away and dies of enervation or cachexia.

In retrospect, traditional medicine has not been able to understand one single "disease".

Presentation German New Medicine® by Dr. med Ryke Geerd Hamer, Madrid 2005

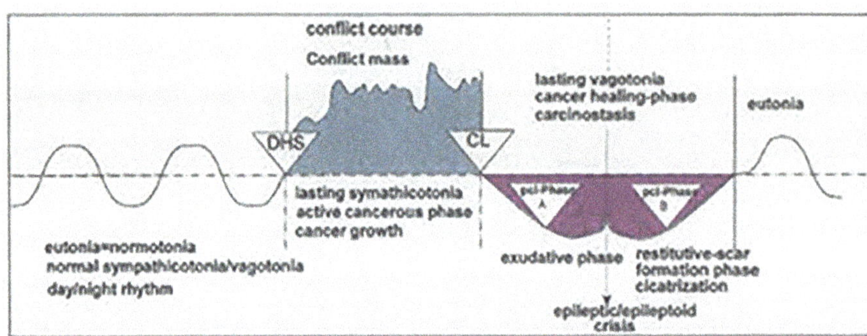

The diagram above shows that with the DHS the normal day-and-night rhythm switches into lasting sympathicotonia. The conflict resolution (CL) initiated the phase of lasting vagotonia. The vagotonic phase is interrupted by the so-called epileptic or epileptoid crisis which occurs at the deepest point of the healing phase. This crisis (a sympathicotonic spike) indicates a crucial turning point during the phase of vagotonia.

Every disease that has a conflict resolution involves a conflict active phase and a healing phase. And every healing phase – if not interrupted by a relapse – has an epileptic or epileptoid crisis, i.e. a turning point occurring at the deepest point of vagotonia.

This **epileptic or epileptoid crisis** is an event that Mother Nature has practiced for millions of years. It is a crisis, which runs simultaneously on all three levels. The purpose of this crisis at the highest point of the healing phase is to get the organism back to normality. What we generally call an epileptic seizure with muscle convulsions is only a specific type of epileptic crisis, which occurs after resolving a motor conflict.

An epileptoid crisis occurs in every disease but with some variations in each. "Epileptoid" means that there are no tonic-clonic muscle-cramps as in motor conflicts but other symptoms. Each type of biological conflict or disease has its own specific type of epileptoid crisis.

Mother Nature created quite a trick for this meaningful event. In the middle of the healing phase, the patient all of a sudden suffers a recurrence of his conflict. In other words: he experiences the conflict for a short time (as a conflict active relapse) all over again, including cold hands, cold sweat and all the symptoms of the conflict active stress phase. This also explains the strong angina pectoris pain during the heart attack.

The epileptoid crisis often presents a real clinical challenge as, for example, the lysis of pneumonia, the heart attack following a territorial conflict, the right cardiac infarction with pulmonary embolism, the loss of consciousness following a separation conflict, or diabetes and hypoglycemia.

For example, a patient suffering a cardiac infarction with a preceding conflict activity of more than 9 months has only a small chance of survival with standard medical treatment. Not one single patient – so we learned from our Vienna heart attack study - survived who was conflict active over a territorial conflict for more than 9 months of average conflict activity. With the so-called "Syndrome" (water-retention) involved the situation is different. Today, we can reduce the risks by treating the patient already 3-6 weeks prior to the epileptic crisis, i.e. prior to the expected heart attack.

- 9 -

A most important criterion in the German New Medicine is the **handedness** of the patient. Without establishing whether the patient is right-handed or left-handed we cannot work in the GNM. Besides identifying the laterality, it is equally important to know the patient's age, gender and hormonal situation, e.g. if a woman is postmenopausal, on the birth control pill, if her ovaries were removed or treated with radiation, if the patient is on chemotherapy, is on hormone drugs, etc.

The easiest way to establish our laterality is the clapping test = clapping as one would when applauding ....

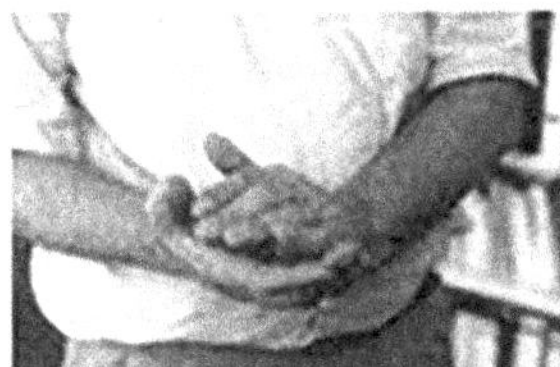

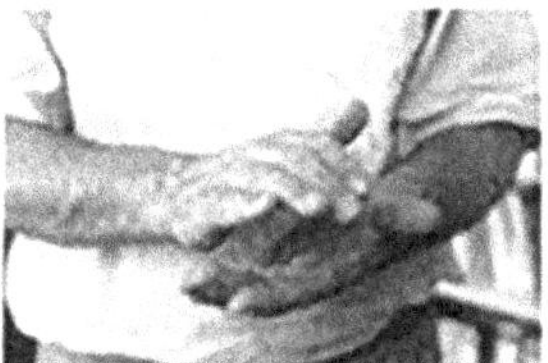

.... the upper hand is the leading hand that determines our biological laterality. If the right hand is on top, the person is right-handed; if the left hand is on top the person is cerebrally left-handed. This test is essential in order to identify on which brain hemisphere a person operates. There are many re-trained left-handers, who think that they are right-handed.

Left- and right-handedness starts in the brain, more precisely in the cerebellum. In the brain stem laterality is insignificant. In other words, the development of the cerebellum starts already with the first cell division and with it the differentiation of right- and left-handedness. Compared to right-handedness, the left-handedness transfers the conflict to the opposite brain hemisphere. The left-handers are differently "poled" from the psyche to the brain.

In the German New Medicine, neglecting to ask a patient whether he is right- or left-handed is considered a big mistake, because the laterality is of utmost importance to understanding the correlation of the conflicts to the brain (HH) and to the cancer or necrosis on the organ. Our laterality determines the "path" on which the conflict corresponds with the brain as well as which type of "disease" a patient can suffer with what type of conflict.

In the cerebellum, for example, the conflicts impact each hemisphere in correspondence to a certain conflict theme. For example: when a woman is right-handed, a mother-child-worry conflict always impacts on the right hemisphere of the cerebellum affecting the glands of her left breast. Even if she suffers another conflict for another child or a mother-child conflict with regards to her own mother, the conflicts still impact on the same are of the cerebellum.

But we have to make a distinction for the case that a mother no longer or only partly views her child as a "child" but more as a partner. In this scenario the conflict would impact the opposite brain hemisphere of the cerebellum and the breast cancer would manifest itself on the right breast, because the left side of the cerebellum is linked to the right side of the body, the "partner" side. Not only a spouse, friend, father or brother is considered a partner but also a sister, the mother-in-law, the neighbor, etc.

Presentation German New Medicine® by Dr. med Ryke Geerd Hamer, Madrid 2005

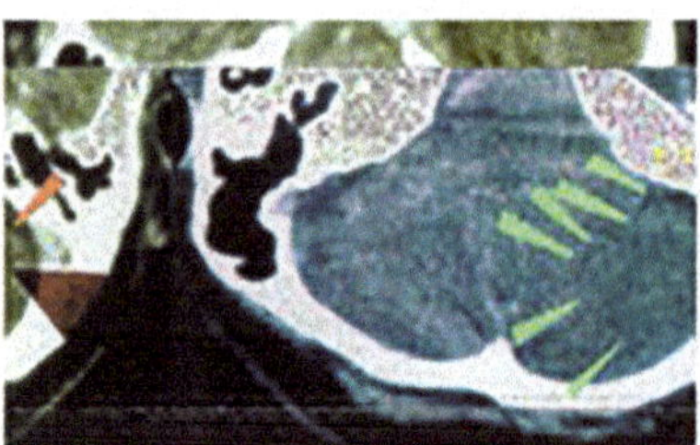

CT-picture
breast cancer (adenoid)

right cerebellum for the left breast (glands)

mother/child - or child/mother-worry conflict for right-handed woman.

An example: A mother suffered a mother/child-worry conflict because her child ran into a car and is seriously injured. The mother blames herself ("Had I only kept him by my side."). From this moment on the patient has cold extremities, she is unable to sleep, she loses her appetite, she loses weight and dwells constantly on the conflict, even more so if she is not able to talk about her conflict.

During this conflict active phase, while the mother constantly thinks of what had happened, we see in her left breast (provided she is right-handed) a multiplication of breast gland cells, commonly called breast cancer. In addition to the cancerous growth we find in the brain in the area ("computer" relay) of the right cerebellum, which controls the left breast, a sharp ring configuration as an indication of conflict activity, in other words, as a sign that the Meaningful Special Biological Program is active.

The so-called breast gland tumor continues to grow as long as the conflict is active. The resolution of the conflict can only occur when the child recovers. It is at this moment that the breast tumor stops growing.

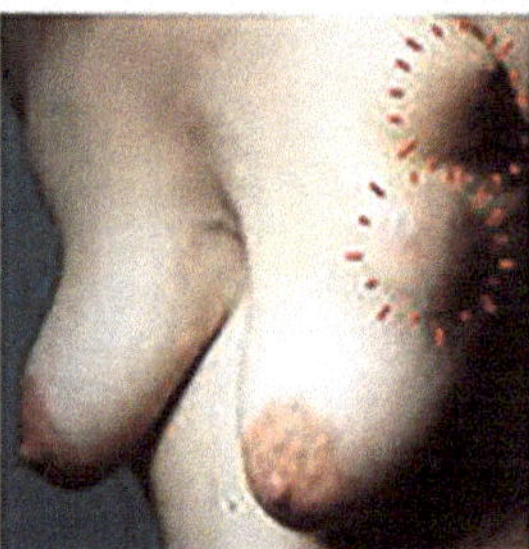

Patient with adenoid breast cancer
a) mother/child conflict or
b) child/mother conflict

In comparison: the conflict content of the so-called intra-ductal mamma carcinoma with its control centre in the cerebral cortex is a separation conflict with ulceration in the milk ducts during the conflict active phase, and swelling and redness of the breast during the healing phase.

When two conflicts impact in the cerebellum, one in each hemisphere (for the right and for the left breast), then we speak of a "Schizophrenic Cerebellum Constellation". This "Constellation" results in severe emotional disturbances of paranoid-delusional nature, however, without affecting logical thinking. Patients describe this state of mind as feeling emotionally burned out, feeling void of any emotions, being unable to have any feelings (so-called "asocial paranoia").

- 11 -

What is commonly coined schizophrenia is an "emergency response of the organism" when the individual sees no way of resolving the conflicts. It has already been hypothesized that schizophrenia ("split brain/ thoughts") has something to do with the two brain hemispheres not vibrating in the same rhythm. But nobody ever considered that this is caused by two different active biological conflicts although, with hindsight, it is so apparent.

Despite the fact that most psychiatric clinics are equipped with CT-scanners, nobody ever noticed anything. Why? Because a psychiatrist doesn't know anything about brain scans and a neuro-radiologist is not interested in biological conflicts.

CEREBELLUM – ORGAN – RELATION

Typical Schizophrenic Cerebellum Constellation

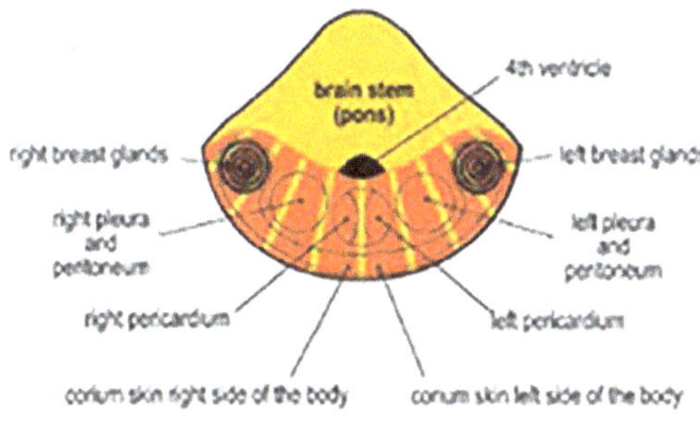

THE THIRD BIOLOGICAL LAW

The ontogenetic system of Meaningful Special Biological Programs (MSBP) of cancer and of cancer-equivalent diseases

Embryology generally divides the development of the embryo into three so-called germ layers: the endoderm (inner germ layer), the mesoderm (middle germ layer) and the ectoderm (outer germ layer), which develop already in the initial stages of embryo growth. All organs derive from these three embryonic layers. Every cell and every organ of our body can be ascribed to one of these germ layers.

The 3rd biological law of the German New Medicine classifies all so-called diseases according to their relation to a specific germ layer. By classifying all types of growths, swellings, and ulcers according to their germ layer correspondence we find that all "diseases" that relate to the same germ layer share special features (concerning the mesoderm we have to differentiate between the cerebellum-controlled and cerebral medulla-controlled mesoderm)

As a result of evolution, to each of these germ layers belongs

- a specific part of the brain
- a specific type of conflict
- a specific location in the brain
- a very specific histology
- specific germ layer related microbes

In addition: every so-called disease or MSBP has, in evolutionary terms, a very specific biological meaning.

All cells and organs that derive from the inner germ layer have their brain relay or control center from which they are directed in the brain stem, the oldest part of the brain.

BRAIN STEM - ORGAN - RELATION

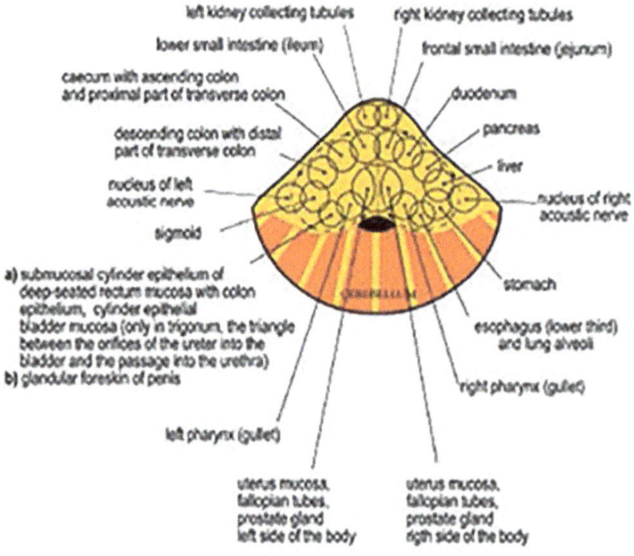

left kidney collecting tubules
right kidney collecting tubules
lower small intestine (ileum)
frontal small intestine (jejunum)
caecum with ascending colon and proximal part of transverse colon
duodenum
descending colon with distal part of transverse colon
pancreas
liver
nucleus of left acoustic nerve
nucleus of right acoustic nerve
sigmoid
a) submucosal cylinder epithelium of deep-seated rectum mucosa with colon epithelium, cylinder epithelial bladder mucosa (only in trigonum, the triangle between the orifices of the ureter into the bladder and the passage into the urethra)
b) glandular foreskin of penis
stomach
esophagus (lower third) and lung alveoli
right pharynx (gullet)
left pharynx (gullet)
uterus mucosa, fallopian tubes, prostate gland left side of the body
uterus mucosa, fallopian tubes, prostate gland rigth side of the body

There is a clear order to their location, for they begin dorsally on the right with diseases of the mouth and the nasopharyngeal area and then continue counterclockwise along the gastro-intestinal canal, ending with the sigma and the bladder.

Histologically, and without exception, all carcinoma are adeno-carcinomas. All organs that derive from this germ layer generate cell augmentation during the conflict active phase with the formation of compact tumors, e.g. in the liver, in the colon, in the lungs.

Presentation German New Medicine® by Dr. med Ryke Geerd Hamer, Madrid 2005

All cells and organs that derive from the outer germ layer have their control center in the cortex of the cerebrum, which is the youngest part of the brain.

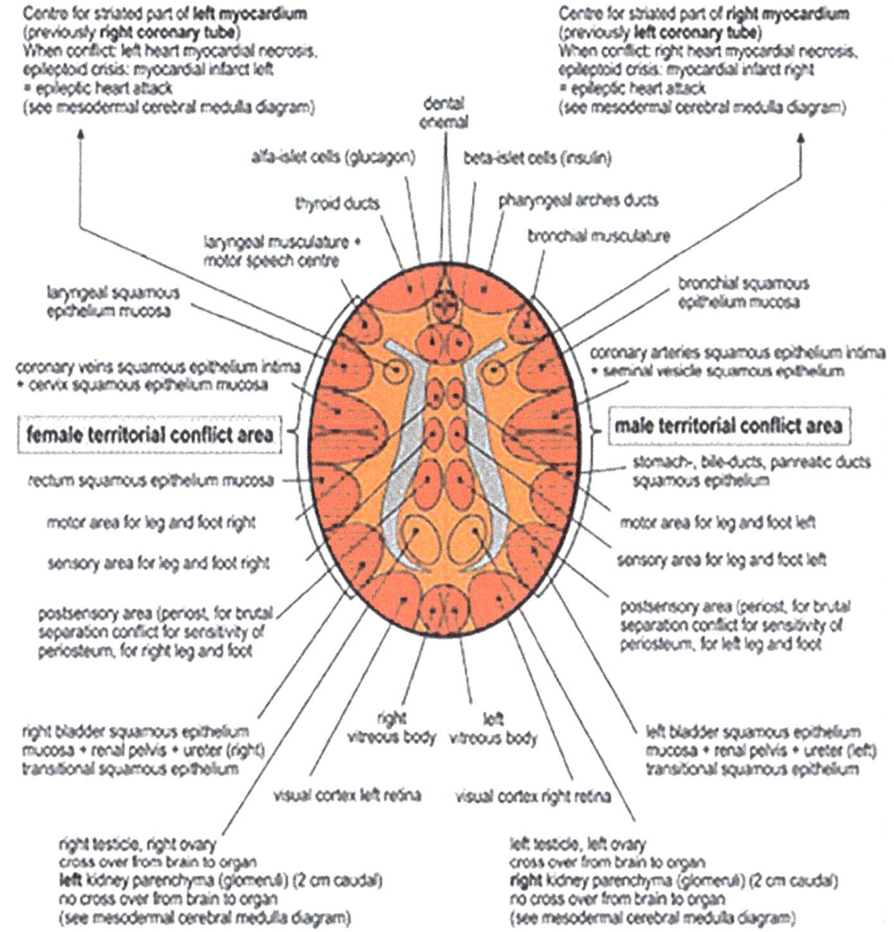

In the case of cancer, they all generate cell loss in form of ulcers in the conflict active phase or biologically meaningful functional changes (partly improvement of function, partly impairment of function, e.g. motor paralysis, diabetes, etc.). During the healing phase the ulceration is being replenished and the organ function re-established.

- 14 -

Concerning the middle germ layer we differentiate between an old and a new group.

CEREBELLUM – ORGAN – RELATION

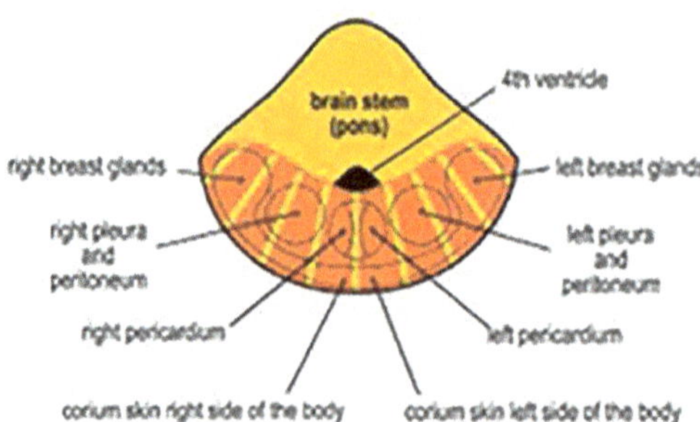

All cells and organs that belong to the new group of the middle germ layer have their control center in the cerebral medulla. In the case of cancer, these cells and organs generate necroses or holes in the tissue during the conflict active phase, e.g. in the bone, the kidney, or the ovaries.

CEREBRAL MEDULLA – ORGAN – RELATION

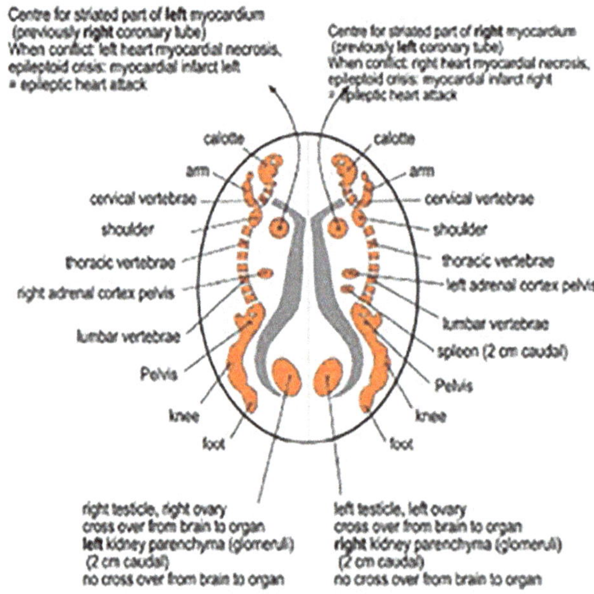

Cerebrum-controlled mesodermal organs make necroses or osteolyses during the conflict active phase. During the healing phase the lost tissue is replenished.

Presentation German New Medicine® by Dr. med Ryke Geerd Hamer, Madrid 2005

Here we can clearly see that cancer is not the result of wildly proliferating cells but rather a meaningful and even predictable process in full accordance with ontogenesis.

			biological meaning		
endoderm (inner germ layer)	fungi, myco-bacteria, Tbc	Hamer Focus in **brain stem** ca-phase: adeno-Ca (tumor: tissue plus) pcl-phase: Tbc tumor degradation	ca-phase	**old brain** cell augmentation	yellow = brain stem ENDODERM
mesoderm (middle germ layer)	bacteria, mycobacteria Tbc	Hamer Focus in **cerebellum** ca-phase: adenoid-Ca (tumor: tissue plus) pcl-phase: Tbc tumor degradation	ca-phase		orange/yellow-striped = cerebellum MESODERM
	bacteria	Hamer Focus in **cerebral medulla** ca-phase: necrosis-Ca (tissue minus) pcl-phase: necrosis restitution (more tissue than before)	at the end of pcl-phase	Cerebrum [illegible]	orange/red-striped = cerebral medulla MESODERM
ectoderm (outer germ layer)	with or without viruses [illegible]	Hamer Focus in cerebral cortex ca-phase: epithelium ulceration (tissue minus) pcl-phase: repair with reconstruction of ulcerated area	ca-phase		red = cerebral cortex ECTODERM

This is the reason why the origin and pathogenesis of cancerous diseases could not be classified and understood. The Iron Rule of Cancer and the Law of the Two Phases of every disease provides us for the first time with a systematic order that applies to all of medicine.

THE ONTOGENETIC SYSTEM OF TUMORS MEANINGFUL SPECIAL BIOLOGICAL PROGRAMS OF NATURE

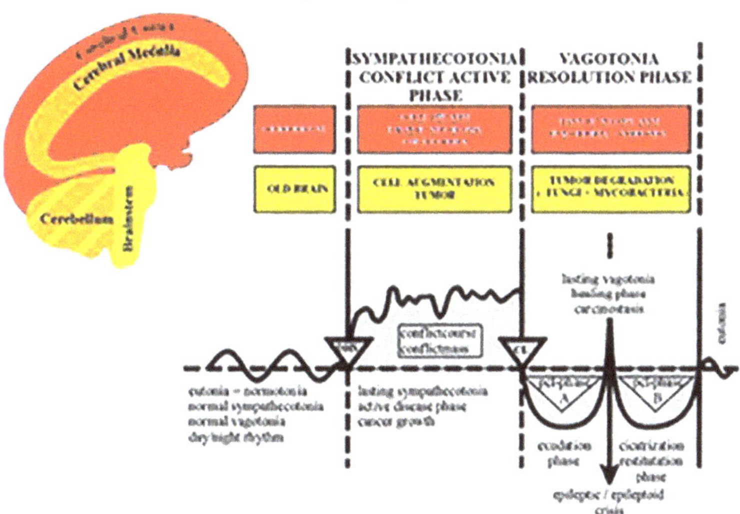

(The lower part of the diagram refers to the diagram of the 2nd Biological Law)

- 16 -

The diagram shows two different groups: The red cerebrum group generates cell loss during the conflict active phase (ca-phase). During the healing phase the necroses or ulcera are replenished with swelling and the formation of cysts.

The yellow old brain group generates the formation of tumors during the ca-phase. During the healing phase the tumor is being decomposed with the help of myco-bacteria (Tbc) provided that they were already present when the DHS occurred.

In medicine this ontogenetic system, specifically that of tumors, is comparable to the significance of the periodical system of elements in the natural sciences. It provides a comprehensive contextual overview for all medical disciplines.

THE FOURTH BIOLOGICAL LAW

The Ontogenetic System of Microbes

Until now, microbes have been considered as the cause of so-called infectious diseases, something entirely understandable because microbes are always present in infectious diseases. However, this view is incorrect, for all infectious diseases are preceded by a conflict active phase, which we have been overlooking.

The point in time that triggers the activity of microbes is not determined by exterior factors (as erroneously assumed) but is rather controlled entirely from our computer brain.

Microbes are not our enemies but our loyal helpers. They start to work on our orders, on the orders of our organism, directed from our brain, and each germ layer-related organ or tissue is in correspondence with specific germ layer-related microbes.

When the functions of our organs were programmed into the different brain relays, the functions of microbes were also programmed into our computer brain. Microbes are all more or less specialists not only in terms of the organs they work on but also with regards to how they work.

According to the Law of the Two Phases of all diseases (provided there is a resolution to the conflict), all microbes "work" without exception only in the second or healing phase, starting with the conflict resolution (CL) and ending with the completion of the healing phase. Myco-bacteria (Tbc) start already multiplying at the moment of the DHS but start their work only when the conflict has been resolved. The body produces the exact amount of microbes necessary to break down the now superfluous tumor.

The classification of microbes is in full accordance with their ontogenetic age:
Fungi and myco-bacteria (Tbc), the oldest microbes, only work on brain stem-controlled endodermal organs.
Myco-bacteria (Tbc) work also on cerebellum-controlled old brain mesodermal organs
Bacteria work on cerebral medulla-controlled new brain mesodermal organs.
Viruses (if they exist at all) are the youngest microbes that work only on cerebral cortex-controlled organs.

THE ONTOGENETIC SYSTEM OF MICROBES

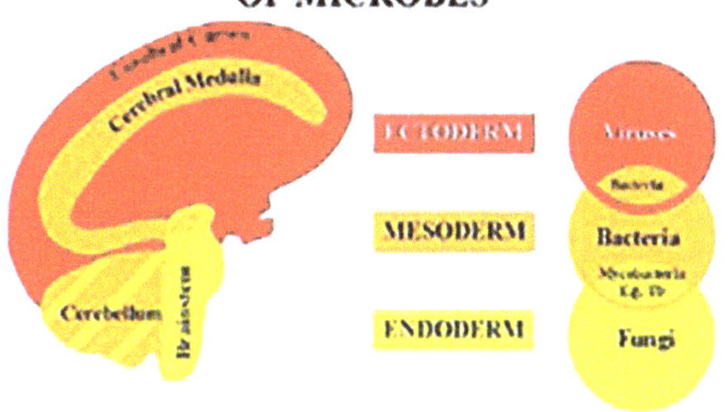

Correlation between

BRAIN - BLASTODERMIC LAYERS - MICROBES

We considered microbes as something "malignant" that has to be eradicated. This was pure nonsense because we badly need these microbes. In fact, we need all microbes available in our environment because if microbes such as myco-bacteria (Tbc) are absent, for instance due to hygienic reasons, our tumors cannot be decomposed during the healing phase – with disastrous consequences for a number of tumors.

Let's look at the example of a thyroid carcinoma: if the conflict has been resolved and the tumor cannot be broken down, more amounts of thyroxine are being produced, a useless process, biologically speaking. Or a colon carcinoma: if there are no myco-bacteria present, the growth can suddenly cause considerable complications and has to be surgically removed.

Now we understand that microbes play a vital role within the Meaningful Special Biological Program. Microbes developed with and for us. They are an essential component of Nature's laws. Since we were not aware of this, we blindly tried to eradicate these beneficial helpers with antibiotics or sulfonamides.

The so-called "immune system", commonly viewed as our body's line of defense in destroying "malignant" cancer cells and "malignant" microbes, just as in a major battle, does not exist in that sense. Acting on our brain's orders, the allegedly pathogenic microbes become a-pathogenic microbes that retreat in our organism and are only re-activated if they are needed.

Pretty much everything, which we had been doing as conventional physicians, was nonsense. Because Nature's natural laws cannot function if we, as the sorcerer's apprentices, randomly eliminate some factors.

The notion of microbes or metastases crawling around in our blood vessels (where they were never found) is nonsense.

The tale of **metastases** is an unproven and unprovable hypothesis. To this day there has never been a single observation of a cancerous cell in the arterial blood of a cancer patient. If cancer cells were able to "swim" to distant organs, they would have to do so via the arterial blood stream because venous and lymphatic vessels only run to the centre, i.e. the heart.

In the German New Medicine, so-called „metastases"(which do not exist) are often the result of the panic suffered through a diagnosis shock (iatrogenically induced) when a new DHS triggers a new biological conflict.

Let's take as an example the case of the patient with breast cancer whose child was seriously injured after having been hit by a car. Let's assume that after three months in hospital the child has finally recovered. In a right-handed woman a tumor will now be detectable in her left breast. Now she is told that her entire breast has to be removed otherwise there would be the danger that the malignant cancer cells will "spread" into the immediate environment or cause metastasis in a distant organ. In order to prevent this from happening, Chemotherapy should be administered as soon as possible in order to kill these malignant cancer cells.

Faced with this devastating diagnosis as well as with the planned intervention and the negative prognosis, the young mother can suffer the following new conflict shocks:

1. a "disfigurement conflict" resulting in a melanoma at the site of the amputated breast
2. a "self-devaluation conflict" ("I am useless there", "I am worthless there") resulting in osteolyses in the area of the amputated breast
3. an "attack conflict" against the left side of the chest where the operation will take place resulting in a pleura mesothelioma of the left pleura.
4. a "death fright conflict" resulting in lung nodules (adeno-carcinoma)

The melanoma and the lung nodules are soon noticeable. Since the child recovered, the "distant metastasis" in the right lateral cerebellum, the so-called Hamer Focus, is also healing! The osteolyses as well as the pleural effusion are also only noticeable in the healing phase after the conflict has been resolved.

We see that the metastasis fairy tale is an unproven and unprovable theory. So is the myth that cancerous cells change into another cell type while traveling through the blood (where it has never been observed). For example, a colon cancer cell that forms a cauliflower-shaped compact tumor in the colon (endoderm), supposedly travels all of a sudden to the bones (mesoderm), where the cells now cause the loss (!) of bone tissue (osteolysis). This theory is pure nonsense and nothing short of medieval dogmatism.

What is disputed is not the fact of a secondary or third carcinoma but the assessment and interpretation of these facts.

The same applies to so-called **tumor markers**. Since conventional medicine makes no difference between the conflict active phase and the healing phase of a disease, markers were developed which show an increased value in the conflict active phase or, at another point in the healing phase. As a result correct facts lead to false diagnoses. In fact, all "healing phase markers" could be called "vitality markers".

THE FIFTH BIOLOGICAL LAW

The Quintessence

Every so-called disease has to be understood as part of an evolutionary Meaningful Special Biological Program of Nature.

The 5th biological law is truly the quintessence. It turns the entire concept of medicine on its head. When we look at the three germ layers separately, we realize that they are biologically meaningful and that what we commonly call a "disease" is in fact not a senseless error of Nature that has to be fought but that every disease is a meaningful event. When we realize that so-called diseases are no longer "malignant", that they no longer have to be understood as a failure of Nature or as God's punishment but rather as part of a Meaningful Special Biological Program (MSBP) then these MSBPs become exceedingly significant.

Let's take, for example, adenoid breast cancer with proliferation of breast gland tissue during the conflict active phase. The biological purpose is clearly to aid, for instance, an injured infant by providing more milk. The mother's organism is trying to cope with the situation. As long as the conflict is active, the tumor will continue to grow to maintain the increased milk production. In this case, the biological meaning lies in the conflict active phase.

In our so-called civilized countries these processes often occur when the woman is not breastfeeding. If a woman who is not nursing suffers a mother/child-worry conflict, the growing breast gland tumor imitates the purpose of wanting-to-provide-more-milk to the baby even if the child is no longer an infant.

This is different from a water- or fluid conflict (new brain mesoderm): during the conflict active phase we observe the necrosis of kidney tissue and elevated blood pressure, which serves the purpose to compensate for the tissue loss in the kidney and thus ensure the elimination of adequate amounts of urine and of urinary substances. During the healing phase a capsule is formed at the site of the necrosis, which is filled with water. This is called a kidney cyst. Inside this cyst a steady cell multiplication process is taking place. At the end of this period, after approx. 9 months, a hard cyst is formed with its own blood supply system. This cyst which started out as a tumor attaching itself to the surrounding tissue eventually becomes detached and participates in the urine production of the kidney. In this case the biological meaning is in the healing phase, i.e. with functional improvement of the tissue involved.

The MSBP has a meaningful biological purpose, or the MSBP is trying to accomplish something that is biologically meaningful. The biological meaning is, as we have seen, either in the conflict active phase or in the healing phase. Mother Nature took the liberty to realize both but always in accordance with the different groups of germ layers.

With cerebrum-controlled carcinoma the biological purpose is in the conflict active phase. Contrary to the cell augmentation of old brain-controlled organs, the cell proliferation that takes place during the healing phase is a repair process during which the lost squamous epithelium tissue is replenished. Since nobody really understood that process, the restitution of the necrotized or ulcerated area during the healing phase was also interpreted as cancer or as a sarcoma.

This explains why we could not understand the true nature of cancer as long as we were unable to understand all these correlations, specifically the evolutionary development of the response programs to our conflicts.

"La medicina sagrada" turns everything around, nothing is correct any more – except the facts.

Not only does each MSBP have its specific biological meaning, but the combination of MSBPs, as we see in "Schizophrenic Constellations", also has a biological purpose, sort of a "meaning beyond the meaning". This has no transcendental, ideological or spiritual connotation but simply means that in case of a hopeless situation Mother Nature created the possibility to open a new dimension for the individual as a chance to master the difficult situation. The German New Medicine also offers new ways of therapy for mental disorders (psychoses).

The 5th biological law completes the German New Medicine. For the first time we can understand in all modesty not only that all of nature is in order but that every single process in nature has a meaning. We recognize with awe that what we previously called "diseases" are neither senseless errors of Nature, which have to be repaired by sorcerer's apprentices nor are they malignant or pathological.

THERAPY in the German New Medicine requires common sense. Be it cancer or any other so-called diseases (which I cannot adequately address in this short time), therapy starts with eliminating the patient's panic by explaining the "context" (the pathogenesis and progression of his disease), something of which he is most likely already aware of. The German New Medicine is diametrically opposed to the therapy of conventional medicine: "*There is nothing we can do for you; this has to be treated with radiation or chemo; we have to administer morphine; we have to cut into the healthy tissue.*"

Radiation therapy, based on the criteria of the German New Medicine, is totally useless for it is founded on the theory that symptoms have to be eliminated in order to prevent metastases.

Selling **chemo treatment** as a therapy is most likely the biggest fraud in the entire history of medicine. Whoever masterminded this chemical torture as "therapy" deserves a monument in hell. Chemotherapy, a treatment with cytotoxic agents aimed at preventing cell multiplication, is equal to exorcism. It is well known that these toxins destroy the bone marrow and affect the sexual organs, which may lead to temporary or constant infertility.

The chemo-pseudo-therapy has no effect at all on tumors, which are controlled from the old brain since the cytotoxic drug amplifies the sympathicotonus and therefore actually accelerates cancer growth – which makes the whole procedure outright criminal. With cerebrum-controlled cancers chemotherapy is downright idiotic. Of course, any healing process can be instantly interrupted with chemotherapy (at the expense of deteriorating bone marrow) regardless which part of the brain controls the disease. But the alleged "successes" are the result of a prevention of the healing process, labeled as "malignant" by conventional medical doctors.

With intra-ductal breast cancers, for example, chemotherapy can stop the swelling of the healing breast. Basically, all that stopped was the healing process, based on the illusion to halt the growth of a tumor, which is not even a tumor.

What about the effect of chemotherapy and radiation on the brain?

The special power of our brain to cope with biological conflicts is based on the ability to heal the HH (brain lesion). As we know, the brain is able to do that by creating a brain edema during the healing phase. With the edema the brain cells are stretched, in other words the HH swells up. By applying chemotherapy or radiation the healing process is stopped and the swollen brain area shrivels. The edema disappears but the HH is by no means healed. After the chemo or radiation round is over the organism immediately tries to trigger the healing process again, in other words it starts to re-fill the HH with edematous fluid. With every chemotherapy or radiation treatment the synapses, the connection between nerve cells, stretch and then shrink again. Eventually this initiates the life threatening "accordion effect".

Operations are in the German New Medicine not categorically dismissed. Surgery has to be used with common sense.

Morphine is catastrophic for every patient. Nature has not foreseen such an intervention. Since morphine and its derivatives are available, we think that we can stop the pain and at the same time get healthy. This is a wrong assumption because morphine alters the entire brain, the patient's morale diminishes and without willpower he lets himself be "put to sleep".

Medical treatment is not only a domain of conventional medicine. In the German New Medicine medication is used to avoid complications during the natural healing process. All remedies with a positive symptomatic effect should be applied for the benefit of the patient and based on the criterion whether the doctor would administer it to his own wife.

It is self-evident that with the help of the German New Medicine patients who have not yet undergone any treatment have the best chance to complete recovery.

Conventional medicine which has been boasting its supposed scientific merit must take a step back and ask itself if it has not left the path of a true natural science a long time ago. But the very fact that fundamental natural laws are now known for the first time (as they have in other disciplines of natural sciences) would grant medicine a unique chance to become a natural science in the truest sense of the word.

Closing Remarks

The participants of this congress had good intentions and nominated me for the Prize of Asturia. I am most grateful for the recognition. But an award, my dear friends and former colleagues, always involves two sides: someone who awards the prize and someone who accepts it. However, the Prize of Asturia for Medicine comes with a heavy debt: In April of this year the prize was awarded to Professors Gallo and Montagnier for their "discovery" of the so-called "AIDS virus", which in reality does not exist. The presence of an HIV Virus has never been established in AIDS patients. Montagnier himself conceded at a congress in Barcelona 10 years ago that he had never observed the presence of an AIDS virus. Now he is giving the lie to himself and lets himself be awarded.

The main argument against "AIDS" as a disease in itself are the findings of the Ontogenetic Systems of Tumors and the derived Ontogenetic System of Microbes. Nobody has ever observed typical symptoms after a so-called HIV infection, as are commonly associated with measles and rubella. If a patient tested HIV-negative and if he was taken ill with, for example, cancer, rheumatic fever, sarcoma, pneumonia, diarrhea, tuberculosis, herpes or any other neurological symptoms or disorders, then these would commonly be regarded as normal diseases according to popular opinion. However, if this same patient tested HIV positive, then all these symptoms would be considered malignant "AIDS" symptoms, or even "AIDS metastases" pointing to the imminent and agonizing death of this poor "AIDS" patient. It must have something to do with the patient's psyche if someone falls seriously ill only after having been told to be HIV-positive.

Has no physician ever been able to fathom what goes on in a patient who is brutally confronted with this devastating diagnosis? And is it not quite strange that "AIDS", which is thought to be a viral disease, progresses entirely differently from all other viral diseases. Those are commonly considered as overcome in the presence of a positive antibody test result.

You must forgive me, but I am a very practical man. It is certainly interesting to enter into a theoretical discussion of "AIDS", but in the meantime those poor people are being terrorized and killed by "AIDS" –

Presentation German New Medicine® by Dr. med Ryke Geerd Hamer, Madrid 2005

exactly as is the case with cancer. Those who do not wish to publicize the true correlations and contexts of cancerous diseases and those who have kept me locked up in jail are the same who masterminded the fatal immunodeficiency disease "AIDS", conveniently driving a second nail – after cancer – into the coffin of those patients "condemned to death", and ultimately granting the perpetrators even more power.

Please forgive me, but I feel I am out of place among such a set of scientists. But I do not wish to close all doors – for the benefit of my patients and your patients. After long deliberation I have decided to accept the prize under the following conditions:

1. I will be granted the official permission to practice my profession as a doctor of medicine.
2. More explicitly, this renewed permit will allow me to practice the German New Medicine – a discipline that received 30 official verifications.

My friends and all who know me can attest to the fact that I am neither megalomaniac nor arrogant but rather a humble and kind person. I would therefore consider it the ultimate treason of our patients if I accepted an award for my vanity without ensuring that the conditions of my patients are fully met.

Something must happen now!
We all must act!
It is the responsibility of us all!
Let us rise and work together to put an end to this crime.

This is what I ask of you!

For more information about German New Medicine®, visit http://germannewmedicine.ca

Codex:

The Agent/Catalyst, for the chemicalisation of all populations and our Earth.

Governments as consumers, are conned at every Trade Summit.

The FDA and TGA have sold their souls to Big Pharma's world domination economy, which entails;

Peddling toxic chemicals to Farmers and various Medical Associations, promoting progress as a war, on peoples sovereign choice and all things natural…

Marketing and mainstream media used to disseminate false hope and investment in our own ultimate destruction.

Reverse engineering, and Damage to our DNA.

Perhaps in engineering blind consumers, they hope to perpetuate this economic Cauldasac (loop)?

Pity the, Oh So Entitled, dependent, indoctrinated nation, that is

Unaware of the deals hidden in full view.

COMBATTING THE CODEX ALIMENTARIUS

Billions of people will suffer from degenerative diseases due to poor nutrition and limited access to health supplements if the powerful global corporations behind the new Codex standards are allowed to "harmonise" the world.

by Gregory Damato, PhD
© September 2008
Email:
info@quantumenergywellness.com
Website:
www.quantumenergywellness.com

POPULATION CONTROL UNDER THE GUISE OF CONSUMER PROTECTION

The Codeath, sorry, Codex Alimentarius Commission is a very misunderstood organisation. Most people have never heard of it, and those who *have* heard of it may not understand the true reality of this extremely powerful trade organisation. According to the official Codex website (http://www.codexalimentarius.net), the altruistic purpose of this commission is in "protecting health of the consumers and ensuring fair trade practices in the food trade, and promoting coordination of all food standards work undertaken by international governmental and non-governmental organizations". The Codex Alimentarius (Latin for "Food Code") is regulated under a joint venture between the Food and Agriculture Organization (FAO) and the World Health Organization (WHO).

Brief History of Codex

The history of Codex began in 1893 when the Austro-Hungarian Empire decided it needed a specific set of guidelines by which the courts could rule on cases dealing with food.[1] This set of regulatory mandates became known as Codex Alimentarius. It was effectively implemented until the fall of the empire in 1918.

At a meeting in 1962, the United Nations (UN) decided that Codex should be re-implemented worldwide in order to "protect" the health of consumers. Two-thirds of funding for Codex emanates from the FAO, and the other third comes from the WHO.

In 2002, FAO and WHO had serious concerns about the direction of Codex and hired an external consultant to determine its performance since 1962 and to designate which direction to take the trade organisation.[2] The consultant concluded that Codex should be scrapped immediately. It was at this time that big industry stepped in and exerted its powerful influence. The updated outcome was a toned-down report asking Codex to address 20 concerns within the organisation.

Since 2002, the Codex Alimentarius Commission has covertly surrendered its role as an international public health and consumer protection organisation. Under the helm of big industry, the surreptitious purpose of the new Codex is to increase profits for the global corporate juggernauts while controlling the world through food.

Codex Inequalities

The most dominant country behind the agenda of Codex is the United States, whose primary purpose is to benefit the large multinational interests of Big Pharma, Big Agribusiness, Big Chema and the like. At the latest meeting in Geneva, Switzerland (30 June to 4 July 2008), the US became the chair of Codex[3] and now will exacerbate the distortion of health freedom and continue to promulgate misinformation and lies about nutrients and genetically modified organisms (GMOs) while fulfilling its tacit population-control agenda. One reason why the US continues to dominate Codex is because other countries falsely believe that it possesses the latest and greatest food safety technology; hence, whatever the US asks for, its allies (Australia, Argentina, Brazil, Canada, Indonesia, Japan, Malaysia, Mexico, Singapore and the European Union) follow suit nearly every time.

The fact that Codex meetings are held all over the world is also no accident and allows the US to maintain its tight grip on the Codex agenda because the less economically viable countries are not able to attend. The governments of many of these countries (such as Cameroon, Egypt, Ghana, Kenya, Nigeria, South Africa, Sudan and Swaziland) realise that Codex has been altered from a benevolent food organisation to one that is fraudulent, lethal and illegitimate.

> **...no country is safe from these mandatory international guidelines, regardless of what government agencies are saying in order to quell pre-emptively any potential public uprising.**

Health Freedom Threats

While the mainstream media are busy with their esoteric agenda of driving fear into the hearts of the world's populace by focusing on terrorism, global warming, salmonella outbreaks and food shortages, the real threats are surreptitiously becoming a reality. Soon, every single thing you put into your mouth, including water (with the exception of pharmaceuticals, of course), will be highly regulated by the Codex Alimentarius Commission.

The Codex standards are a complete affront to people's freedom to access clean, healthy food and beneficial nutrients, yet these regulations have no legal international standing. Why should we be worried? These soon-to-be mandatory standards will apply to every country that's a member of the World Trade Organization (WTO) (presently there are 153 members). If countries do not follow these standards, then crippling economic and trade sanctions may be imposed on them, although countries may be able to avoid the standards of Codex through the implementation of their own international standards.

Some government-run agencies, like the Therapeutic Goods Administration (TGA) in Australia, are informing the public that the vitamin and mineral guideline of Codex will not affect their country. For example, the TGA had this to say: "The proposed Codex Guidelines for Vitamin and Mineral Food Supplements will *not* apply in Australia and will have *no impact* on the way these types of products are regulated in Australia."[4]

The bottom line is that no one knows what types of laws will be passed before Codex harmonisation occurs, and no country is safe from these international guidelines, regardless of what government agencies are saying in order to quell pre-emptively any potential public uprising. Many alternative health activists believe this may be a method to confuse and obfuscate the Codex issue until it is too late.

Some Codex standards which are proposed to take effect in the near future, and which will be completely irrevocable once initiated, include:[5]

• *All* nutrients (e.g., vitamins and minerals) are to be considered toxins/poisons and are to be removed from *all* food because Codex prohibits the use of nutrients to "prevent, treat or cure any condition or disease".

• *All* food (including organic) is to be irradiated, thus removing all "toxic" nutrients from food (unless consumers can source their food locally). The precursor to Codex harmonisation in this area began in the USA in August 2008 with the clandestine decision to mandate the mass irradiation of all lettuce and spinach in the name of public health and safety. If the safety of the public was the main concern of the US Food and Drug Administration (FDA), then why were people not alerted to this new practice?

• Nutrients allowed will be limited to a Positive List developed by Codex; it will include such "beneficial" nutrients as fluoride (3.8 mg daily), sourced from industrial waste.

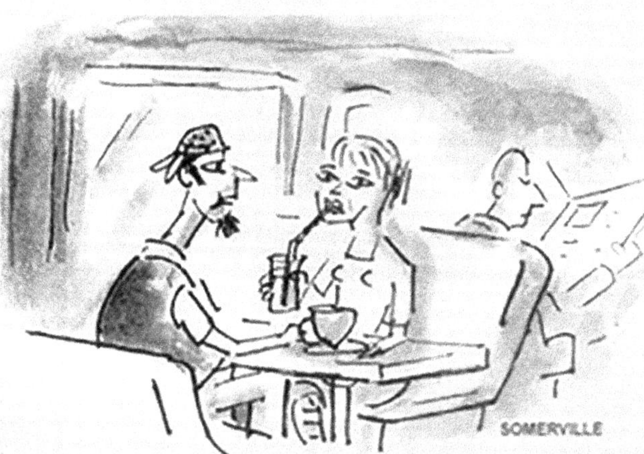

"I did my university degree online, met my girlfriend on FaceBook, got married live-streaming on YouTube and make a living buying/selling on eBay. I'm just worried I won't find a cemetery website I can be buried in."

16 • NEXUS www.nexusmagazine.com OCTOBER – NOVEMBER 2008

• *All* nutrients (e.g., vitamins A, B, C, D, zinc and magnesium) that have any positive health impact on the body will be deemed illegal in therapeutic doses under Codex and are to be reduced to amounts negligible to health, with maximum limits set at 15 per cent of the current Recommended Dietary Allowance (RDA).[6] You will not be able to obtain these nutrients in therapeutic doses anywhere in the world, even with a prescription.

Potentially permissible *safe* levels of nutrients under the Codex are not yet set in stone. Some probable examples based on the European Union (EU) system may include:

– Niacin: upper limit of 34 μg (micrograms) daily (effective daily doses range from 2,000 to 3,000 μg).

– Vitamin C: upper limits of 65 to 225 μg daily (effective daily doses range from 6,000 to 10,000 μg).

– Vitamin D: upper limit of 5 μg daily (effective daily doses range from 6,000 to 10,000 μg).

– Vitamin E: upper limit of 15 IU (international units) of alpha tocopherol per day, even though alpha tocopherol by itself has been implicated in cell damage and is toxic to the body (effective daily doses of mixed tocopherols range from 10,000 to 12,000 IU).

• It will most likely be illegal to give *any* advice on nutrition (including in written articles posted online and in journals as well as oral advice to a friend, a family member or anyone). This directive applies to any and all reports on vitamins and minerals and all nutritionists' consultations. This type of information may be considered a hidden barrier to trade and may result in economic trade sanctions for the involved country.

• *All* dairy cows on the planet are to be treated with Monsanto's genetically engineered recombinant bovine growth hormone (rBGH).

• *All* animals used for food are to be treated with potent antibiotics and exogenous growth hormones.

• Deadly and carcinogenic organic pesticides, including seven of the 12 worst (e.g., hexachlorobenzene, toxaphene and aldrin), which were banned by 176 countries (including the US) in 1991 at the Stockholm Convention on Persistent Organic Pollutants,[7] will be allowed back into food at elevated levels.

• The Codex will allow dangerous and toxic levels of aflatoxin (0.5 ppb) in milk. Aflatoxin, produced in animal feed that's gone mouldy in storage, is the second-most-potent (non-radiation-related) carcinogenic compound known.

• Use of growth hormones and antibiotics will be mandatory on all livestock, birds and aquacultured species meant for human consumption.

• The worldwide introduction of unlabelled and deadly GMOs into crops, animals, fish and plants will be mandated.

• Elevated levels of residue from pesticides and insecticides that are toxic to humans and animals will be allowed.

The Population Control Agenda

In 1995, the FDA adopted an illegal policy which stated that international standards (i.e., Codex) would supersede US laws governing all food, even if these standards were incomplete.[8] Furthermore, in 2004, the US passed the Central America Free Trade Agreement (illegal under US law, but legal under international law) that requires the US to conform to Codex.[9]

Once these standards are adopted, there is no way to return to the standards of old, but countries can adopt ones that are considered higher than those of Codex. An example of this would be the European Supplements Directive. Once Codex compliance begins in *any* area, as long as any country remains a member of the WTO, it is totally irrevocable: the standards cannot be repealed, changed or altered in any way, shape or form.[10, 11, 12]

> **Population control for money is the easiest way to describe the new Codex Alimentarius, which in effect is being run by the US and primarily controlled by Big Pharma...**

Population control for money is the easiest way to describe the new Codex Alimentarius, which in effect is being run by the US and primarily controlled by Big Pharma with the aim of reducing the world's population from its current estimate of 6.692 billion to a *sustainable* 500 million—an approximate 93 per cent reduction. Interestingly enough, before the arrival of Europeans in America, the Native American population in the US was around 60 million;[13] today it hovers around 500,000, or an approximate 92 per cent reduction as a result of government policies of genocide, starvation and poisoning.

Codex is similar to other population control measures undertaken clandestinely by governments of the western world; for example, the introduction of DNA-damaging and latent immunosuppressive agents in vaccines (e.g., weaponised avian flu and AIDS), aspartame, chemtrails, chemotherapy for cancer *treatment* and RU486 (the abortion pill funded by the Rockefeller dynasty).

FAO and WHO have estimated that by the introduction of just the vitamin and mineral guideline alone, within 10 years a *minimum* three billion deaths will result.[14] One billion of these deaths will be due to starvation, and two billion as a result of preventable and degenerative diseases of undernutrition, e.g., cancer, cardiovascular disease and diabetes.[15,16]

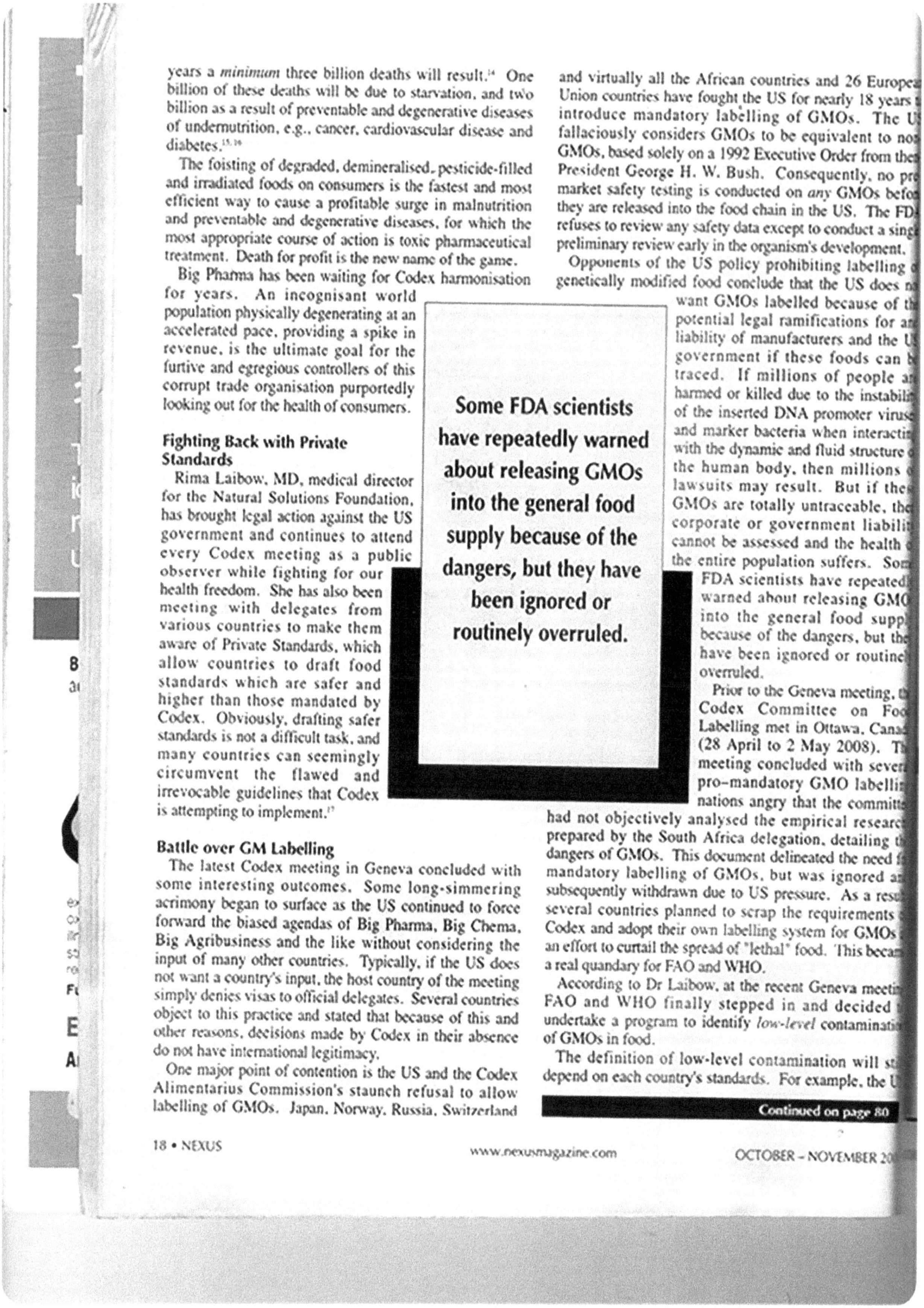

The foisting of degraded, demineralised, pesticide-filled and irradiated foods on consumers is the fastest and most efficient way to cause a profitable surge in malnutrition and preventable and degenerative diseases, for which the most appropriate course of action is toxic pharmaceutical treatment. Death for profit is the new name of the game.

Big Pharma has been waiting for Codex harmonisation for years. An incognisant world population physically degenerating at an accelerated pace, providing a spike in revenue, is the ultimate goal for the furtive and egregious controllers of this corrupt trade organisation purportedly looking out for the health of consumers.

Some FDA scientists have repeatedly warned about releasing GMOs into the general food supply because of the dangers, but they have been ignored or routinely overruled.

Fighting Back with Private Standards

Rima Laibow, MD, medical director for the Natural Solutions Foundation, has brought legal action against the US government and continues to attend every Codex meeting as a public observer while fighting for our health freedom. She has also been meeting with delegates from various countries to make them aware of Private Standards, which allow countries to draft food standards which are safer and higher than those mandated by Codex. Obviously, drafting safer standards is not a difficult task, and many countries can seemingly circumvent the flawed and irrevocable guidelines that Codex is attempting to implement.[17]

Battle over GM Labelling

The latest Codex meeting in Geneva concluded with some interesting outcomes. Some long-simmering acrimony began to surface as the US continued to force forward the biased agendas of Big Pharma, Big Chema, Big Agribusiness and the like without considering the input of many other countries. Typically, if the US does not want a country's input, the host country of the meeting simply denies visas to official delegates. Several countries object to this practice and stated that because of this and other reasons, decisions made by Codex in their absence do not have international legitimacy.

One major point of contention is the US and the Codex Alimentarius Commission's staunch refusal to allow labelling of GMOs. Japan, Norway, Russia, Switzerland and virtually all the African countries and 26 Europea Union countries have fought the US for nearly 18 years t introduce mandatory labelling of GMOs. The U fallaciously considers GMOs to be equivalent to no GMOs, based solely on a 1992 Executive Order from the President George H. W. Bush. Consequently, no pr market safety testing is conducted on *any* GMOs befo they are released into the food chain in the US. The FD refuses to review any safety data except to conduct a sing preliminary review early in the organism's development.

Opponents of the US policy prohibiting labelling o genetically modified food conclude that the US does n want GMOs labelled because of th potential legal ramifications for an liability of manufacturers and the U government if these foods can b traced. If millions of people ar harmed or killed due to the instabili of the inserted DNA promoter viruse and marker bacteria when interacti with the dynamic and fluid structure o the human body, then millions o lawsuits may result. But if the GMOs are totally untraceable, the corporate or government liabili cannot be assessed and the health o the entire population suffers. Som FDA scientists have repeatedl warned about releasing GMO into the general food suppl because of the dangers, but the have been ignored or routine overruled.

Prior to the Geneva meeting, t Codex Committee on Fo Labelling met in Ottawa, Cana (28 April to 2 May 2008). T meeting concluded with sever pro-mandatory GMO labelli nations angry that the committe had not objectively analysed the empirical researc prepared by the South Africa delegation, detailing t dangers of GMOs. This document delineated the need f mandatory labelling of GMOs, but was ignored a subsequently withdrawn due to US pressure. As a resu several countries planned to scrap the requirements o Codex and adopt their own labelling system for GMOs an effort to curtail the spread of "lethal" food. This beca a real quandary for FAO and WHO.

According to Dr Laibow, at the recent Geneva meeti FAO and WHO finally stepped in and decided t undertake a program to identify *low-level* contaminati of GMOs in food.

The definition of low-level contamination will st depend on each country's standards. For example, the U

Continued on page 80

Combatting the Codex Alimentarius

Continued from page 18

currently allows for up to 10 per cent (the highest of any country under Codex) of GMO *contamination* of organic foods and, amazingly, still allows them to be labelled as "USDA Certified Organic". Some governments, such as the European Union, allow only 0.9 per cent contamination, while others permit merely 0.1 per cent.

However, the FAO and WHO's use of the term "contamination" simply does not describe the GMOs as being mixed in with normal food. This term is also very noteworthy, as most research on the dangers of GMOs can no longer be denied.

The US, of course, vehemently objected to such a designation, but this time to no avail.

Although FAO and WHO have not gone so far as to require mandatory labelling of GMOs, their recognition that GMOs can contaminate food is a huge win for health freedom.

Expanding that requirement to mandatory labelling is the next logical step, but this is still a work in progress.

Take Action against Codex!

The only way to avoid the death-for-profit agenda is to fight back by disseminating knowledge to everyone you know.

It does not matter whether they are still asleep or hypnotised by the enslavement of daily life or too busy to pay attention: *the time to wake up is now*.

The US government and the collaborating media have been trying to distract the world while all these egregious and mandatory standards are covertly passed.

It is time to take action, and you can do so by going to the website of the Natural Solutions Foundation, which can be found at www.healthfreedom usa.org, and following the latest updates on Codex. You can also sign a legal citizen's petition at the web page http://www.healthfreedomusa.org/index.php?page_id=184.

It is very important that swift and vociferous action be taken now. Times are changing very rapidly, and unless we all come together on this issue we may have to start thinking about growing our own food in the near future to avoid calculated extermination.

Here are more contacts for action against the Codex:

• Australia

You can send an email to the Department of Agriculture and Food in Western Australia or the Minister for Agriculture in your respective state. For example, in WA the email address is enquiries@agric.wa.gov.au.

The Therapeutic Goods Administration can also be contacted online via its website http://www.tga.gov.au/contact.htm.

• New Zealand

You can use the NZ Health Trust's

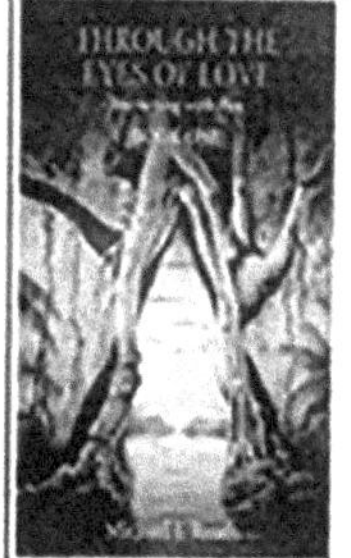

THE CHICKENPOX VACCINE

PROMOTING A CONTINUAL CYCLE OF TREATMENT AND DISEASE

Chickenpox vaccinations in the USA have lowered the incidence of the disease, but may shift chickenpox outbreaks to older age groups and increase the risk of shingles.

by Gary S. Goldman, PhD

PO Box 847
Pearblossom CA 93553, USA
Email: pearblossominc@aol.com
Websites:
http://www.MedicalVeritas.com
http://www.drgoldmanonline.com/

INTRODUCTION: First Do No Harm—to Pharmaceutical Industry Profits?

Prior to the acceptance of the chickenpox vaccine by the US Food and Drug Administration (FDA) on March 17, 1995, chickenpox was considered a rather mild disease. According to the Centers for Disease Control and Prevention (CDC), approximately 12,000 of four million (or 0.3 per cent of) cases of chickenpox in the United States each year resulted in hospitalisation (mainly due to infected lesions), and approximately 50 cases among children (0.0013 per cent) and another 50 out of 200,000 cases among adults (0.025 per cent) resulted in death. In other words, the risk of a child contracting and dying from chickenpox was less than the risk of being struck and killed by lightning (about 89 cases per year in the United States).

Chickenpox (or varicella) and shingles (also known as herpes zoster) are related diseases: both are caused by the varicella-zoster virus (VZV). Once a child contracts chickenpox, the virus goes dormant or inactive for a period (usually decades) and can reactivate later as shingles. Unlike chickenpox where the rash appears in different stages of development over many parts of the body, the shingles rash is often localised and occurs on one side of the body. The rash seems to arise in one or two adjacent regions of the skin (called dermatomes) along nerve routes. Shingles pain often begins with an area of the skin becoming sensitive to the touch or to clothing prior to the eruption of the rash. The pain from shingles can be excruciating and the nerve damage (known as post-herpetic neuralgia or PHN) can last long after the rash has disappeared. Shingles in children is generally more mild than in adults.

When a child becomes infected with chickenpox, the immune system is activated and cell-mediated immunity (CMI) is boosted. This boost to the immune system helps protect against further episodes of chickenpox and helps suppress the reactivation as shingles. In fact, each time a child (or adult) with a previous history of chickenpox comes into contact with another child infected with chickenpox, this outside exposure—whose source is often unknown (and chickenpox is most contagious one to two days before the outbreak of the rash)—boosts the cell-mediated immunity to VZV, which in turn helps to suppress the onset of shingles.

The United States became the first country to adopt a Universal Varicella Vaccination Program, with the recommendation to vaccinate every healthy child 12 months or older who was susceptible to chickenpox. By promoting high varicella vaccination rates, including the states mandating varicella vaccination of school-age children, chickenpox cases in many communities had declined 50–80 per cent within five to 10 years of licensure of the vaccine in 1995. On the surface, this seemed good news. While the protective immunity derived from vaccination appeared to be long term and was touted as lasting 20 or more years, this statistic was based primarily on the experience of varicella vaccination in Japan where only one in five (or 20 per cent of) children were vaccinated. Thus, vaccinees continued to be boosted for 20 years due to their periodic exposure to other unvaccinated children who continued to demonstrate a high incidence of natural chickenpox.

Since the effectiveness of the vaccine was increased when vaccinees were exposed to other children with natural chickenpox, as cases of natural chickenpox decreased it might also be expected that the protective effect of the vaccine might decline over a period of years, creating the need for a booster dose. Without such a booster dose, vaccinated children may in time become susceptible to varicella when they are older and subject to more adverse complications of chickenpox. If the chickenpox vaccine wears off in adulthood, women who contract natural chickenpox in their first or second trimester of pregnancy could also pass on their infection to the developing foetus, potentially causing congenital varicella syndrome—currently a rare disorder in which the newborn has severely malformed limbs or other distinctive abnormalities. Also, a mother who has been vaccinated may not pass on sufficient maternal antibody protection to her newborn, leaving the child susceptible to acquiring chickenpox during the first months of life.

It should also be considered that 90–95 per cent of the adult population with a previous history of chickenpox presently no longer receives periodic exposures (boosts) through contact with children with chickenpox. Thus, their cell-mediated immunity gradually wanes (declines), increasing their risk of shingles.

Merck Inc., the manufacturer of the varicella vaccine, has developed a "shingles vaccine" (at US$150 per dose) to substitute for the immunologic boost that occurred naturally in the community, especially during annual outbreaks of chickenpox. The vaccine, Zostavax®, was approved in 2006 for use in adults 60 years and older. If we ignore the medical costs in treating adverse reactions associated with Zostavax and consider only the cost of the vaccine itself, the cost of preventing one case of shingles is US$8,850 and the cost of preventing one case of moderate to severe PHN is $150,000.

Have important research data concerning deleterious effects of the varicella vaccine been selectively omitted or suppressed from published research and reports? Has the effectiveness of the varicella vaccine decreased as cases of natural chickenpox have become rare? Have adults experienced an increased risk of shingles disease? As an "insider" who served as a research analyst and studied varicella for eight years and herpes zoster for almost three years, I address these important questions.

Have important research data concerning deleterious effects of the varicella vaccine been selectively omitted or suppressed from published research and reports?

PART I: Seemingly Good Results from First Five Years of Study

It was January 2000 and I was very ıuch enjoying a sixth year as research ıalyst for the Varicella Active rveillance Project (VASP), based at ·h Desert Hospital in Lancaster, California. This project was of three in the nation that had been funded by the CDC ınta, Georgia) to study varicella—commonly known as enpox. The CDC was interested in our collecting data from 300 reporting sites (including public and private schools, centres, physicians, medical centres and hospitals in the to determine the effect that the recently introduced vaccination program had on the 300,000 inhabitants of Valley, a geographically distinct high-desert community of two main cities (Lancaster and Palmdale) and other cities, located approximately 60 miles north of Los alifornia.

two sites selected by the CDC were located in West ı, Pennsylvania, and Travis County, Texas. These d chickenpox cases from just a *sample* of the many healthcare facilities in their respective regions. ntelope Valley site collected reports from virtually le schools and healthcare locations in its region. ›pe Valley project was more suited for uncovering developing trends and disease patterns from reports of chickenpox cases submitted to the project every two weeks, 26 times during each study year.

With great enthusiasm and optimism, we documented in our project how varicella disease decreased by 72 per cent in Antelope Valley, from 2,934 verified and reported cases in 1995 to just 836 cases in 2000. My superiors from the Los Angeles County Department of Health Services (LACDHS) encouraged me to submit these data and to develop other analyses for publication. In cooperating with that directive, I received credit as a co-author for the project data supplied to the CDC, which were summarised along with data from the other two sites and subsequently published in the February 6, 2002 edition of the *Journal of the American Medical Association*.[1]

I continued to investigate various trends in the reported data and desired to explain the reason why the number of varicella cases had a seasonal variation: usually the highest number of cases occurred in the late spring or early winter. My model was able to predict the observed variation in cases by considering the outside air temperature and school enrolments (or population density). During the warm weather (e.g., summer months) and school breaks (e.g., holidays), varicella transmission was seen to be reduced. Using daily weather temperature data and daily average enrolments provided by the fully cooperating schools, I developed a computer simulation or model which estimated the number of cases of varicella expected to be reported each month. When compared to the actual historical figures, the estimated figures closely agreed. The CDC assigned one of their epidemiologists to refine this analysis further, a manuscript was written—crediting me as lead author—and the study was presented by the CDC epidemiologist internally at the CDC and later at a medical conference.[2]

Second Doses of Chickenpox

Interestingly, other project data indicated that the number of varicella patients reporting a *second* case of chickenpox increased from about five per cent in 1995 to 12 per cent in 2001. One hypothesis accounting for the occurrence of a second case of chickenpox concerns the possibility that an individual was exposed to a second varicella strain that differed significantly from the strain associated with his/her first encounter (e.g., the two strains were heterologous). Those data and analyses were provided to the CDC, and again I received co-authorship credit for a manuscript on this subject, which was published in *Pediatrics* in June 2002.[3]

Breakthrough Chickenpox among Vaccinated Children

When a child breaks out in a chickenpox rash 42 or more days following varicella vaccination, this is referred to as "breakthrough" chickenpox. Initially, the percentage of cases reported with natural chickenpox far outnumbered the breakthrough cases among vaccinees. As chickenpox vaccine became more widespread in the community, the situation reversed—with the majority of cases consisting of vaccinated children experiencing breakthrough disease.

VASP Collects and Publishes Valuable Data and Results

The VASP continued collecting valuable data, which have been published or presented at various conferences; I received co-authorship credit on some of these papers.[4-8] I considered it a privilege to be a part of the team, which included three others in our local office: a project director and two research assistants.

In January 2000, I was encouraged when my earlier suggestion to collect cases of shingles (herpes zoster) was adopted and added to the chickenpox data collection. In retrospect, we should have been collecting shingles cases from the onset of the project in order to have a consistent methodology for determining baseline incidence rates that could be used in year-to-year comparisons. Numerous studies dating from as early as 1965 had alluded to a potential link between the two diseases: that a decrease in chickenpox incidence could give rise to an increase in shingles (see summary of references in Appendix 1 of my complete paper at http://www.MedicalVeritas.com/FULLNEXUS.pdf).

PART II: Vaccine Causes a Rash of Controversy: CDC Requests a Special Study be Conducted

Up to this point, everything seemed to be going well. I was receiving positive feedback, and a letter from the LACDHS commended all of our efforts. However, things began to change when the CDC asked our project to conduct an additional study among middle-school (7th–8th grade) students to determine the percentage who had not had chickenpox—in other words, those who were considered still susceptible to the disease. Surveys were provided to each school, asking the relevant questions in order to allow computation of the percentage of susceptible students by age and race. With the approval of the project director, an additional question was added to the survey, inquiring if the student had ever had shingles and, if so, the age at which the outbreak occurred. This was intended to provide some baseline data on shingles incidence among children and adolescents in the Antelope Valley region.

After analysing several thousand questionnaires, I wrote a manuscript that addressed varicella susceptibility as well as the incidence of shingles. To my surprise the CDC claimed that the study was not designed to determine shingles incidence, and neither the LACDHS nor the CDC expressed interest in publishing or discussing the results pertaining to shingles. The manuscript discussing varicella susceptibility was published word for word as I had written it, with only minor changes to a few sentences.[9] The remainder of the manuscript on shingles was simply discarded.

My manuscripts discussed preliminary data describing potential deleterious effects of the Universal Varicella Vaccination Program.

No Follow-up Allowed on Recurring Shingles Cases

While preparing another annual report, I had identified 10 cases where individuals reported a *second* case of shingles. I computed the incidence of recurrent shingles in the same manner as had been done in another peer-reviewed article and requested permission from my superiors to conduct a telephone interview with each of these 10 cases to assess whether or not they had some pre-existing or underlying condition that might have suppressed their immune system. Despite our calling 10,000 parents/caregivers of children with chickenpox, no permission was granted to contact these 10 individuals. Further, this analysis was also deleted from the annual report without explanation.

Suppression of Reports Leads to Resignation

At the beginning of 2001 and again in 2002, after one and two years of shingles data collection, I submitted manuscripts for review by my superiors and subsequent approval for publication by the CDC. These manuscripts discussed preliminary data describing potential deleterious effects of the Universal Varicella Vaccination Program. (The biological mechanism supporting these observations had already been explained in the scientific and medical journal literature; see references in Appendix 4 of my complete paper at http://www.MedicalVeritas.com/FULLNEXUS.pdf.) Unlike previous analyses of the positive aspects of vaccination, these manuscripts were treated very differently. By October 2002, I felt that I could no longer conduct research objectively; and with the submitted manuscripts still pending formal review, I resigned from the VASP, citing my ethical compromise.

In my letter of resignation, I stated: "Whenever research data and information concerning potential adverse effects associated with a vaccine used in human populations are suppressed and/or misrepresented by health authorities, not only is this most disturbing, it goes against all accepted scientific norms and dangerously compromises professional ethics."

Notice to "Cease and Desist" from Publication

Following my resignation, I submitted final versions of four manuscripts that had been awaiting review for the past one to two years during my employment to both the LACDHS and the CDC, notifying them of pending publication and making inquiry as to whether other individuals desired authorship credit. When there was no response, I submitted the manuscripts for publication. All four manuscripts were peer reviewed and published in *Vaccine*, a medical journal based in the UK and known throughout Europe.[10-13]

Following the acceptance of the first three manuscripts,[10-12] I received a letter from the Los Angeles County legal department on behalf of the LACDHS, requesting that I "cease and desist" publication in a medical journal. My attorney filed a response citing the possibility of litigating based on state and federal False Claims Acts and calling upon Dr Philip R. Krause, lead research investigator at the FDA's Center for Biologic Evaluation and Research, to testify as an expert witness in support of my findings. The "cease and desist" issue appeared to have ended with no further response forthcoming from the LA County legal department.

CDC Intervenes and Slurs Author's Reputation

However, prior to publication of the fourth manuscript and after I had received a letter of acceptance from the editor of *Vaccine*, the CDC attempted to block publication of this manuscript by calling the Life Sciences editor of Elsevier, which oversees publication of *Vaccine*. Again my attorney intervened, asking the CDC if it served on the editorial board of *Vaccine*. After a year's delay, the manuscript was finally released for print publication in May 2005. The basic analysis for this manuscript had been outlined in 2001 while I was serving as research analyst.[13]

The CDC next attempted to slur my reputation by stating that I was merely a "data manager having no input into the studies". In reality, I was responsible for submitting the background material suggesting that herpes zoster be included in active surveillance beginning with the new project cycle starting in January 2000.

The CDC then wrote a letter for publication to *Vaccine*, additionally expressing dissatisfaction with the first three manuscripts but providing criticisms with respect to only one of those manuscripts.[11] I happened to be perusing the publicly available online list of manuscripts to be published in *Vaccine* when I located the CDC's letter and wrote to the editor of *Vaccine*, stating that it was customary to allow the author an opportunity to provide a related rebuttal. The editor agreed that this was ethical procedure and within several days I submitted a point-by-point rebuttal to each of the specious arguments that the CDC had presented in its letter. My attorney communicated with the CDC legal department, which agreed that my characterisation as a "data manager with no input into the studies" was untrue; and so a correction was made prior to publication of the CDC letter, which appeared with my rebuttal immediately following.[4]

The historical fact was that in addition to developing the entire project's database and overseeing data entry, I implemented numerous statistical programs (including capture-recapture with 95 per cent goodness-of-fit-based confidence intervals, or CIs, as described by Dr E. B. Hook and Dr R. R. Regal), analysed and summarised household contact information, studied breakthrough varicella, lesion severity, vaccine efficacy, seasonal incidence patterns, outbreaks among schools, and much more. I also participated in project presentations and on-site seminars at the CDC, and provided suggestions regarding methodology. I wrote the preliminary justification for adding herpes zoster to the active surveillance and contributed much more than act as a "data manager with no input into the studies".

Table 1: Vaccine efficiency (efficacy) by year, 1997 to 2002, in households with contacts less than 20 years old and verified cases of chickenpox reported in 5–18 year olds, Antelope Valley, California.

Year	Vaccine Efficacy (95% confidence interval)	Verified Cases of Chickenpox
1995	—	1,290
1996	—	1,201
1997	86.7 (75.0–92.9)	1,095
1998	93.7 (83.2–97.7)	92
1999	95.7 (82.7–98.9)	330
2000	85.5 (73.9–92.0)	485
2001	73.9 (57.9–83.8)	442
2002*	58.4 (13.7–79.9)	Figure n/a

* Efficacy based on verified cases reported January through June (half-year) only.

I considered I had certainly fulfilled all my ethical obligations and responsibilities. But then the CDC published a new article on contagiousness of varicella in household settings.[7] This research article stated that the vaccine was highly effective and that the efficacy (effectiveness) of the varicella vaccine did not significantly change over the period 1997 to 2001.

I recalled having collected these data and transmitted them to the CDC to permit independent analysis. Early in 2002, I had performed a data analysis of vaccine efficacy and placed my report in a notebook containing other manuscripts awaiting review.

Just like the other manuscripts discussing shingles, this manuscript was not reviewed and the summary of vaccine efficacy by year was also deleted from the annual report without explanation. The results and trends that I had previously derived and confirmed with a CDC data manager were so very different from those currently presented in the CDC article that I was compelled to publish a fifth manuscript in the peer-reviewed *International Journal of Toxicology* (July–August 2005).[8] This manuscript demonstrated how important trends in the data had been masked in the CDC's article and other presentations concerning the incidence of herpes zoster.

PART III: What the Public Was Not Supposed to Know: Chickenpox Vaccine Effectiveness Declines

The CDC's contagiousness article states: "...finding no trend, we conducted subsequent analyses for the 5-year period [1997–2001]". Yet, interesting trends became apparent when using the exact same database; the vaccine effectiveness was stratified or computed by each year.

With reference to Table 1, notice that the vaccine efficacy increased to a high of 95.7 per cent in 1999, and then decreased to 73.9 per cent and 58.4 per cent in 2001 and 2002 respectively. The initial increase in vaccine effectiveness or efficacy demonstrates the "honeymoon" effect, whereby there is a relatively brief period following the introduction of the chickenpox vaccine during which time vaccinated children receive additional immune boosting by virtue of their contact with children having natural chickenpox. During 1999 and thereafter, the number of children reported as having natural chickenpox dramatically declined (along with the boosting effect), and this contributed to the statistically significant downward trend in vaccine effectiveness.

There is a legitimate concern that vaccinated children will be left unprotected and may prove to be susceptible to chickenpox as adults, when chickenpox can be a more serious illness if contracted then.

VASP/CDC Reports are Misleading

Civen et al.[9] report an incidence of shingles of 40 per 100,000 among children in Antelope Valley, where vaccine coverage exceeds 80 per cent. These authors also report incidence of shingles of 45 per 100,000 among individuals aged 10 to 19 years, a group which is largely unvaccinated but has had a previous experience of natural chickenpox. Notice there is hardly a difference in incidence rates between these groups despite differences in their vaccination status.

There are two fundamental problems with the manner in which these figures were derived. First, Civen et al. assume that 100 per cent of shingles cases are voluntarily reported to VASP. This assumption is rarely true in any study. Because there were two reporting sources (schools and healthcare providers), a statistical technique known as "capture-recapture" can be used to quantify the percentage of underreporting, which was estimated to be about 50 per cent. Without adjusting for underreporting, incidence rates reported by the VASP merely reflect the case ascertainment and cannot be compared to other studies.

Second, Civen et al. present what is called an average (or mean) of a bimodal incidence rate. To illustrate why this is statistically invalid, consider that when the same data are stratified by vaccination status, this yields an estimated rate of 22 cases of shingles per 100,000 among vaccinees and 223 per 100,000 among children with a previous history of natural chickenpox. Combined, the weighted average of these two very different incidence rates is 52 per 100,000; however, this rate is not representative of the rate in either of the two diverse groups.

Reporting the single figure masks the high trend in shingles incidence among unvaccinated children with a previous history of natural chickenpox—which could have major implications for adults, 90-95 per cent of whom have had previous histories of chickenpox. Also masked is the positive statistic that shingles among vaccinees is currently 1/10th (22/223) the risk in children with a previous history of natural chickenpox based on the above figures.

Interestingly, the CDC reports 2.6 cases of shingles per 100,000 doses using the VAERS (Vaccine Adverse Event Reporting System) database. This database is notorious for reflecting only 5–10 per cent of the actual adverse events, since reporting to VAERS is voluntary and not enforceable.

CDC's Criticisms Unfounded

My manuscripts were initially criticised for presenting preliminary shingles data and analyses based on the collection of two years of data among a population of 318,000, of which 118,685 were individuals under the age of twenty. Yet, when the data supported its agenda, the CDC utilised a very small study (Behavioral Risk Factor Surveillance System, BRFSS) that consisted of only 4,916 and 3,123 respondents aged one to 19 years in 1999 and 2000 respectively. The sample size was too small in this study for any valid conclusions to be drawn. Any statistician would agree that there was insufficient statistical power to state "No increase in shingles has occurred". Yet, this is precisely what the CDC related to other research and media sources. Unlike the situation involving the role that temperature and school enrolment played on the seasonality of chickenpox, suddenly the CDC epidemiologist assigned to assist on that study became unavailable to assist with investigations concerning shingles.

When this occurs, the vaccinated child is subject to the higher incidence of shingles that is associated with the natural chickenpox virus ...

Increased Shingles Risk Among Adults

In Antelope Valley, shingles cases among adults 20 years and older increased 17.7 per cent from 237 cases reported in 2000 to 279 in 2001. The 370 shingles cases reported in 2002 represented an increase of 32.6 per cent over those reported in 2001 and 56.1 per cent over those reported in 2000. In 2005, the CDC presented corroborating data from a large population study that demonstrated a 90 per cent increase in adult shingles during a period of increasing vaccination coverage (1998–2003).

Breakthrough Cases Not Easily Recognised

While chickenpox outbreaks may appear to be greatly reduced, very light breakthrough cases are no longer easily recognised as chickenpox and appear as "insect bites" or other localised rashes. Children are becoming infected with the wild-type or natural chickenpox virus when exposed to either a child with natural chickenpox or an adult with shingles. When this occurs, the vaccinated child is subject to the higher incidence of shingles that is associated with the natural chickenpox virus which then dominates the attenuated vaccine (or Oka) strain.

Varicella Hospitalisations and Deaths have Decreased

While hospitalisations and deaths due to chickenpox have decreased after the introduction of the varicella vaccine program, the impact on shingles has not yet been considered. It is estimated that there are three times as many hospitalisations and four to five times as many deaths from shingles as from chickenpox. Therefore, a small increase in the number of shingles cases could offset the cost-benefit of eliminating four million cases of chickenpox—at least until the entire adult generation dies out and has been replaced by vaccinees. Since those children receiving only one vaccine may be susceptible as adults, hospitalisations and associated costs could increase in the future since there is 20 times more risk of complications in chickenpox cases among adults compared to children.

Adverse Events Mitigate against Discovery of the True Costs and Benefits of Varicella Vaccination

Varicella vaccination is generally considered safe but there are usually no pre-screening tests to determine whether an adverse reaction is likely to occur. The literature contains a surprising number of adverse reactions following varicella vaccination, including vaccine-strain herpes zoster (HZ) in children and adults.

The Advisory Committee on Immunization Practices (ACIP) states: "Vaccine Adverse Event Reporting System (VAERS) data are limited by underreporting and unknown sensitivity of the reporting system, making it difficult to compare adverse event rates following vaccination reported to VAERS with those from complications following natural disease. Nevertheless, the magnitude of these differences makes it likely that serious adverse events following vaccination occur at a substantially lower rate than following natural disease."

Since follow-up is not conducted, it may be argued that some reports may not be attributed to or associated with vaccination, and therefore the true rate of adverse events is essentially unknown. Nevertheless, adverse reactions reported in VAERS have typically been shown to be only five per cent or 10 per cent of the true rates. The lot number associated with each vaccine is recorded in the VAERS database. However, the CDC and FDA have never required the vaccine manufacturers to divulge publicly the number of vaccines contained in a given lot. This prevents researchers from determining "hot lots", since calculation of the number of adverse reactions per lot is not possible.

Table 2 presents a comparison of the number of adverse reactions reported to VAERS for the varicella vaccine with four other different vaccines. The high mean of 2,980 reports per year is attributed to the hepatitis B vaccine, followed next by a mean of 2,350 reports per year attributed to varicella vaccine. The first report of an adverse reaction following varicella vaccination was filed with VAERS (ID 74221) on May 26, 1995. This three-and-a-half-year-old boy from Georgia, who had no pre-existing conditions, received a dose of varicella vaccine on May 12, 1995. He developed convulsions the following day, was hospitalised and reportedly recovered.

Many physicians consider vaccination extremely safe, and parents or patients are not provided with information regarding potential adverse outcomes. Since varicella disease is relatively benign, only a few serious adverse reactions might offset the intended benefits.

A post-marketing evaluation by Black et al. concluded that the varicella vaccine is safe based on VAERS reports. Admittedly, the spontaneous reporting in general and VAERS in particular are unreliable. Thus it is illogical for the FDA and the CDC to acknowledge these limitations, yet state that VAERS serves "to reassure the general public concerning the safety of a new vaccine"—basing assessment of the safety of the varicella vaccine only on an analysis of VAERS.

Clinical descriptions of five different serious adverse effects that followed varicella vaccination, as well as scientific literature concerning other adverse reactions and vaccine-related complications, are provided in the appendices of my complete paper (see http://www.MedicalVeritas.com/FULLNEXUS.pdf).

Table 2: VAERS reports associated with varicella, DTaP, hepatitis B, Hib and MMR vaccines through December 2003.

Vaccine type	No. of reports	Date of first report	Duration (years)	Mean cases/year
Varicella	20,004	12 May 1995	8.5	2,350
DTaP[a]	23,886	2 Apr 1992	11.4	2,080
Hep B[b]	41,708	25 Jan 1990	14.0	2,980
Hib[c]	25,060	2 Jan 1990	14.0	1,790
MMR[d]	31,132	17 Nov 1989	14.0	2,220

a. Diphtheria and tetanus toxoid and acellular pertussis
b. Hepatitis B
c. *Haemophilus influenzae* type b
d. Measles–Mumps–Rubella

Source information from US Government VAERS database, 1990–2003, http://www.medalerts.org/vaersdb

PART IV: Conclusions

Prior to the universal chickenpox vaccination program, 95 per cent of adults experienced natural chickenpox (usually as school-age children), which was usually benign and which resulted in long-term immunity.

This high percentage of long-term immunity has been compromised by mass vaccination of children, which provides at best 70–90 per cent immunity that is temporary and of unknown duration—shifting chickenpox to a more vulnerable adult population, where it carries 20 times more risk of death and 15 times more risk of hospitalisation compared to children.

Add to this the adverse effects of both the chickenpox and shingles vaccines as well as the potential for increased risk of shingles for an estimated 30 to 50 years among adults.

The Universal Varicella (chickenpox) Vaccination Program now requires booster vaccines that are less effective than the natural immunity that existed in communities prior to licensure of the varicella vaccine. Routine vaccination against chickenpox has produced continual cycles of treatment and disease.

Rather than information being presented so that the parent or public is truly informed, only selective information from studies is typically chosen for publication.

Data, analyses, results and conclusions that are supportive of a vaccine are desired by the sponsoring agency to promote vaccination; while deleterious aspects are often rarely investigated and, in the few instances where they are objectively pursued by conscientious scientists and researchers, the results are often suppressed because these are seen as having a potentially negative impact on vaccination uptake rates.

Rather than depicting a true cost-benefit scenario, public health officials in increasing numbers appear to be unduly influenced by conflicts of interests with the pharmaceutical industry itself and the pursuit of profits regardless of the negative impact and adverse consequences to public health. These considerations are not limited solely to the Universal Varicella Vaccination Program, but to other vaccination and drug programs as well. What has been previously outlined represents merely the tip of the iceberg.

Cost-benefit analyses of varicella vaccination appear optimistic, but they fail to factor in the resulting deleterious effects. Analyses of the Universal Varicella Vaccination Program in the US have also failed to consider the potential effect on the closely related shingles disease.

Outside exposures to children with natural chickenpox previously contributed a significant immunologic boosting effect that helped suppress or postpone the reactivation of VZV as shingles among adults. In the US where vaccination coverage is increasing, and since natural chickenpox has been dramatically reduced in many communities, immunologic boosting via periodic exposures to children with natural chickenpox is becoming rare, causing a need for booster chickenpox vaccinations in children (recommended at four to six years) and shingles vaccinations among adults.

There was a time not so long ago when parents could place their implicit trust in their healthcare provider to make the best informed choices with respect to recommended interventions and procedures. With conflicts of interest plaguing the current healthcare system, studies often report flawed conclusions that are biased toward promoting pharmaceutical products. Public health policies based on study outcomes that are not objectively obtained and which have been manipulated toward promoting vaccination based on flawed underlying assumptions of vaccine policies are surfacing with greater frequency—demonstrating the need for parents to exercise caution, do careful research and take a more prominent role when it comes to making healthcare decisions for themselves and their loved ones.

A key that a problem exists is seen in the statistic from the US Department of Education, indicating that the number of cases of autism among individuals aged six to 21 in US schools increased from 12,222 in 1992–1993 to 118,602 in 2002–2003, an overall increase of 870 per cent.

Furthermore, despite its spending the most income per capita on healthcare, the US is ranked lower than many industrialised nations in infant mortality, at 6.63 deaths per 1,000 live births, and is even ranked lower than some countries that are relatively poor, including Cuba at 6.45 per 1,000, according to a 2005 estimate. Public health officials claim the causes are largely unknown.

The journal *Medical Veritas* (where *veritas* is Latin for "truth") was started in April 2004 to assist in the goal of providing research that is free from conflicts of interest with the pharmaceutical firms and fostering the belief that a better-informed public will help to ensure better medical practice.

Continued on page 79

The Chickenpox Vaccine: Promoting a Continual Cycle of Treatment and Disease

Continued from page 24

About the Author:

Gary S. Goldman graduated with honours in 1977 from California State University, Fullerton (CSUF), with a double major: a BS Engineering (electronics emphasis) and a BS Computer Science. He holds a PhD in Computer Science, gained in 1981 from Pacific Western University in Los Angeles, California, USA.

In 1980, as Vice-President of Systems Development at Cascade Graphics Development, he developed the first microcomputer-based computer-aided drafting (CAD) system (prior to the well known AutoCad product). Dr Goldman holds a US patent (#4,223,255, granted in September 1980) for a micro-programmed, high-efficiency motor-in-a-wheel called "Power Wheel", for use in electric vehicular applications. This invention was featured on the front cover of the Fall 1980 issue of *Science and Mechanics*.

For 30-plus years, Dr Goldman has served as a computer consultant, responsible for the automation of a wide variety of businesses, improvements in production and conversion of databases. He has authored and presented numerous manuscripts contributing to engineering and computer science disciplines and enjoys writing heuristic programs.

Dr Goldman served for eight years (from January 1995 until his resignation in October 2002) as Research Analyst for the Varicella Active Surveillance Project in Antelope Valley, in a cooperative project with the Centers for Disease Control and Prevention (CDC, Atlanta, Georgia). A new book based on his research, *The Chickenpox Vaccine: A New Epidemic of Disease and Corruption*, by Mark Orrin, is available at the web page http://www.injectionbook.com/chickenpoxvaccine.html. The book was an award-winning finalist in the Current Events: Political/Social category of the National Indie Excellence 2007 Book Awards.

Presently, Dr Goldman serves as a consulting computer scientist and is on the board of directors of Pearblossom Private School, Inc., which provides distance education to over 5,000 independent study students each year in grades K through 12 throughout the USA (see website http://www.PearblossomSchool.com). He is also Editor-in-Chief of the peer-reviewed journal *Medical Veritas: The Journal of Medical Truth* (http://www.MedicalVeritas.com). He has served as a reviewer for the *Journal of the American Medical Association*, *Vaccine* and *The American Journal of Managed Care*. He is included on the Editorial Board of *Research & Reviews in BioSciences*. His biography is included in *Who's Who in Science and Engineering* (Marquis, 8th Edition, 2005–2006) and *Who's Who in the World* (Marquis, 23rd Edition, 2006).

Dr Goldman has recently contributed 18 articles, presentations and abstracts (nine in which he served as the lead author) on varicella vaccination, herpes zoster, capture-recapture techniques as well as other vaccine-related topics; the majority of the articles were published in peer-reviewed medical journals in the US and UK between 2000 and 2006. He can be contacted by email at pearblossominc@aol.com or via his website http://www.drgoldmanonline.com/.

Editor's Note:

Due to space constraints, we are unable to publish the complete version of this paper with appendices including case studies, endnotes and references; it is available as a PDF document at the web page http://www.MedicalVeritas.com/FULLNEXUS.pdf.

#Excerpt from Viera Scheibner Ph.D. book reference from page 183.

7

POLIO VACCINES: leukæmia, cancer, simian retroviruses and AIDS

Everybody remembers, or has heard of, the 1949-50 epidemic of polio in Australia and in many other countries. It is commonly quoted to scare parents into vaccinating their children. Even those parents who decide not to vaccinate against whooping cough, diphtheria, tetanus and measles usually make a concession and vaccinate against polio. After all, who would want their child exposed to the risk of paralysis?

However, only very few know that that famous 1950s polio epidemic has a quite different, and much more sinister, background.

In 1950, Dr McCloskey published an article in The Lancet "The relation of prophylactic inoculations to the onset of poliomyelitis."

He wrote in the introduction that "*Early in the epidemic, attention was directed to a few patients who had been given an injection of pertussis vaccine, or of a mixture of diphtheria toxoid and pertussis vaccine, shortly before the onset of their symptoms.*

"The parents of these children were naturally inclined to blame the inoculations for the development of the disease, though their medical attendants either dismissed the probability of any causal relationship, or else considered the effect to be due to a radiculitis caused by the vaccine... Considerable evidence, however, will be presented to show that such an association has existed in this epidemic."

The British Medical Journal 1950 (1 July) published an article by Hill and Knowelden on Inoculation and Poliomyelitis. The authors wrote, among other things, that during the progress of the diphtheria

143

immunisation campaign, begun in 1942, there have been occasional and sporadic cases of paralysis reported following the injection of an antigen: *"This paralysis has sometimes been limited to the limb in which the injection was made; sometimes it had involved other limbs as well... In most cases a diagnosis of poliomyelitis was made."*

The same issue of the British Medical Journal published another article, by MacCallum, on clinical poliomyelitis in association with peripheral inoculation of prophylactics. The author wrote that: *"Stools have been obtained less than 21 days after the onset of the illness in a number of children included in some of the recent observations, and the poliomyelitis virus has been isolated by monkey inoculation from each of the five children whose stools have so far been tested. The rhesus monkeys used all developed a disease similar to experimental poliomyelitis, and lesions pathognomonic of the disease were found in the brain and (spinal) cord at necropsy."*

The affected children were given smallpox, diphtheria-pertussis and/or tetanus injections prior to the onset of poliomyelitis.

The same journal (BMJ 29 July) published an article by Banks and Beale (1950) titled "Poliomyelitis and immunisation against whooping-cough and diphtheria" reporting on a number of paralytic polio cases which occurred in 1947, 1948 and 1949, following pertussis and diphtheria inoculations, with a preponderance of upper-arm paralysis (most inoculations in London being done in the arm, rather than in the leg). The interval between the last injection and the onset of paralysis in the majority of cases was between nine and 14 days.

Leake (1950), in his letter to the Editor of the Journal of the American Medical Association, summarised the published data confirming the occurrence of paralysis after a variety of vaccine injections including pertussis, diphtheria and typhoid-paratyphoid.

Perhaps not surprisingly, an American study of similar associations between injections of vaccines and paralytic polio by Bell (1950) [quoted in Leake(1950)] discounted any suggestion of similar association between diphtheria and pertussis inoculations. However, the author nevertheless cautioned against administration of any inoculations during the polio seasons, as well as against strenuous physical activity, and unaccustomed sunning and chilling.

At least one American study, by Anderson and Skaar (1950), concluded that *"In poliomyelitis patients who have received some antigen during the month prior to onset there is a high degree of correlation between site of paralysis and site of injection. Such cases tend to show a different distribution of paralysis and a more severe paralysis than do comparable children immunised two to six months previously, immunised in previous years or never immunised."*

Martin (1950) collected data on 17 cases of paralysis after diphtheria vaccine injections in which paralysis occurred in one limb within 28 days of the injection. In almost all cases the diagnosis of poliomyelitis was made. It is very unlikely that the relationship would have been totally coincidental, especially considering the great number of papers reporting the same observations.

Geffen (1950) reported the occurrence of poliomyelitis in recently inoculated children in the Metropolitan Borough of St Pancras and London. Paralysis tended to occur in the injected limb.

Wyatt (1981) dealt with the repeated observations of provocation poliomyelitis after a number of procedures.

He reviewed data from literature starting with Hans Kern's report published in 1914 on the occurrence of poliomyelitis in institutionalised children in Germany. Of 22 children suffering congenital syphilis, five developed polio after being treated with Neosalvarsan, Salvarsan and other drugs.

The period from injections of Neosalvarsan to illness was from five to 21 days, and from six to 31, and two to 14 days, after an injection of Hg-salicyl-Kur in individual cases of paralysis.

A further seven cases were reported in Germany after similar treatment between 1921 and 1926. Some authors reported provocation polio after injections of alum-precipitated diphtheria and pertussis vaccine.

Many other similar cases were reported. Likewise, many authors reported polio after tonsillectomies.

Increased risk of contracting polio following tonsillectomy

Paffenbarger (1957) presented convincing evidence for a statistic[al] association between previous tonsillectomy and increased risk [of] contracting poliomyelitis, specifically the bulbar form. Although th[e] timing of onset of symptoms varies, the association is most prominen[t] within one month after surgery.

The reported observations were based on: 1. an epidemic of typ[e] 1 poliomyelitis in Olmsted County, Minnesota, in 1952, when 215 cases developed among 49,000 residents, an attack rate of 438 per 100,000; 2. the reported poliomyelitis outbreak in metropolitan Washington DC, during an endemic year, 1954, when 155 paralytic cases, representing infections with all 3 virus types occured among nearly 1,500,000 residents; 3. 113 cases from the St Louis encephalitic epidemic in Hildago County, Texas, in 1954, when over 500 cases developed among 160,000 residents, an attack rate exceeding 310 per 100,000.

Over half of those poliomyelitis patients whose illness began with bulbar symptoms had undergone tonsil removal, as compared with remarkably uniform proportions approximately fourth in the control groups which did not undergo tonsilectomy.

Lambert (1936) described a campaign to treat yaws in Samoa with neoarsphenamine administered by two or more injections. In 1932 some 36,000 persons were treated this way. The first case of paralysis occurred a week after the second yaws injection. All patients first seen had paralysis in the lower limbs and all had double buttock injections. Paralysis occurred in all 37 villages where the yaws campaign was conducted. Although Lambert had a very convincing account of provocation poliomyelitis, he rejected the connection despite all natives claiming the connection.

Wyatt (1981) also commented on a connection between small pox vaccination and paralysis. These observations were ignored because there was no obvious connection between the two and because a *"fuss over these observations would have disturbed the smallpox vaccination program."* The same author commented on the Brodie-Park and Kolmer polio vaccine accidents in 1935. He wrote that *"It has always been assumed that the cases of poliomyelitis associated with the Kolmer and Brodie-Park vaccines were caused by virus incoculation as in the Cutter incident of 1955."*

In another paper Wyatt *et al.* (1992) examined the effect of prior injections on the pattern and severity of paralytic poliomyelitis by a retrospective analysis of cases recorded in an outpatient clinic in South India. Of 262 children with acute polio, 176 had received unnecessary injections less than 48 hours before paralysis and 12 had received diphtheria-pertussis-tetanus provocative injections. There was a considerable association between the injected arm and localisation of paralysis. After injections there was greater likelihood of death or lack of recovery of muscle strength.

In a more recent paper, Wyatt (1993) called for campaign to banish all unnecessary injections.

Polio — the Disease and Immunity to It

The above reports of polio, undoubtedly triggered by injections of a variety of antigens and other foreign substances, are of great interest, especially after years of experience with mass immunisations. First of all, they give credence to opinions expressed several decades ago by such authors as Jungeblut and Engle(1932), who believed that polio may, after all,be of endogenous origin.

These authors realised that the occurrence of infection is obviously dependent upon a delicate balance between the virulence of the invading micro-organism and the receptivity of the host. They wrote that with *"high virulence of the ætiologic agent, differences in individual predisposition of the host will frequently be obscured; a low innate susceptibility to a disease, on the other hand, may virtually obliterate the infectious character of its incitant. A rational analysis of resistance or susceptibility must, therefore, allocate in each instance proportionally a greater or lesser importance to specific immunologic and nonspecific physiologic factors.*

The lack of natural resistance frequently is synchronised with fluctuations in the regulatory influence of non-specific physiologic elements, such as age, sex, heredity, diet and endocrine activities."

Polio represents an extreme example of an infectious disease in which lack of susceptibility to the disease is so widespread that only under particular environmental circumstances does it ever assume epidemic proportions. According to these authors, support for their conclusions comes from innumerable instances of epidemics, for instance the epidemic in Brooklyn in which, in 469 cases of 500, it was impossible to establish contact with a previous case (*op. cit.*).

Jungeblut and Engle (1932) recognised a strong seasonality of polio incidence. They also stressed that because clinical cases of polio are numerically far too few they cannot account for the universal natural immunty of the adult population.

However, Paul *et al*. (1932) emphasised the importance of minor illnesses occurring during an epidemic ("Heine-Medin" disease of uncharacteristic sporadic colds or diarrhoeas occurring in summer).

The formation of antibodies against certain infectious diseases, and some non-infectious agents, is essentially an expression of an endogenous, hereditarily fixed maturation process, rather than the result of exogenous influences, which reaches its climax around puberty. Paul *et al*. (1932) talked about serologic ripening and the age-dependent development of agglutinins. They reasoned that a gradually increasing number of negative reactions to the Schick and Dick tests through adolescence occurs also with dysentery toxins. Under extreme climatic conditions, such as occur in the tropics or subtropics and in arctic regions, negative reactions to the Schick and Dick tests may develop with puberty while clinical diphtheria and scarlet fever occur only very sporadically.

The viricidal power of blood develops with maturity both in monkeys and man, despite a low incidence of clinical polio (the 'hundred monkeys' syndrome?).

Jungeblut and Engle (1932) also discussed the differences in polio-virus neutralising power of serum of different blood groups from normal human adults. One half of group A sera were capable of neutralisation when tested in the usual quantities while 80% of group B sera possessed this property. Group O sera behaved similarly to group A, with one half neutralising. Thus the genetic factor was infinitely more important than any hypothetical contact factor in influencing neutralisation capacity of a person's serum.

A similar relationship was ascertained between blood group and neutralising power in serum of convalescent patients. Group B sera neutralise at many times higher dilution than do group A sera.

In persons of blood group A, a constitutional inability to form diphtheria antitoxin after recovery from that disease has been described by Nowak (1931) [quoted by Jungeblut and Engle (1932)].

Jungeblut and Engle (1932) quoted the work of Draper (1932) who methodically observed an endocrine deficiency in children stricken with poliomyelitis. It is known that after puberty the incidence of polio declines earlier and more abruptly in females than in males. Pregnant women show remarkable resistance to polio; babies receive certain circulating hormones, charactertistic of adult age, with the maternal blood . However, Anderson et al., (1952) stated that poliomyelitis has frequently been recorded during pregnancy, indicating increased susceptibility to recognisable infection.

A premenstrual drop in bactericidal power of blood has been described by Geller (1930) [quoted by Jungeblut and Engle (1932)].

Previously, Aycock (1926) acknowledged an apparent discrepancy between the theory of spread through direct person-to-person contact and observations in the field and epidemiologic incidence of scant direct contact. There is a great number of comparatively mild forms of polio which escape recognition, and a relatively large proportion of healthy carriers. Taken together, these are largely responsible for the spread of the virus.

Support for the endogenous origin of polio comes also from such examples as the incidence of three paralytic cases in a camp of 60 boys or simultaneous occurrence of cases within the same families.

Hudson *et al.* (1936) discussed at some length the factors of resistance and immunity in experimental poliomyelitis. They wrote that efforts to induce immunity in humans have been based on *"classic principles effective in other infectious states, and insufficient attention has been paid to the basic difficulties and to factors of the host's resistance to this particular virus."*

They concluded that the upper respiratory tract is the portal of entry of the polio virus and at the same time a certain degree of resistance is manifested by the nasopharyngeal mucosa. The intestinal mucosa was an effective barrier to infection by virus administered directly into isolated intestinal loops.

The spleen played a definite role in inducing resistance to the virus. Neutralising antibodies were formed in monkeys "vaccinated" with certain preparations, but their presence was not an indication of effective protection of the animal to intranasal virus. Natural or artificially induced menstruation and physiologic maturation did not lead to a demonstrable viricidal property of the blood.

They also wrote that, after entering the olfactory nasal tract, the virus migrates intracellularly through the central nervous system to the "loci of predilection" in the cord, and sensitises the nervous tissues in some way so that it is resistant to re-exposure to the virus. The neutralising antibodies in the natural conditions are thus an indication of specific sensitisation by extra-neural stimulation after nerve cell migration of the virus. Antibodies induced artificially are not necessarily a measure of nerve tissue resistance.

The authors warned that artificial immunisation of humans, either active or passive, should take into account the distinctness of the central nervous system in the pathogenesis of polio and the significance of certain factors of resistance imposed as a barrier to the virus between the vascular and central nervous systems.

Sub-lethal doses were made fatally infective through damage to the cerebral cortex by starch injections. This phenomenon may provide a theoretical explanation for the occurrence of poliomyelitis after injections as discused above.

Epidemiology of poliomyelitis

The epidemiology of poliomyelitis is equally as interesting as the questions of immunity to it. Nathanson and Martin (1979) considered many of the salient epidemiological features of polio enigmatic. Apparently, polio appeared as an epidemic disease some 100 years ago in northern Europe and the United States. It is basically a disease of infancy, and practically all individuals experience infection at some time during their lives. There was a steady decrease in the incidence of polio while the age distribution rose dramatically in both areas. While there was an upward trend in age, there was no upward trend in incidence. After decades of constant incidence there was only a dramatic upsurge of incidence in 1945-1954. This may be partly accounted for by the reporting of non-paralytic cases.

However, there is a more plausible explanation, namely intensified vaccination with a variety of vaccines leading to provocation poliomyelitis as documented above.

Vaccination trials with poliovirus vaccines, based on monkey neural tissues, were carried out in the 1930s. The trials were condemned because of marked side effects and fatal cases associated with administration of these vaccines. However, the work resumed some 20 years later and resulted in the production of the Salk polyvalent vaccine. A large trial with the Salk vaccine was organised by the poliomyelitis vaccine evaluation center of the University of Michigan, Ann Arbor, Michigan (Francis *et al.* 1955).

During the trial, one syringe was used for five children. Concerns about the possibility of transmitting infectious diseases or serum hepatitis because of this led several areas to organise their own clinics using individual syringes for each child. Some doctors objected to the fact that the vaccines contained dead monkey kidney tissue. However, nobody did anything about it.

In this trial, over 1,000,000 children were injected with three doses of the Salk vaccine between 1 May and 1 December 1954. One hundred and twenty nine cases of "presumed" poliomyelitis occurred during the trial period, including three weeks after the third injection: 90 cases in the vaccinated group and 39 cases in the placebo controls. However, because the 90 cases occurred during the vaccination period between May 1 and two weeks after the third injection, they were excluded from calculations.

Of 749,236 placebo control children, 428 developed poliomyelitis; of 1,080,680 vaccinated children, 585 developed polio. The corrected figures are 428 plus 39 (467) and 585 plus 90 (675).

The authors of the report stated that there were 57/100,000 cases of polio among the vaccinated and 54/100,000 among the unvaccinated. So the rate of polio was slightly higher in the vaccinated than in the unvaccinated. When the complete figures are calculated (including the 90 which were excluded) the rate of cases of polio in the vaccinated children is even higher.

Based on their own figures, the trial showed a total failure of the Salk polio vaccine to protect against poliomyelitis.

Despite this, in April 1955 six pharmaceutical companies obtained licences for production of inactivated poliovirus vaccines. Within 14 days of the release of the vaccine a large number of babies (94), their parents (126) and other contacts (40) were reported to have contracted paralytic polio from the vaccine (the "Cutter incident") encompassing a period from 25 April to the end of June 1955 and described in detail by Nathanson and Langmuir (1963a, b c).

Vaccination was halted for two weeks but resumed again in May. Polio epidemics continued occurring in the United States despite a high proportion of the population being vaccinated. During a 1959 epidemic in Massachusetts, 77.5% of the paralytic cases had received three or more doses of inactivated vaccine. Similar disappointing results were reported from many other countries where the Salk vaccine was used on a large scale: Czechoslovakia, Hungary and Israel. The quality of the vaccines had been very uneven and generally low. Not only were the vaccines ineffective, they continued causing paralytic poliomyelitis at the time when there were no epidemics with the wild virus.

Contamination of Polio vaccines by Animal Tissue

A new menace appeared when polio vaccines proved to be contaminated with a great number of animal (simian) retroviruses, called SV1 to SV40. Of these, SV40 was the most researched. Rustigian *et al.* (1955) established that monkeys carry a great number of viruses such as B virus, foamy agent, measles-like virus, hæm-adsorption viruses, LCM virus, arboviruses and a great variety of miscellaneous viral agents.

Hull and Minner (1955) and Hull *et al*. (1958) extensively studied viruses found in normal monkey kidney cell cultures and called them simian viruses or SV. They were classified into four groups based on the kind of cytopathic changes induced in monkey kidney cell cultures infected with these viral agents. Twenty eight of these viruses were grouped into serological types and an additional 24 unidentified viruses were recorded.

Malherbe and Harwin (1957) distinguished seven different types among the simian agents or SA viruses recovered from vervet kidney.

According to Sweet and Hilleman (1960) a new simian virus has been encountered repeatedly. This virus was unique among simian viruses because it did not cause detectable cytopathic effects in the rhesus or cynomolgus kidney cell culture from which it was derived, but instead grew and caused marked cytopathic changes in cell cultures of other species. The virus was recognised by McClelland in the course of safety testing of vaccines and was subsequently called vacuolating SV40 virus.

At about the same time another virus was isolated from laboratory chimpanzees with coryza and was called respiratory syncytial (RS) virus (Morris *et al*. 1956). Soon it was established that a number of these viruses caused cold-like symptoms in adult human volunteers. Needless to say, they formed prominent contaminants in polio vaccines and were soon detected in children, causing respiratory tract infections in babies and small infants vaccinated with polio vaccines.

Parrot *et al*. (1961) published results of serologic studies over a 34-month period of children with bronchiolitis, pneumonia and minor respiratory diseases. Their data confirmed an ætiologic relationship between RS virus and respiratory tract illness, particularly *"relatively severe lower respiratory tract illness in children"*.

Chanock *et al*. (1961) recovered respiratory syncytial virus from 57% of young infants with bronchiolitis or pneumonia during a 5-month period. The virus was also recovered from older infants and children with pneumonia or bronchiolitis and from a significant proportion (12%) of young patients with a milder febrile respiratory disease. The outbreaks lasted from three to five months. They established that RS virus represents a major pathogen during early life. Soon, these animal viruses spread and were recovered from cases of common cold in human adults [Hamparian *et al.* (1961)].

Melnick and Stinebaugh (1962) and many others confirmed that SV40 vacuolating virus was a "viable contaminant" of killed and live virus vaccines grown on rhesus and cynomolgus kidney cultures. They wrote that it appears that *"the virus has been injected as a live contaminant of formalinised polio vaccines and adeno-vaccines into hundreds of thousands, if not millions, of persons, and especially babies, and that it has been fed in active form together with live poliovaccine to groups equally as large"*.

The authors however emphasised that in spite of the large numbers of persons injected or fed the virus, not *"a single human illness has been attributed to this agent."*

That belief can no longer be sustained.

Human Illness Associated with Simian Virus

ZuRhein and Chou (1965) found numerous spherical randomly distributed virus particles in tissues infected with any number of papova viruses (for more detail see below) including SV40 in human cerebral demyelinating disease. Demyelination resulted from the cytocidal effect of the virus on oligodendroglia.

Weiner *et al.* (1972) reported on isolation of virus related to SV40 from patients with human demyelinating disease: progressive multifocal leukoencephalopathy. Shah *et al.* (1972) tested four groups of donors for the presence of SV40 reacting antibodies. Vaccines have been required since 1961 to be produced free of SV40. However, SV40 neutralising antibodies were found in some tested babies born after 1964. The authors did not even consider that this may have shown that the vaccines are very much not free of the S40 virus – they were looking for sources of the infection in humans other than the vaccines.

Baguley and Glasgow (1973) reported on the incidence of subacute sclerosing panencephalitis (SSPE) which occurred from

1956 to 1966 in the northern half of the North Island of New Zealand. It was 100 times greater than expected. Mass vaccination of primary-school children with Salk vaccine from 1956 onwards was blamed for this major outbreak because the vaccine used *"is likely to have contained live SV40 virus"*. The authors concluded that *"the administration of Salk vaccine in New Zealand was related to the appearance of S.S.P.E."* and that *"The idea that an unusual reaction to measles infection is the sole cause of S.S.P.E. is not consistent with the observation in New Zealand"*.

In 1962 Eddy *et al*. identified oncogenic substance in rhesus monkey kidney cell culture as the simian SV40 virus. Both Eddy *et al*. (1962) and Girardi *et al*. (1961) confirmed that SV40 virus causes tumours in hamsters inoculated in the neonatal period with vacuolating virus SV40.

Rabson *et al*. (1962) demonstrated that oncogenicity of SV40 was not restricted to hamsters. Fraumeni *et al*. (1963) reported on the oncogenicity of SV40 in humans introduced into the body with injections of inactivated Salk poliomyelitis vaccine. They quote several authors who clearly demonstrated alterations of human tissue cultures infected with SV40.

Shein and Enders (1962) observed a reproducible "epitheloid transformation" characterised by abnormal growth pattern, greatly accelerated growth rate and chromosomal aberrations in human kidney tissue cultures. Koprowski *et al*. (1962) recorded similar transformation during SV40 infection of organ cultures of adult human skin and buccal musosa. Rabson *et al*. (1962) produced a strain of rapidly multiplying pleomorphic cells in human thyroid tissue *in vitro* with SV40 which grew rapidly, with large amount of virus persisting and demonstrated intranuclear virus in 5% of these cells. Eddy *et al*. (1962) demonstrated multiplication of SV40 in continuous line cultures of human cancer cells.

Melnick (1962) invented the term 'Papova' viruses for a group that includes "pa(pilloma)", "po(lyoma)" and "va(cuolating)" (SV40) viruses. These are all de-oxyribonucleic acid (DNA) viruses. Other similarities include a slow growth cycle with multiplication inside the cell nucleus, an ability to cause chronic and latent infections in their host and a capacity to induce tumours in their natural and/or host species.

Although the authors played down these findings, they nonetheless quoted Innis (1968) who established that from 1955 to 1959 the leukæmia mortality rate per 100,000 rose from 3.5 to 3.8 for children 5-9 years old and from 2.2 to 2.5 for children 10-14 years old. The leukæmia mortality for those states using vaccine containing SV40 was generally greater than that for the states whose vaccine was free of SV40. Their figure 2, nevertheless, shows a major increase in deaths from cancers other than leukæmia in children under 12 months of age and 5-9 years of age, and an increase in leukæmia deaths in under one year, 5-9 years of age and in the 1-14 yearsage groups.

In 1973 Shah *et al.* confirmed a high prevalence of antibodies to BK virus, an SV40-related papova virus, in residents of Maryland. The prevalence of antibodies increased from 50% to 100% between the ages of three to 10-11 years and then declined to 67% in the age group 35 years or older. Shah *et al.* (1972) also confirmed that SV40 neutralising antibodies were found in 3.2% of tested sera (9 children) of Maryland children born during or after 1964. This was established despite the fact that vaccines were required to be free of SV40 since 1961. Indeed, in 1992 (Kyle) published in The Lancet an article proposing a link between contaminated polio vaccines in treatment by homosexual men of genital herpes, popular in the late seventies, and the simultaneous outbreak of AIDS in American homosexual men. Reverse transcriptase analyses of released vaccine have shown positive for such simian viruses up to 1985 and the author urges that a critical look should now be taken at all such vaccines and "*... the results should be made public*".

Contaminated Poliovirus Vaccines and the Causation of AIDS

By far the most competent and veritable summary of the dangers of the oral polio vaccine and the origin of AIDS is that published by Louis Pascal. He is the epitome of the independent scholar, a person without formal affiliation to a university or a research institution.

His paper, ***"What happens when science goes bad. The corruption of science and the origin of AIDS. A study of spontaneous generation"*** was finally published by the University of Wollongong as a Working Paper (No.9) in 1991, after a number of research journals rejected or simply ignored his submissions.

In his paper, Pascal demonstrated that AIDS originated in the Belgian Congo as a direct result of mass oral polio vaccination while the vaccine was conatminated with a simian immunodeficiency virus (SIV). The special strains of polio virus that had been carefully bred to lack neurovirulence, but that would nevertheless induce immunity, retained the ability to revert to their former neurovirulence by passage from one person to another. Also, and very importantly, the manufacturing procedure almost guaranteed contamination with foreign viruses which could not be killed without also killing the polio virus and ruining the vaccine.

In late 1957, in the eastern part of the Belgian Congo, and especially in the early part of 1958 in Ruanda-Urundi, the world's first mass vaccination campaign using live polio vaccine was conducted. A few months later, the same batch of the vaccine was used in Leopoldville, the capital of the Belgian Congo, 900 miles (almost 1500 km)west of the sites of the first vaccination campaign.

Almost immediately, contaminating viruses began emerging (in addition to the SV1-40 group referred to above). Indeed, Pascal quoted Hilary Koprowski, who manufactured the very batch of vaccine used in these two African campaigns, writing that "If indeed somebody were to poke his nose into the live virus vaccine, he might find a non-polio virus in all the preparations currently available."

He also added that this presented no real problem because people were exposed to many viruses every day in their food.

Pascal correctly pointed out that Koprowski was wrong on 3 counts.

Firstly, if vaccines could not be made free of contamination, they should be abandoned or the contaminants pronounced harmless. Koprowski was hardly a disinterested party, because in the first instance he would have had to renounce years of work.

Secondly, the contaminating viruses were monkey viruses and humans are not daily exposed to monkey viruses. Also the fact that these contaminated vaccines were fed to infants less than 30 days old (or even just 48 hours old), increases the danger, since their immature immune systems presented much less of an obstacle to a foreign virus than a mature immune system would have. (Infant animals are generally used in experiments for just this reason).

Thirdly, new viruses starting in "virgin" populations without prior immunological experience are often particularly virulent and contagious.

In 1985 the first of the simian immunodeficiency viruses was identified in rhesus monkeys, one of the three main species whose tissues were used to culture the polio vaccine. Since then, the SIVs have been found in the two other species — cynomolgus and African Green monkey — as well. All of these SIVs are closely related to each other and are the closest-known relatives of the HIV. Pascal quite correctly highlights *(op. cit.)* that the conclusion was immediately drawn that transfer from a monkey to a human of one of these viruses had caused AIDS. *"And how was it transmitted? Why, through a monkey bite, of course!"*

Pascal also raised ethical and moral questions in asking why neither the scientific community nor the reporters raised these questions much earlier to prevent the spread of the SIVs through vaccines.

Instead, both the World Health Organisation and the health authorities in the so-called developed countries are still pushing, and indeed intensifying, a general mass vaccination of human infants.

Billi Goldberg (1993) ascertained that in the late 1950s and early 1960s, poliovirus vaccines grown on diploid lines from human embryonic tissues (attenuated and killed) were acceptable only when grown in primary monkey kidney *"since such tissue was presumed to have no malignant properties."* A human diploid line was inoculated with the CHAT strain type 1 poliovirus cultured and attenuated in monkey kidney, a source of simian viral and retroviral contamination. Between August 1958 and April 1960, more than

75,000 children uder five years in Leopoldville (Belgian Congo) were given the vaccines prepared at the Wistar Institute. The vaccine was squirted into the back of the child's throat. As shown in other experiments [Morris et al. (1961)], *"Subclinical viral infection may be initiated by spraying of contaminated vaccines into the nasopharyngeal cavity if the vaccine enters the respiratory system."* And *"Retroviral infection of recipients of nebulised contaminated vaccine remains a possibility."*

Myers et al. (1992) asked whether as a "starting point for enquiry, HIV might simply be SIV adapting to a human host." "The notion is less far-fetched in 1992 than it was merely a few years ago" concluded Goldberg (1992).

Salk (1955) discussed considerations in the preparation and use of poliomyelitis virus vaccine. The motivation to write this article came from the "Cutter incident"(see below). In April 1955 the polio vaccine preparations caused " ... *subsequent development of paralytic poliomyelitis. 146 cases of paralytic polio developed in vaccinated children and their contacts within a short period of time. This demanded a very intensive re-examination of the theoretical and practical implications of vaccine preparation, testing, and use ...*

"It has been realised always that the preparation of a safe poliomyelitis vaccine would, at the beginning at least, require adherence to detail such as is not demanded for the preparation of any other immunising agent.

"It was recognised, too, that there must be incorporated into the vaccine preparation process itself a test for safety, which we refer to as the 'margin of safety', of such degree that the most sensitive tests upon a sample of each successive batch would be negative for living virus unless something unexpected had occurred, unknowingly, in the process of manufacture, or in subsequent handling, or in testing; it would follow that such would not be expected to occur but rarely."

And, also:

"The relative infrequency of severe paralysis under natural circumstances requires, above all else, that the vaccine must be free, insofar as it is possible to create such a preparation, of the capacity

to induce the disease that it is intended to prevent; nor should a vaccine for poliomyelitis cause such side effects as would make its use undesirable. If either the direct effects associated with its use, or incidental side-effects to any constituent, are of such nature as to make one prefer the chance of escaping the paralytic disease, one would not have a practically useful immunising agent."

And further

" ... *The objective in the preparation of a poliomyelitis vaccine cannot include the knowing or wilfull acceptance of a risk that is tangible,.or measurable to any degree. Any risk that is involved, so long as it is recognised, must be corrected, whatever may be its cause."*

Every point in this proclamation has been violated and there is no guarantee that it does not continue to be violated. Children receiving any of the polio vaccines continue contracting paralysis from the vaccine. The wide-spread incidence of chronic ill health, an endless stream of respiratory infections, usually resisting all treatment, occurring in small children and the continuing high incidence of child leukæmia and cancer are themselves the evidence that not all is healthy in the kingdom of vaccines.

The continued contamination of polio vaccines with animal viruses is of special concern. Goffe *et al*. (1961) pointed out that the vacuolating virus (SV40) which was resistant to formaldehyde occurred potentially in all polio vaccines, since until 1961 none of them was checked for this virus. It was also only one of many viruses and other agents lurking *"hitherto undetected"* in the monkey kidney tissue culture preparations. Despite these warnings, the authors considered oral administration of polio vaccines safer since they thought the alimentary tract may serve as a selective screen.

Gerber *et al*. (1961) reported on inactivation of vacuolating virus (SV40) by formaldehyde. Their studies showed there was a residual viable fraction of SV40 throughout the entire 14 days of observation. SV40 also showed a remarkable thermostability as evidenced by full retention of infectivity during heating without formaldehyde at 37 degC for a period of 14 days.

Randomly selected samples of poliomyelitis and adenovirus vaccines were tested for the presence of viable SV40: four of eight polio vaccines and three out of three adenovirus vaccines produced characteristic cytopathic changes in all subculture tubes. An isolate from each positive vaccine was identified by serum neutralisation tests.

The repeat tests with different lots of monkey kidney gave similar results. All subcultures derived from positive vaccines showed characteristic cytopathic changes between the seventh to the tenth day. They also found that the course of treatment of SV40 with 1:4,000 formaldehyde was characterised by a biphasic reaction. The major portion of the viral population was inactivated progressively at a slightly slower rate than poliovirus. The second phase of the curve indicated the persistence of a residual fraction which resisted inactivation.

When tested for more than ten days there was a marked delay in the appearance of cytopathic effects (CPE) caused by formaldehyde-treated SV40. In most cases CPE did not appear until the 11th day and the final infectivity titers were reached on the 13th and 14th days. The amount of viable SV40 depended on the concentration of this agent before formaldehyde treatment. The degree of contamination of the seed virus inoculum with SV40, the total incubation period of the kidney cell cultures during vaccine production and specific variations in the manufacturing process may also influence the final concentrations.

Sweet and Hilleman (1960) confirmed that, following injection of two doses of polio or adenovirus vaccines, a high percentage of persons developed relatively high antibody titers to SV40.

Results of studies by Shah (1973), Weiner *et al.* (1972), Baguley and Glasgow (1973) and others show that millions of children were indeed infected with SV40 during the course of vaccination with formalinised polio and adenovirus vaccines, with tragic long-term consequences. Baron *et al.* (1961) reported on more sensitive methods developed to test the commercial vaccines. They were able to detect viable virus in one out of every 23 commercial vaccines.

Polio vaccination, leukæmia and cancer

Girardi *et al.* (1973) confirmed that the oncogenic effect of SV40 was especially pronounced in younger individuals. Innis (1965) wrote in his letter to the editor of The Lancet that

"Since antigenic stimulation is known to cause hyperplasia of mammalian lymphoreticular tissue and since such hyperplasia may, in some strains of mice, proceed to malignant neoplasia, the possibility that a similar mechanism could operate in children submitted to the repeated antigenic stimulation inherent in immunisation seemed worth investigating."

He looked at immunisation status of 59 (out of 65) patients with leukæmia and compared it with that of patients admitted for different illnesses and concluded that

"The difference between the state of immunisation of leukæmic and non-leukæmic children may therefore be regarded as significant ... and the logical conclusion is that human lymphoreticular tissue, like that of some strains of mice, is possibly provoked to, or conditioned for, neoplasia by antigenic stimulation."

He considered his study a pilot survey indicating a need for further investigation. As an interim measure, he recommended a protection against individual disorders, when indicated, instead of immunisation with triple antigen since "fewer clones would then be provoked to (unnecessary) proliferative activity."

Answering the criticism of his conclusion by Lancaster and Clements (1965) Innis stated:

"Retrospective surveys are not the best means of determining antecedent events, but if mine was valueless, it should be simple to disprove an association between antigenic stimulation (including immunisation) and leukæmia."

In another letter to the editor of The Lancet, Innis continued

"...if the premises on which the deductions are based have been tested and found to be statistically significant, as have those used here, then any valid conclusion from these premises is inevitably true to fact; antigens, including those used for immunisation, are therefore leukæmogenic and carcinogenic in inviduals with the

requisite number of inherited and/or acquired mutant genes in a generative somatic cell."

Dr Scheuer-Karpin (1965) confirmed that antigenic stimulation, such as that provided by chronic and/or recurring inflammatory disease, appeared to be higher in the histories of patients with leukæmia than in the histories of patients with other disorders. The inflammatory diseases included chronic tuberculosis, recurrent discharging inflammation of the ear, nose and throat and urinary tract; chronic bronchitis with bronchial asthma and chronic osteomyelitis.

There was also a higher incidence of eczema and autoimmune disorders in the cases than in the controls. The well-known causal relationship between administration of vaccines and accentuation and susceptibility to a great variety of chronic infections certainly supports Innis's (*op. cit.*) warnings.

Flies Spread Polio Viruses

An interesting article on possible spread of polioviruses was published by Riordan *et al.* (1961). The authors described an experiment in which the oral polio vaccine was administered during a non-epidemic period (February 1958) to a group of Yaqui Indians living in the village of Guadalupe, Arizona.

The intention was to infect a small number of children with attenuated type 1 poliovirus vaccine and to follow the spread of the inapparent infection within the community by testing for the presence of poliovirus in rectal swabs from vaccinees and their contacts; in specimens of fæces from the various privies and the flies trapped in the village.

Six days after the administration of the oral vaccine, seven fly traps were set within the study area and five outside its periphery, but still within the village. The collections were made in the afternoons for about 70 days. Poliovirus types 1 and 3, ECHO 2, and Coxsackie B 5 viruses were isolated consistently from flies trapped both inside and outside the study area. Isolations increased during warm weather.

Type 3 poliovirus was isolated from virtually all the traps at one time or another, so it must have been widely disseminated throughout the village. Type 1 poliovirus was isolated more during the latter part of February and March than at other periods. Many of the strains were tested on monkeys and shown virulent, intermediate and attenuated (from the vaccine). The number of vaccine viruses was small because the number of vaccinated children was small.

In this particular environment it was not uncommon to see food at mealtimes covered with flies so that they could act as disseminators of the enteroviruses.

During the summer of 1958 an outbreak of poliomyelitis occurred among the Blackfeet Indians residing in Glacier County, Montana. 19 cases occurred, of which 18 lived in the reservation. This represented an incidence of 171 cases per 100,000 in a population of 11,100 (Glacier County) while the rate for Indians on the reservation was 640 per 100,000 among the 2,810 residents. The rate of the entire state was 10 per 100,000.

Since 1947 only seven cases of poliomyelitis had been reported to the Montana State Board of Health, so it was highly unusual that so many cases occurred in a population which, due to poor sanitary conditions, usually enjoyed solid immunity to poliomyelitis.

Poliovirus 1 was recovered from 50 per cent of 16 children under the age of 1 and from 69 per cent of children between one and four years. It was not detected in persons 29 and older. Of 19 patients, nine were unvaccinated (mostly adults– four), while one was vaccinated three times, two twice and seven once.

Flies were extremely prevalent, commonly crawling on garbage and fæces scattered outside the homes. The authors demonstrated that vaccination did not prevent infection or produced an intestinal immunity, since over 50% of the children vaccinated three or more times were found to be excreting type 1 poliovirus. There was no evidence of a common source of infection. 90% of individuals tested had neutralising antibodies against all three poliovirus types, irrespective of vaccination status. Considering the above-mentioned circumstances, it is quite clear that vaccination was responsible for this epidemic in the Indian community.

Ashkenazi and Melnick (1962) described an induced latent infection of monkeys with vacuolating SV40 papova virus. They wrote that like other papova viruses, SV40 can establish latent infections. The virus has infected and transformed human cells, even producing chromosome changes in them. In hamsters, huge fibrosarcomas, larger than the host individual, are produced.

The authors induced a latent infection by a variety of routes in African primates with vacuolating SV40 virus. Virus was recovered from the urine of all four baboons inoculated parenterally, but not from three baboons infected by intranasal or oral administration of the virus. Kidney biopsies were obtained three to eight months after infection, when virus was no longer recoverable from the urine. The latent infection developed and the virus was recovered in four out of five previously positive monkeys in a second biopsy six to eight months after infection.

Black and Rowe (1962) described changes in morphology and growth characteristics by SV40 in human tissue such as buccal mucosa, skin and human embryonic kidney cultures. During the experiment, by the 18th to 20th day, a small number of multinucleated cells 2- 4 times the size of normal cells were seen in the inoculated tubes. During the first 30 days after inoculation, slow "non-specific" degeneration of all cellular types occurred. By the 34th day cellular proliferation and progressive increase in acidification was observed in the virus-inoculated tubes. During the next 30 days these areas spread over most of the glass which was covered by tissue culture medium. In places, the cell sheet was several layers thick.

From about the 50th to 55th day after inoculation, parts of the sheet underwent necrosis followed by re-growth of epithelial tissue. This resulted in patches of epithelial re-growth alternating with areas of fibroblastic tissue growing in a disorganised, criss-cross fashion.

When these altered cells were transplanted into hamsters 4-6 weeks old they produced local tumours in 3-4 weeks. Qualitative as well as quantitative chromosomal changes were also noted in response to SV40 infection.

 # excerpt from Robert S Mendelsohn MD book reference from page 182.

8
If This Is Preventive Medicine, I'll Take My Chances with Disease

A fellow doctor once wrote and asked me how the medical profession "might play an inspirational and practical role in the quest for world peace."

My answer was: "Go out of business."

We've already seen what a disaster curative medicine has become, but so-called preventive medicine is just as dangerous. In fact, the juggernaut of Modern Medicine's drive for power over our lives is preventive medicine. It's no secret what mayhem power-hungry institutions—including governments—can get away with hiding behind the intention of "preventing" trouble. Modern Medicine gets away with even *more*. For example, the Defense Department explains the billions it spends by forwarding the old "we're protecting you from camels" routine. Though a great portion of those billions is no doubt wasted money, at least the Defense Department can point to the virtual absence of camels as evidence that *some* of the money is spent on worthwhile activities.

Modern Medicine can't even make that claim. There's no way

141

anybody can justify the billions of dollars we spend every year on "health care." We're not getting healthier as the bill gets higher, we're getting sicker. Whether or not we have national health insurance is, at best, irrelevant and, at worst, one of the most dangerous decisions facing us in the years ahead. Because even if all doctors' services were free, disease and disability would not decrease.

I wonder if we can really expect anyone to ask whether more of what we already have too much of will do us any good. Modern Medicine has succeeded in teaching us to equate *medical care* with *health*. It is that equation which has the potential to destroy our bodies, our families, our communities, and our world.

We've already seen how much of what Modern Medicine describes as "preventive" medicine is not only ineffective but dangerous. The sacrament of the regular physical exam exposes you to the whole range of dangerous and ineffective procedures. From this "act of faith" you receive the absolution of the priest—if you're lucky. First you have to give him a full confession, a complete and honest history including things your wife and best friends don't even know. Then he'll pass the ceremonial stethoscope over your vital parts—a stethoscope that has a good chance of not working properly. The doctor will check your orifices, further the humiliation by having you give a bottle of urine to the nurse, hit you ceremoniously on the knee with a rubber hammer, and pronounce you saved!

Or write out your penance in Latin.

Or—if your sins have been legion—send you to a specialist for really sophisticated punishments.

Screening programs could be called a Comedy of Errors if the results weren't so often less than funny. The tuberculin test, for example, was originally very valuable as a method of identifying people who required further investigation for tuberculosis. But the current very low incidence of tuberculosis means that the test has instead become used as a method of "preventive management." This means that in order to prevent the possible one case out of 10,000 or more, potent and dangerous drugs such as INH are given for months and months to people who are so-called "primary reactors." There is also considerable psychological damage that can result when a person becomes a social pariah because friends and neighbors find out that he or she is a positive reactor. Doctors now have to caution mothers against letting neighbors and even relatives know that a child has had a positive tuberculin test, since the test doesn't usually indicate communicability in a child.

If you follow the sounds of medical-governmental drum-beating in favor of a "preventive" procedure, you'll more often than not find yourself in the midst of one of the Church's least safe and effective sacraments. For instance, with some immunizations the danger in *taking* the shot may outweigh that of not taking it!

Diphtheria, once an important cause of disease and death, has all but disappeared. Yet immunizations continue. Even when a rare outbreak of diphtheria does occur, the immunization can be of questionable value. During a 1969 outbreak of diphtheria in Chicago, four of the sixteen victims had been "fully immunized against the disease," according to the Chicago Board of Health. Five others had received one or more doses of the vaccine, and two of these people had tested at full immunity. In another report of diphtheria cases, three of which were fatal, one person who died and fourteen out of twenty-three carriers had been fully immunized.

The effectiveness of the whooping cough vaccine is hotly debated all over the world. Only about half of its recipients benefit, and the possibility of high fevers, convulsions, and brain damage is too high to ignore. So great are the dangers that many public health authorities now prohibit the use of the vaccine after age six. Meanwhile, whooping cough itself has almost completely disappeared.

Whether or not the mumps vaccine is advisable is also in doubt. While the vaccine definitely lowers the incidence of mumps in those who receive it, it does so at the risk of exposing them to the dangers of mumps later on after the immunity has worn off. Furthermore, diseases such as mumps, measles, and German measles—for which vaccines have been developed over the past few years—don't have the dread implications of smallpox, tetanus, and diphtheria. Contrary to popular belief, measles cannot cause blindness. Photophobia, which is merely a *sensitivity* to light, can be treated as parents years ago did: by pulling down the windowshades. Measles vaccine is supposed to prevent measles encephalitis, which is said to occur in one out of 1,000 cases. Any doctor who has had decades of experience with measles knows that while the incidence may be that high among children who live under poverty and malnutrition, among well-nourished middle and upper class children the incidence is one in 10,000 or even one in 100,000. Meanwhile, the vaccine itself is associated with encephalopathy in one case per million and more frequently with other neurologic and sometimes fatal conditions such as ataxia (discoordination), retardation, hyperactivity, aseptic meningitis, seizures, and hemiparesis (paralysis of one side of the body).

German measles or rubella vaccine remains controversial in that there is little consensus regarding the age at which people should be immunized. Vaccine for rubella may also do more harm than good, since there is a risk of arthritis arising from the drug which, although temporary, may last for months. In the United States, rubella vaccine is given to children rather than to women contemplating pregnancy. It's debatable whether this does any good in protecting unborn fetuses since the rate of deformed babies born to mothers with obvious, diagnosed rubella varies from one year to the next, from one epidemic to the next, and from one study to the next.

Immunization isn't the only factor determining whether or not a person contracts a disease. Numerous other factors such as nutrition, housing, and sanitation all figure strongly. Doubts persist as to whether the whooping cough (pertussis) vaccine has really had much to do with the decline in that disease—as well as to whether the vaccine would pass Food and Drug Administration standards if introduced today.

Sometimes the vaccine itself can trigger the disease. In September, 1977, Jonas Salk testified along with some other scientists that of a handful of polio cases which had occurred in the United States since the early 1970s most were likely the byproduct of the live polio vaccine which is in standard use here. In Finland and Sweden, where the killed virus is used almost exclusively, there have been no cases of polio in ten years. No one who lived through the 1940s and saw children in iron lungs, saw a president confined to his wheelchair, or who was forbidden from using public beaches for fear of catching polio, can forget the frightening spectre raised in our minds. Today, when the man credited with stamping out polio points to the vaccine as the source of the handful of cases which do exist, it's high time to question what we are gaining by using the vaccine on an entire population.

The mad vehemence of Modern Medicine is nowhere more evident than in the yearly influenza vaccine farce. I can never think about flu shots without remembering a wedding I once attended. Strangely enough, no grandparents were among the participants and no one seemed to be over age 60. When I finally asked where all the old folks were, I was told they had all received their flu shots a few days before. They were all at home recovering from the shots' ill effects!

The entire flu shot effort resembles some massive roulette game, since from one year to the next it's anybody's guess whether the strains immunized against will be the strains that are epidemic. We were all afforded a peek at the real dangers of flu vaccines when in 1976, the Great Swine Flu Fiasco revealed, under close government and media surveillance, 565 cases of Guillain-Barre paralysis resulting from the vaccine and thirty "unexplained" deaths of older persons within hours after receiving the shot. I wonder what would be the harvest of disaster if we kept as close a watch on the effects of all the other flu shot campaigns. Dr. John Seal, of the National Institute of Allergy and Infectious Disease, says, "We have to go on the basis that any and all flu vaccines are capable of causing Guillain-Barre syndrome."

Again, besides children and old people, women are more vulnerable and, therefore, more often abused by the medical profession. No good evidence exists that screening for breast cancer does anybody any good. Yet doctors have whipped the populace into such a frenzy over breast cancer "prevention" that what I can only call "Alice-in-Wonderlandish" events start to occur. Consider the suggestion that the danger of breast cancer and other female-associated cancers is so great in some families that surgical removal of breasts and ovaries should be performed as a preventive measure! Another example of this sort of "preventive surgery" is the current practice of vaginectomy (removal of the vagina) in adult women who have no symptoms but whose mothers received DES during their pregnancies. Women should be very careful what they tell their doctors about themselves or their family. You never know what he might want to remove from your body in order to "protect" you! Men, on the other hand, probably don't have to be so careful, since doctors will never start surgically removing penises to protect men from anything.

Of course, besides the fact that these "preventive measures" are ineffective and harmful, doctors do further harm by withholding information that might *really* prevent disease. I'm thinking of the four causes of breast cancer which all women *should* know about. I'd be willing to wager that very few of the women who do know these four causes found out about them from their doctor. The four ingredients in the recipe for breast cancer are: small number of children or no children at all, bottle-feeding rather than breastfeeding, use of the Pill, and use of post-menopausal hormones such as Premarin.

Another campaign carried on against women in the name of "prevention" is the widely promulgated notion that women over thirty shouldn't have children. When I was in medical school, I was taught that women should not have babies if they're older than forty-five. By the time I was an intern, it was down to forty. When I was a resident, thirty-eight. Ten years ago it was down to thirty-five. And now it's hovering between thirty and thirty-two. The reason usually given by doctors for restrictions on the age of a mother is that something happens to the eggs of a woman as she gets older, they get worn out and tired. So we have *"tired egg"* syndrome causing deformities in babies. You never hear anything about "tired" *sperms*.

Actually, age has nothing to do with whether a mother gives birth to a deformed baby. A study at Johns Hopkins revealed that the incidence of dental and medical *x-rays* in mothers who have given birth to Mongoloid children is seven times as high as in mothers of comparable age who have given birth to normal children. This study has been backed up by other studies, too, so the *real* cause of deformed babies is associated with age only in that older women—if they haven't been careful—have exposed themselves to more medical, dental, therapeutic, and largely useless x-rays.

At the other end of life, women are told not to have babies if they're too *young!* Teenage pregnancies have a bad reputation, but again, the real threat has nothing to do with the age of the mother. Teenage pregnancies get their bad reputation from the fact that most of them occur in poor women. If a middle or upper class, well-nourished and cared for teenager gets pregnant, she has as good a chance—maybe better—as anyone of having a healthy baby.

Modern Medicine's brand of preventive medicine is so dangerous that we really should abandon the term. There's nothing wrong with the idea that people should take care of themselves so that they won't get sick, but Modern Medicine's concept of prevention is as far from that as you can get. Preventive medicine performed by the Church is as oppressive and dangerous as "curative" medicine—maybe more so, since doctors *use* the shield of preventive medicine to hide any number of truly *aggressive* procedures.

In the first place, Modern Medicine does not address itself to health. Most doctors don't know how to describe a healthy person. The most they can come up with is, "This is normal." Furthermore, since the doctor can run the patient through an incredible arsenal of tests, the limits of what is "normal" are practically all-exclusive. There's always going to be *something* wrong with you, because the doctor doesn't get anything out of the situation if you're "normal," or healthy.

Public health doctors were once held by their colleagues in very low esteem. They dealt with sanitation and other basic items that tended to keep people *away* from doctors. However, since public health doctors have adopted *screening* as their primary activity, they're now held in very high esteem because they are the *procurers* of Modern Medicine. They *deliver* patients instead of keep them away.

Modern Medicine doesn't believe that a person *can* do anything about staying healthy, since doctors believe that disease is just a curse inflicted anonymously and warded off not by concrete actions but by symbolic sacraments that bear no relation to the real world.

And because Modern Medicine recognizes no sins but those against its laws, everyone comes into the world with the original sin of potential disease. Doctors *assume* you're sick until you prove otherwise. You cannot be cleansed merely by "claiming" to be healthy and symptom-free. You have to go through the exam, the proof of your immunizations, and the "confession" of your and your family's history. Doctors make judgments just like other priests. When you are questioned during the "confession," and asked whether you've ever had venereal disease, do you know what the doctor writes down if you say you've never had VD? He writes: "Patient *denies* VD." There are no other diseases that doctors are taught to write "patient *denies*."

If a doctor practices *real* preventive medicine, his patients are going to be healthier and will therefore require fewer visits to his office. You can see right away that this is as contrary as you can get to Modern Medicine's idea. The Church is primarily interested in its authority, so anything that lessens it—such as fewer visits to the doctor—is taboo. Modern Medicine thrives on disease, not health. The more frightened people become of all the disease "out there" waiting to strike them down *randomly*, the more susceptible they are to the come-ons and put-downs of Modern Medicine.

One of the mechanisms doctors use to enhance the general frenzy is the Blame The Victim game. It's *your fault* if you're sick, *not* because of disease-producing habits you developed and refused to exchange for health-producing ones, but because you didn't receive the sacraments of Modern Medicine soon enough or at all. Though a doctor will never give up and declare a patient "in God's hands" until he has exhausted his supply of potions, mutilations, and sacrifices, a patient sometimes goes all the way to God sooner than expected. Even when the worst occurs, doctors never admit that it was the sacrament that killed. Using their semantic privilege they turn it around and make it the victim's fault. *He was too far gone.*

If you believe in Modern Medicine, you believe that you never really can *expect* health. You never really know what to expect, since disease is a random process. You live in a neurotic state of tension, fear, and guilt, anesthetized against your responsibilities and powers. You are primed to be passively taken over by the nearest will stronger than your own.

The fact that patients often don't take their medicine drives doctors up the wall. Patient compliance is a very big research field, because Modern Medicine wants to improve its methods of getting patients to do what it tells them. The ideal would be a constant electronic monitoring system that would allow the doctor to keep tabs on the "compliance" of every patient, with perhaps an optional electronic buzzer or "cattle" prod to remind the patient to take his medicine. Until this kind of enforcement of doctor's orders becomes socially acceptable, Modern Medicine has to satisfy itself with keeping the flock in line through more conventional, indeed *medieval,* methods.

When enough people are radicalized by too good a look at a religion, that religion goes on the defensive and institutes a *theology.* To prevent heretics from unsettling a comfortable status quo, church fathers *freeze* the religion's beliefs and practices and invent or exaggerate the importance of already existing mythology. By harking back to previous successes, the doctor-priest glorifies contemporary practices by giving them the aura of divine revelation. Then, to protect the priest's interpretation of the divine, Modern Medicine declares itself infallible.

Argue with that and you're a heretic. Anything outside the narrow sight of Church Law, any treatment not part of standard procedure, is termed unorthodox, thereby banishing it to a netherworld of suspicion*.

I've already discussed how Modern Medicine neutralizes effective preventive action by ignoring true causes of disease. The same

*Modern Medicine has grown so corrupt that not only does its Vision fail to inspire faith and devotion, but its sacraments and symbols cannot move people to a better life. So Modern Medicine has started to become *more than defensive.* It must rely on *force* to maintain itself and grow. As its spiritual authority has diminished, Modern Medicine has grown more oppressive and violent. What was once the option of a free people is becoming an enforced obligation.

We have a Medical Inquisition.

The first, seemingly innocuous, sign of an inquisition is the selling of indulgences. By promoting the selling of indulgences, a church admits that it has lost any rightful claim on people's imaginations and hearts. When you can *buy* your blessings, a religion motivates you not to good works but to whatever will allow you to purchase your place in "heaven."

mechanism by which we are taught that heart disease is a matter of chance rather than diet and lifestyle is also used to divert our gaze from other causes of disease, namely, *political* causes.

Most of the diseases which are killing us nowadays are the result of "pollution" of our physical, political, economic, community, family, and individual psychological environments. True preventive medicine cannot ignore these issues when addressing a problem of health, yet doctors declare the problems strictly medical, thus solvable through the sacraments of the Church of Modern Medicine.

One of my favorite examples of this process is lead poisoning. Doctors are taught in medical school that the cause of lead poisoning is *pica*. Pica is defined as any abnormal appetite for non-food substances. In this case, the offending substance is lead. Where do the children get the lead? From windowsills and various parts of a building where paint is peeling. As long as we believe that, we don't recognize the root cause of lead poisoning, which is that *the child is eating paint off the windowsills because there's no food in the refrigerator.* Even in the days of interior lead-based paint, middle and upper class children never got lead poisoning. Why should they eat paint? They can go to the refrigerator when they're hungry!

If we are allowed to see the real cause of lead poisoning as hunger, we either must write off the children in danger or decide to address the problem at its roots, since the medical treatment of lead poisoning is mostly ineffective and often dangerous. Once you decide to get at the roots of the problem of lead poisoning, you open a closet full of medical-political skeletons. After you look at hunger, you have to look at lead in the air from fuel burning, lead in toothpaste,

The Church of Modern Medicine passed that point long ago. Medical insurance is the doctor's version of indulgences. Whereas most traditional religions never demanded more than ten percent, the Church of Modern Medicine's price tag on its blessings and sacraments increases faster than anything else in the marketplace. You buy *future blessings* because Modern Medicine tacitly admits it can't maintain your health, so you're going to need these blessings someday. This lets the doctor off the hook and puts you on it. The doctor can't lose and you can't win, because you're tricked into believing that you're going to get sick no matter what you do. What a way to go through life! What a spiritual inspiration!

Besides, medical insurance has accomplished little in terms of protecting the patient. After all, considering the deductibles, a hospitalized patient today is likely to spend just as much money as a few decades ago before insurance. The almost exclusive effect of medical

and lead in baby formula. It's so much simpler to blame the mother for letting the child suck on paint. Of course, it also makes the political climate much more amenable to the growth of Modern Medicine.

Medical sanction and promotion of birth control at all costs and small families doesn't serve any proven medical purpose, but it sure serves the interests of the industry-government complex. Once again, women and children are on the wrong end of the process. Many women *must* work in an outside job merely to make ends meet in the household. That strikes me as a political-economic problem more than anything else, since the head of a household—man or woman—should be able to support the family without the other adult having to go to work. Facing *that* problem requires taking on some of the basic inequities of our society. So we call in the doctors to medicalize the situation. Since large families require a mother (or father) to stay around the house longer before going to seek employment, doctors declare small families better than large ones. Then, doctors supply the apparatus needed to keep families small and put less strain on the institutions that like to maintain economic and political control, institutions that would have to yield some power if it suddenly became an issue that one wage-earner per family was simply not enough anymore.

Large families require more *time* and *money*, but they also provide a *support* for their members, which ultimately makes them more independent of the government and the industrial employer. If a man has brothers, sisters, aunts, uncles, and parents close-by, he can count on their support if conditions on the job make working more unhealthy than not working. But when the family is small and iso-

---

insurance has been to enhance the income of the providers.

Like the medieval Inquisition, the Medical Inquisition assumes you're guilty. External acts of health will not sway your doctor. The fact that you can run marathon distances will only make your doctor suspicious of you, and won't convince him that you're healthy. He's more likely to warn you against hurting yourself. Also like the medieval Inquisition, all your business with the Church is secret—even from you. Try getting copies of your medical records.

The medieval Inquisition was not accountable for its actions. Neither is the Medical Inquisition. If the medieval Inquisition executed or tortured a witness to death, no matter. There was probably something sinful about him anyway. If in the course of your treatment your doctor kills you because of stupidity, negligence, or just plain malevolence, your family will need the best lawyer money can buy to have a chance of getting justice. If your

lated from relatives, there is no such cushion at home. The nuclear family best serves the interests of the employer, since the worker has enough responsibility to require employment, but not enough to motivate him to exceed the limits acceptable to industry. When the *home* is strong, however, job, hospital, and government have less chance of appropriating the will of the people. Doctors promise a woman "liberation" from her biology, but deliver her into the hands of far less considerate slavers. Doctors don't really address the problem of what causes cancer. They declare a "War on Cancer" which is a futile assault on symptoms. Identifying the pollution of our air, water, food, and lifestyle would require the same kind of political action Modern Medicine mustered to elevate immunizations, fluoridation, and silver nitrate to the level of Holy Waters enforced by law.

Because Modern Medicine is the Church of Death, the stronger its influence on society, the worse off all human elements will be. A public order brought about through the tools of Modern Medicine will resemble the peace of the cemetery. Wherever Modern Medicine gains significant influence in the life of a community, that community is more often than not harmed rather than helped. Government food programs dictated by nutritional experts, for example, assault minority communities by forcing them to eat "standardized" American food, which may be intolerable to their habits as well as their biology. In school lunch programs and nutrition programs for older people, little attention is paid to cultural, familial, or religious food traditions. Modern Medicine simply says that everybody needs the Big Four: vegetables and fruits, grains, meats, and dairy products. We know, of course, that many cultures cannot tolerate cow's milk because of enzymatic deficiencies. We also know that

---

doctor kills you because the recognized sacred treatment he uses on you is bogus though no one will admit it, then the best lawyer in the world won't be able to get justice. This happens thousands of times each day.

Most people have some idea of the dictionary definition of the Inquisition: the detection and punishment of heretics. What isn't obvious in the definition is that the Inquisition was actually a very effective tool for enforcing Church law and maintaining the Church as a cultural and political force. The effect was to keep the Church a potent force in people's lives and the life of the culture. You just couldn't get from one end of life or society to the other without paying your dues to the Church.

Try getting from one end of life to the other without paying your dues to Modern Medicine. No one passes through without being dipped or splashed with the already men-

traditional cultural diets are quite nutritious, since they have developed over hundreds of years of adaptation. American nutritional habits, however, are dictated by a variety of considerations, some of which are healthy, but most of which are not.

Communities also are damaged by mass screening programs designed to isolate carriers of certain racially-associated diseases. Screening for Tay-Sachs disease has been controversial within the Jewish community because of its effects on the morale and behavior of anyone who is identified as a carrier. The same is true within the black community, which must endure the invasion of community health officers screening for sickle cell anemia.

The first ingredient in my recipe for turning a healthy community into a slum is to build a hospital right in the middle of it. Once the hospital has established a beachhead, Modern Medicine can launch its first attack, which is against the family. If I were out to destroy family ties among the poor, the first thing I would do is hospitalize them for childbirth and make sure they gave their children formula instead of breastmilk. At the University of Illinois Hospital about thirty years ago, ninety-nine percent of the new mothers were breastfeeding. Today it's down to one percent.

Next, I would institute family planning in poor neighborhoods. I'd hire a whole bunch of poor people to teach contraception to other poor people. The federal government started to do all this twenty-five years ago with the intentions of preventing illegitimacy and venereal disease. What has been the result after twenty-five years? The poor people have more illegitimacy and venereal disease than ever before, and family ties are weaker.

The next thing I want to do, once I've softened them up with

---

tioned four Holy Waters of Modern Medicine: immunizations, fluoridated water, intravenous fluids, and silver nitrate. All four of these substances are of questionable safety and value—objectively speaking. Nevertheless, Modern Medicine has elevated them to the sacred. To the faithful, not only do these substances carry great power, but it is "taboo" to question or tamper with them. They are to be treated only with reverence, and they are *maintained* in their holiness by *civil law* as well as the Church of Medicine's law.

An Inquisition makes it easier for a church to discredit and disenfranchise competing churches, simply by declaring the competition's rituals to be heresy. Any group of people, ideas, or practices that can affect health is attacked, including traditional religions and the family.

Inquisition gives Modern Medicine the power it needs to prosecute the competition

forays of infant formula and family planning, is to make the inhabitants of poor neighborhoods—black people—feel inferior. So I institute a sickle cell anemia screening program which identifies one out of seven blacks as carriers. Then I reassure the carriers just as I reassure people with functional heart murmurs, that it doesn't mean anything to be a carrier. Of course, they don't believe it for a minute. They are convinced they've got "bad blood," so they have to be careful about whom they marry, and they let it weigh them down for the rest of their lives.

So much for the poor neighborhoods.

Doctors make sure other segments of society remain poor, too. Discrimination against old people begins with the "curse" on them, which says they will necessarily decline in all talents and abilities which make people worthwhile members of society. Thus medically cursed, the old person is forced to retire and become a ward of the state, or—better still—a ward of the Church as an inmate of a rest home.

Of course, the ultimate goal is that we would *all* become wards of Modern Medicine. Doctors exhibit a dangerous tendency to take advantage of every opportunity to *force* individuals to do things just for the sake of doing them. If doctors didn't want more and more power over the individual, why would more and more medical procedures be showing up as laws? Why should you have to fight with a doctor in order to have your baby at home, breastfeed it, send it to school, or treat its illnesses in any manner you believe effective?

with the force of law behind it. If a doctor "suspects" a child had been the victim of child abuse, the state has given the doctor the power to incarcerate the child in the hospital. What is there to prevent the doctor from suspecting child abuse in any number of situations where the doctor's power is threatened? A lot of people are currently getting around the immunization laws by forging the records or by taking advantage of slack enforcement by school officials. What would happen if both sides got tough at the same time, if the parents publically refused to *submit* and the school refused to *admit?* What's to stop the doctors from accusing the parents of child abuse and taking the children away from them, or, at least, fining them punitively?

In return for the power granted the Inquisition by the state, Modern Medicine does an enormous favor for the state by medicalizing problems that are not medical at all. As John McKnight, Professor of Communications Studies and Associate Director of the Center for Urban Affairs at Northwestern University, has said in his essay "The Medicalization of

I'm not too surprised that normally alert and powerful organizations like the labor unions and the American Civil Liberties Union haven't responded to this threat against our freedom. They fail to acknowledge the problem because they subscribe to the religion of Modern Medicine. Instead of saying that every person is entitled to *not* have an x-ray or an abortion, they say the opposite. They won't notice when the Church requires first older mothers, then all mothers, to submit to amniocentesis to rule out birth defects. They won't notice when the Church forces these mothers to have abortions, either. And when your turn before the Medical Authorities comes up—who knows what for? Maybe you'll need preventive surgery—you'll stand alone.

Whenever a revolutionary group adopts a word, the reactionary group coopts it. This is precisely what Modern Medicine has done with the term "preventive medicine." By making a distinction between preventive medicine and other forms of medicine, the Church controls the concept and *legitimizes* its own obsession with crisis medicine.

If they want to call what they're doing preventive medicine, let them. But let's not call anything *we* do preventive medicine. On the other hand, if they want to label revolutionary procedures according to their own interests, that's OK, too. You can be referred to as child abuser for encouraging mothers to have their babies at home. If necessary, instead of fighting over the words, you should be perfectly willing to be identified as a child abuser. If somebody says

Politics," "The essential function of medicine is the medicalization of politics through the propagation of therapeutic ideology. This ideology, stripped of its mystifying symbols, is a simple triadic credo:

1. The basic problem is you.
2. The resolution of your problem is my professional control.
3. My control is your help.

"The essence of the ideology is its capacity to hide control behind the magic cloak of therapeutic help. Thus, medicine is the paradigm for modernized domination. Indeed, its cultural hegemony is so potent that the very meaning of politics is being redefined. Politics is (usually) interactive—the debate of citizens regarding purpose, value, and power. Medicalized politics is unilateral—the decision of the 'helpers' in behalf of the helped."

that breastfeeding ties down mothers and increases the child's dependency, say you're in favor of mothers being tied down and of children being dependent on their mothers. If anybody says that people who want their food to be pure and natural are nuts, faddists, and extremists, refer to yourself and your friends as nuts, faddists, and extremists. Modern Medicine may label unorthodox doctors as quacks; maybe what we need is more "quacks." Words aren't important. Action is. And the kind of action that's required is nothing less than the destruction of the Church of Modern Medicine.

Across the country there are hundreds of brilliant people performing research on ways to fight and prevent killer diseases such as cancer and heart disease, but because their ways aren't orthodox, they must tread on very light feet if they don't want to be hounded out of town by the Church. Witness the denial of funds to Nobel Laureate Linus Pauling, who simply wanted the National Cancer Institute to grant a modicum of funds to find out if ascorbic acid really provided some benefit for cancer patients—which his earlier research indicated. Witness the fact that more than one doctor I have spoken to has admitted that he would use outlawed cancer therapies on himself or his family. Is this the kind of system you can work within?

People should work to liberate themselves completely from Modern Medicine. It will take an army of heretics with firm resolve to be free of Modern Medicine and with the courage, cunning, and resources to reconstruct society's attitudes towards health and disease.

What's needed is a New Medicine, a new vision of medical care.

From the inventor J Sherridan. Refer to Entelev product information, page 208

> pathway of energy flow and energy production in the respiratory system to: (a) cause a cancer, or (b) cure a cancer.[1]

Jim Sheridan was profoundly affected by the guidance he felt he had received in this dream. As Jim, himself, wrote:

> When I woke up, I felt that I had received my MARCHING ORDERS. 3 years later I bought my first mice and I was on my way in my basement lab. The suggested cure was to make the cancer cell even more primitive – to the point where the cancer cell would lyse.[2]

(The terms "redox", "lyse" and "respiratory enzymes" will be explained in upcoming pages.)

Jim Sheridan dedicated himself to pursuing the goal put forth in his afternoon dream of 1936. It took him many years of hard work and trial and error to develop his formula fully. In fact, he actually worked on the formula from the 1930's until the 1990's. Most of that time, Jim worked on "the project" (as he called it) out of his home after hours, or whenever he had some spare time. He made his living by being employed full-time doing other work. At first, Jim was employed as a chemist at Dow Chemical Company. While working there, he studied law and passed his bar exam, eventually becoming a patent attorney. In 1946, Jim left Dow Chemical to practice law.

At this point, Jim was able to fully stock his laboratory at home where he continued to develop his formula, using mice for testing. He never stopped working on "the project", as he called it. By the early 1950's, he was able to get a private grant to work at the Detroit Cancer Institute where he further improved his formula in a more formal laboratory environment. Jim Sheridan began getting 70-80% positive results on the mice cancers he treated. He kept working on and improving his material and by 1983, he felt that he finally had a formula which could consistently cure about 80% of the cancers it was used on.

Jim Sheridan originally named his product "Entelev", which stems from the classical Greek phrase "Entelechy" (pronounced enteleekee). Jim's understanding was that "Entelechy" translated as "that part of man known only to God", and he added the letters "EV" to represent "electro-valence". Thus, he created the name "Entelev" to mean "the electrovalence of man known only to God". The electrovalence part will be explained in the next section as we look at the theory behind Jim's formula.

Theory

To understand the theory behind Sheridan's formula, we start with the concept that all cancer cells are primarily anaerobic. Cancer cells are not the *only* type of anaerobic cell found in the body, however. In other words, we can have *other* types of anaerobic cells that are not necessarily cancer cells. But any human cell that is anaerobic is unhealthy, or abnormal, and these unhealthy anaerobic cells tend to be involved in illnesses of various sorts. Jim Sheridan believed that cancer cells form from some of these anaerobic cells.

In a nutshell, this is how Protocel works. When a person takes Protocel regularly every day, the formula biochemically lowers the voltage of every cell in the body *just a little bit.* (Actually, for those with technical backgrounds, the more accurate term is "capacitance", but most people understand the term "voltage" better.) This results in a voltage reduction of about 10-15%, and Protocel accomplishes this by depleting ATP energy. Because anaerobic cells obtain their energy by fermentation of glucose, or "glycolysis", instead of by oxidation like normal cells, they operate on a minimum energy level and sustain a lower voltage than normal cells. The slight reduction in voltage caused by Protocel shifts the cancer cells downward to a point below the minimum that cancer cells need to remain intact. When this happens, the cancer cells (as well as other anaerobic cells of the body) break down, or "lyse", into harmless protein. In other words, they cannot hold themselves together anymore and they simply fall apart!

Normal healthy cells of the body, on the other hand, sustain such a high voltage level that the slight reduction in voltage promoted by Protocel does not hurt them. This is why Protocel is deadly to cancer cells but harmless to the rest of the body.

The details of how this happens are somewhat complicated, but the following is a simplified explanation of how Protocel works, using an analogy to "car batteries".

One could say that all the cells of the human body are somewhat like little car batteries in the sense that they must manufacture and deliver energy throughout the cell so that the cell can perform its important functions. This process of producing and distributing energy in each cell is called "cell respiration". (Most of us think of respiration as the process of breathing oxygen, but on a cellular level, the term "respiration" refers to the acquiring and distributing of energy for the cell, not about breathing oxygen.) Every cell in the body can only grow, divide and carry out its specific functions as long as the cell can continue to get sufficient energy to support these functions. This could be likened to how the battery in a car can continue to do it's job only as long as the engine is kept running to resupply the battery with the energy that continually gets used up. If the supply of energy to the car battery is cut off while the energy from the battery is still outgoing, as when a person turns the engine off but leaves the lights on, then the battery energy reserves will be used up and the car battery will eventually "die".

Though human cells are somewhat like car batteries, they are also infinitely more sophisticated. So, when *more* energy is being used up than is getting supplied to the cell through respiration, the cell doesn't immediately "die". Instead, it tries to compensate by transforming itself to need less energy. It does this by making changes in its respiration.

To understand this, we need to know that, central to the respiratory system of each cell, there is something called the "oxidation reduction system". Scientists often refer to this as the "redox system". Though every cell in the body has a redox system, there are gradations of how advanced, or efficient, this redox system is in various types of cells. These gradations could be looked at as the steps on a ladder. Different types of cells in the body could then be represented as different points on this ladder. In Sheridan's own words,

> The oxidation reduction system can be thought of as a ladder, with a different chemical reaction taking place on each step. The respiratory reaction which takes place on each step of this ladder is the same as on every other step in what it produces (i.e. energy for the cell to do its work), but each step is also different from every other step in the sense of how effective the reaction is.
>
> The bottom steps of the ladder involve relatively simple or 'primitive' respiratory reactions. An example of a primitive reaction would be yeast while it is fermenting. Keep in mind that this is still an amazingly complex reaction. It is only 'simple' or 'primitive' compared to the other reactions in the oxidation-reduction system.
>
> The higher steps involve more complex respiratory reactions. The primitive reactions at the bottom of the ladder take place without oxygen being present. The higher respiratory reactions require the presence of oxygen. Generally, for 'reduction' you are moving down the ladder. For 'oxidation' you are moving up the ladder.
>
> Each 'step' on this ladder has a different 'potential'. 'Potential' means a measurable *electrical voltage*, like a small battery would have. Primitive yeast cells which are fermenting will give off a certain amount of electrical energy, i.e. movement of electrons. (We are talking about very *small* amounts of electrical energy.) As you move up toward the top of the ladder you will get increased potential energy. Thus, the potential electrical energy at the top of the ladder is greater than at the bottom. The top of the ladder has a potential of about +0.4 volts while the bottom is about -0.2 volts.[3]

Thus, a normal, healthy aerobic cell would be represented high on the ladder, and anaerobic and primitive cells would be represented lower on the ladder.

According to Jim Sheridan's theory, a healthy cell will maintain a balance of ingoing and outgoing energy and will remain over time in its same position on the redox ladder hierarchy. Short-term drains of energy on cells are usually no problem, and cells can normally regain their balance without serious difficulty. But just like a car battery, if there is a *long-term*, severe drain on the energy of a cell, then there can be a serious problem. In a *chronic* energy drain situation, the balance point of the cell's respiration system will eventually be affected to where the point of balance *will be forced to occur at a lower oxidation reduction level for the cell to survive.*

When this energy balance point is forced to go lower, the cell could be said to move down the redox ladder. And it can continue to move down the ladder until it hits what Jim Sheridan called a "critical point". According to Sheridan's theory, this critical point is the lowest point the cell can go on the redox ladder and still retain its primary similarities to a normal cell. However, at this critical point, the cell is also now on the highest point of the ladder that could be said to apply to primitive cells. In other words, the cell that is forced to move down the redox ladder to survive can get to a point where it is, so-to-speak, straddling the fence between being "normal" and being "primitive".

This is a very interesting point for a cell to be at. At this straddling point, the cell actually becomes quite stable because it is not enough like a normal cell to be differentiated and to function normally, but it is also not enough like a fully primitive cell for the body to know how to get rid of it. It is also at this critical point where the cell may become an anaerobic cancer cell!

Jim Sheridan concluded that it would be very difficult to move a cancer cell *back up* the redox ladder and make it normal again. He devised his formula to work by taking advantage of the fact that the cancer cell sits on the critical point of the ladder, or right on the dividing line between normal cells and primitive cells. By reducing the voltage (or potential) of every cell in the body just a tiny bit, those cells that are sitting on the fence are the most affected. The reduction of potential caused by Protocel effectively reduces their respiration ability just enough to push them *down* the redox ladder to where they are fully in the primitive zone, or even past it. At this point, the cancer cells are not able to produce enough energy to survive, and they subsequently die off and are disposed of by the body. According to Sheridan, the way his formula affects cell respiration is

> . . . by shunting off 'energy units' of the cell as it is working, so the energy is not going through the respiratory system. (An 'energy unit' is two electrons and a proton). Thus, work is being done by the cell, but not respiration . . . . If work is being done, but not respiration, the cell is forced further down the oxidation-reduction ladder. Thus, once respiration is reduced, the cell is forced down completely into the primitive state.
>
> One of the chemicals which reduces respiration is catechol. The natural catechols have many different oxidation-reduction potentials (i.e. the level on the oxidation-reduction ladder where the particular catechol will work or operate.) The trick is to find one that works at the same level as a cancer cell, i.e. at that 'critical point' level.
>
> Entelev/Cancell was developed to act like a catechol, i.e. to inhibit respiration at the critical point.[4]

By following guidance that came to him in a dream, Jim Sheridan was able to develop a truly ingenious way to cause cancer cells, as well as other anaerobic cells of the body, to self-destruct!

Dr. Tony Bell is a Ph.D. chemist who understands on a detailed, technical level how Jim Sheridan's formula works. To put it in simple terms that most of us can understand, Dr. Bell explains that for each cell in the body, the voltage of the cell operates as the cement, or glue, that holds the cell together. Healthy aerobic cells operate on a much higher energy level, or voltage, than do unhealthy anaerobic cells. So, in terms of energy voltage, healthy cells have plenty of energy to spare. But, according to Dr. Bell, cancer cells sit right on the edge of the cliff in terms of voltage, and have very little to spare. When the voltage of a cancer cell is reduced by 10-15% the cell subsequently loses the "cement" that holds it together, and it breaks down into harmless protein that the body can then easily dispose of .

This process of the cancer cells breaking down is called "lysing" and it often results in a clear or somewhat yellowish, egg white-like substance. The body then processes this substance (which is really just "dead cancer cell parts") out through various elimination systems. In other words, when cancer patients use Protocel, this egg white-like material *may* come out of them through any avenue that the body uses to get rid of waste. Thus, people using Protocel for cancer will often see mucousy material in their feces and/or urine, or experience a runny nose or crusty eyes in the morning. Sometimes, people will even cough up mucousy whitish stuff. If any of this happens, it can generally be taken as a good sign since it means that dead cancer cell parts are being ejected out of the body.

One of the wonderful things about using Protocel for cancer is that, because it targets the basic respiratory system of every cancer cell, cancer cells do not seem to be able to mutate to resist it. (At least, there is no type of mutation known so far that can do this.) This is in contrast to treating cancer with chemotherapy, which cancer cells *are known* to mutate around and resist. That's why several chemotherapy agents are so often used at one time, or why sometimes a chemotherapy regimen will work for a while and then have to be replaced by a different one.

In the next section, we will look at seventeen remarkable testimonials of people who have used Entelev, Cancell or Protocel for their cancer. Dr. Bell got interested in Sheridan's formula when one of his own family members came down with cancer, and we'll start with his story first.

Case Stories

Case Story #1 -- Lung Cancer Metastasized to Brain

Dr. Tony Bell first became acquainted with Sheridan's formula (then called Cancell) when his brother, Frank, was diagnosed with cancer in 1989. Frank's cancer was non-small cell lung cancer, the type of lung cancer that smokers typically get. His doctors proceeded with treatment by first surgically removing one of his lungs. Then, in 1990, they found out that the cancer was in Frank's other lung as well, and had also metastasized to his brain. Frank's doctors administered some radiation directed at the brain tumors, but the radiation had little effect, and the tumors remained.

Shortly after the radiation treatments, Frank had a heart attack because his lung cancer had seriously stressed his heart. He survived the attack, but was too ill to undergo chemotherapy at this point. Frank's doctors sent him home and gave him about two months to live. They told the family not to worry about the cancer, because at this point it was probably Frank's heart that would kill him.

Frank then heard about Cancell and asked his brother, Dr. Bell, to look into it for him. Dr. Bell looked into it and didn't think it would work, but told his brother he might as well try it because it wouldn't hurt him. After taking Cancell for a while, Frank told Dr. Bell, "I don't know if the Cancell is working on the cancer or not, but it sure is a lot better than morphine because I'm not in any pain anymore!"

HEALTH SCIENCES INSTITUTE

Private access to hidden cures...powerful discoveries...breakthrough treatments... and urgent advances in modern underground medicine

Billion-dollar drug company nearly squashes astounding research on natural cancer killer

Colon and breast cancer conquered with miracle tree from the Amazon found to be 10,000 times stronger than chemotherapy

Since our inception in 1996, *Health Sciences Institute* has scoured the world to find cutting-edge treatments few people have access to or have even heard about. And sometimes, what we uncover startles even the medical mavericks on our board.

Two months ago, we learned about an astounding cancer-fighting tree from the Amazon that has literally sent shock waves through the HSI network

Today, the future of cancer treatment and the chances of survival look more promising than ever. There's a healing tree that grows deep within the Amazon rain forest in South America that could literally change how you, your doctor, and possibly the rest of the world think about curing cancer.

With extracts from this powerful tree, it may now be possible to...

- conquer cancer safely and effectively with an all-natural therapy that doesn't cause extreme nausea, weight loss, and hair loss
- protect your immune system and evade deadly infections
- feel strong and healthy throughout the course of treatment
- boost your energy and improve your outlook on life

Through a series of confidential communications involving a researcher from one of America's largest pharmaceutical companies, this ancient tree's anticancerous properties have recently come to light. Although not yet tested in human trials, the tree has been studied in more than 20 laboratory tests since the 1970s, where it's been shown to:

- effectively target and kill malignant cells in 12 different types of cancer, including colon, breast, prostate, lung, and pancreatic cancer
- be 10,000 times stronger in killing colon cancer cells than Adriamycin, a commonly used chemotherapeutic drug
- selectively hunt down and kill cancer cells without harming healthy cells, unlike chemotherapy.

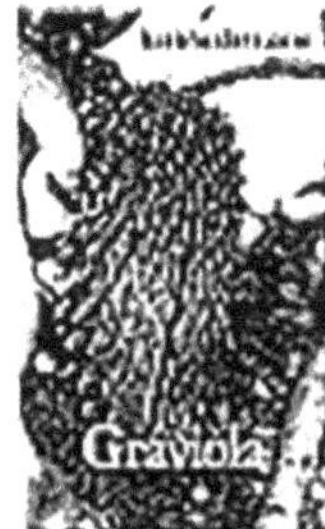

So why isn't every health publication extolling the benefits of this treatment?

Why hasn't it been made widely available throughout the natural-medicine community?

And, if it's only half as promising as it appears to be, why isn't every oncologist at every major hospital insisting on using it on all his patients?

Especially when you consider that since the early 1990s, extensive independent research—including research by one of today's leading drug companies and by the National Cancer Institute—confirms that the tree's chemical extracts attack and destroy cancer cells with lethal precision.
The answer to these difficult questions can only be explained by recounting a disturbing story we recently uncovered. More than anything else we've reported on this year, the story of this Amazon cancer treatment reinforces the need for groups like HSI and illustrates how easily our options for medical treatment are controlled by money and power.

News of this amazing tree was nearly lost forever

A confidential source, whose account we've been able to independently confirm, revealed that a billiondollar drug company in the United States tried for nearly seven years to synthesize two of the tree's most powerful anticancerous chemicals. In the early 1990s,
behind lock and key, this well-known drug giant began searching for a cure for cancer—while preciously guarding their opportunity to patent it and, therefore, profit from it.
Research focused on a legendary healing tree called *Graviola*. Parts of the tree—including the bark, leaves, roots, fruit, and fruit seeds—had been used for centuries by medicine men and native Indians in South America to treat heart disease, asthma, liver problems, and arthritis. Going on little documented scientific evidence, the company poured money and resources into testing Graviola's anticancerous properties—and they were shocked by the results. Graviola was a cancerkilling dynamo. But that's where the story of Graviola nearly ended.

Graviola is 10,000 times stronger in killing colon cancer than Adriamycin, a commonly used chemotherapeutic drug.

The pharmaceutical company had a big problem. They'd spent years trying to isolate and create manmade duplicates of two of the tree's most powerful chemicals. But they'd hit a brick wall. They couldn't replicate the original. And they couldn't sell the tree extract itself profitably—because federal law mandates that natural substances can't be patented. That meant the company couldn't protect its profits on the project it had poured millions of dollars and nearly seven years of research into.

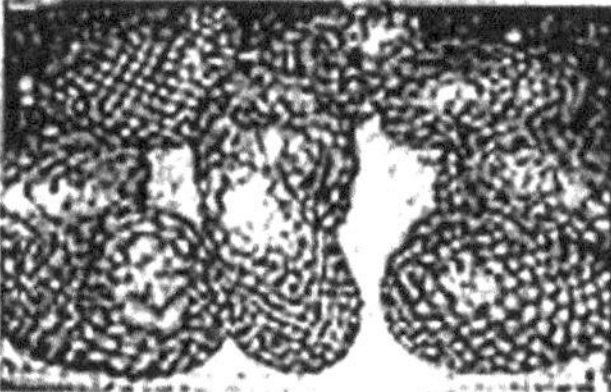

As the dream of big profits evaporated, testing on Graviola came to a screeching halt

After seven frustrating years and without the promise of lucrative sales, the company shelved the project and refused to publish its findings in an independent journal. But one responsible researcher struggled with the decision. While understanding the company's goal of profits, he couldn't accept the decision to hide this unique cancer killer from the world. Following his conscience and risking his career, he contacted Raintree Nutrition, a company dedicated to harvesting plants from the Amazon.

As a result, Raintree went into high gear and began to research related studies published on
Graviola. They discovered that several other teams in the United States (in addition to that of the drug company) had been testing Graviola in vitro (in test tubes). The results supported the drug company's secret findings; Graviola had been shown to kill cancer cells. Encouraged by these early laboratory tests, Raintree hired indigenous Indian tribes in Brazil to grow and harvest the tree. They spent a year on research and development and then began offering Graviola in the United States. They also developed a new supplement called N-Tense, which contains 50 percent Graviola as well as smaller amounts of seven other cancer-killing botanical extracts. (See page 4 for more information on N-Tense.)

Health Sciences Institute came across Graviola and Raintree Nutrition a few months ago while researching *Chanca Piedra*, a natural kidney-stone therapy from the Amazon, that was featured in our September 2000 issue. In the course of our working together, Raintree pointed us toward Graviola. And needless to say, our panels of experts were intrigued by
the possibility of this powerful natural cure for cancer.

Graviola hunts down and destroys prostate, lung, breast, colon, and pancreatic cancers... leaving healthy cells alone

Since November, we've been looking closely into the research to date on Graviola. It appears one of the first scientific references to it in the United States was by the National Cancer Institute (NCI). In 1976, the NCI included Graviola in a plant-screening program that showed its leaves and stems were effective in attacking and destroying malignant cells. But the results were part of an internal NCI report and were, for some reason, never released to the public.1

Since 1976, there have been several promising cancer studies on Graviola. However, the tree's extracts have yet to be tested on cancer patients. No double-blind clinical trials exist, and clinical trials are typically the benchmark mainstream doctors and journals use to judge a treatment's value. Nevertheless, Graviola has been shown to kill cancer cells in vitro in at least 20 laboratory tests that our research has uncovered.

The most recent study, conducted at Catholic University of South Korea earlier this year, revealed that two chemicals extracted from Graviola seeds showed "selective cytotoxicity comparable with Adriamycin" for breast and colon cancer cells. The chemicals targeted and killed malignant breast and colon cells in a test tube—comparable to the commonly used chemotherapy drug Adriamycin.2

Another study, published in the *Journal of Natural Products*, showed that Graviola is not only comparable to Adriamycin—but dramatically outperforms it in laboratory tests. Results showed that one chemical found in Graviola selectively killed colon cancer cells at "10,000 times the potency of Adriamycin."3

Graviola selectively targets cancer cells leaving healthy cells untouched. Chemotherapy indiscriminately seeks and destroys all actively reproducing cells—even normal, healthy ones.

Other promising and ongoing research at Purdue University is supported by a grant from the National Cancer Institute. Purdue researchers recently found that leaves from the Graviola tree killed cancer cells "among six human-cell lines" and were especially effective against prostate and pancreatic cancer cells.4 In a separate study, Purdue researchers showed that extracts from the Graviola leaves are extremely effective in isolating and killing lung cancer cells.5

Perhaps the most significant result of the study cited above from the Catholic University of South Korea, and of each of the others we've found, is that Graviola was shown to selectively target the enemy— leaving all healthy, normal cells untouched. By comparison, chemotherapy indiscriminately seeks and destroys *all* actively reproducing cells—even normal hair and stomach cells. This is what causes such often devastating side effects as hair loss and severe nausea. In this respect, Graviola looks to be a promising alternative or supplement to mainstream treatments.

Patient reports show Graviola and N-Tense help eliminate tumors

From a clinical standpoint, Graviola still has a long way to go. Its properties have only been studied in a test tube. That's why it has yet to become widely known and accepted. The unfortunate truth is that without the promise of huge revenues from a synthesized, patented drug, it's unlikely that any pharmaceutical company will invest the hundreds of thousands (even millions) of dollars it would take to conduct the double-blind, placebo-controlled studies on humans. This is the underlying challenge to substantiating most nutritional therapies. Fortunately, Graviola is a natural substance, so we don't have to wait around for the drug companies. And, thanks to one researcher with a conscience, Raintree Nutrition bravely took the initiative in making this promising cure available.

Only a relative handful of doctors and patients in the United States have been using Graviola and the Graviola-rich botanical supplement N-Tense to fight cancer. Still, according to Raintree Nutrition, the combined therapy has produced some incredible results.

One such case history involved an executive at a high-tech company in Texas. Daryl S. came across Raintree when exploring alternative treatments to cure his prostate cancer. A sonogram and biopsy confirmed that Daryl had more than 20 tumors in his prostate. One doctor recommended surgery. But Daryl thought a cure using this common conventional treatment would come at too great a cost. He didn't want to suffer from impotence and incontinence for the rest of his life.

Instead, he agreed to a far less invasive round of hormonal therapy (to shrink the size of his prostate) and began a rigorous supplement regimen that centered around the Graviola-rich supplement N-Tense. Within two months, Daryl's PSA level had dropped from 4.1 to 0.00. A sonogram and several other gamma-ray tests later confirmed that all the malignant tumors inside his prostate had disappeared.

Seven years of silence broken

We are continuing to work with Raintree and others conducting ongoing research on Graviola. As more scientific and anecdotal evidence comes to light, you'll be among the first to hear about it. However, after seven years of silence and hidden research, we felt it irresponsible not to bring this to you now.

Grown and harvested by indigenous people in Brazil, Graviola is available in limited supply in the United States and distributed only through Raintree Nutrition. But now, you can be among a select few in the entire country to benefit from Graviola. We encourage you, as always, to consult with your doctor before beginning any new therapy, especially when treating cancer.

You can make tea out of the Graviola leaves, obtain the herb alone in capsule form, or benefit from the power of Graviola combined with seven other immune-boosting herbs in Raintree Nutrition's N-Tense capsules.

Based on South American traditional therapies, it's recommended you take one to five grams a day. As a dietary supplement, N-Tense should be taken at 6 to 8 capsules daily.

Graviola and N-Tense are completely natural substances with no side effects apart from possible mild gastrointestinal upset at high dosages (in excess of 5 grams) if taken on an empty stomach.

Despite the mounting collection of laboratory tests and anecdotal reports about this cancer-fighting dynamo, Graviola may always remain an underground therapy!

Graviola has yet to be clinically tested on animals or humans. And because Graviola is a natural product, it can't be patented. Without the promise of exclusive sales and high profitability, it will likely never again draw the attention of a major drug company or research lab. So we may never see a double-blind clinical study on the tree that's reported to help defeat cancer.

But there's no doubt about it—the early laboratory tests and anecdotal reports about Graviola are *very* exciting. And if you've been diagnosed with cancer, you and your doctor should look at all the available treatment options. Graviola may just provide the help you've been looking for that could make all the difference in beating cancer.

Note: We are carefully tracking the success of Graviola use among our members. Please write to us describing your experiences with this important treatment.
Send to: **Graviola Project**, *Health Sciences Institute*,
819 N. Charles St., Baltimore, MD 21201.

Graviola fights more than cancer...

While the research on Graviola has focused on its cancer-fighting effect, the plant has been used for centuries by medicine men in South America to treat an astonishing number of ailments, including:

hypertension	influenza	rashes	neuralgia	arthritis
rheumatism	high blood pressure	diarrhea	nausea	dyspepsia
ringworm	scurvy	malaria	dysentery	palpitations
nervousness	insomnia	fever	boils	muscle spasm

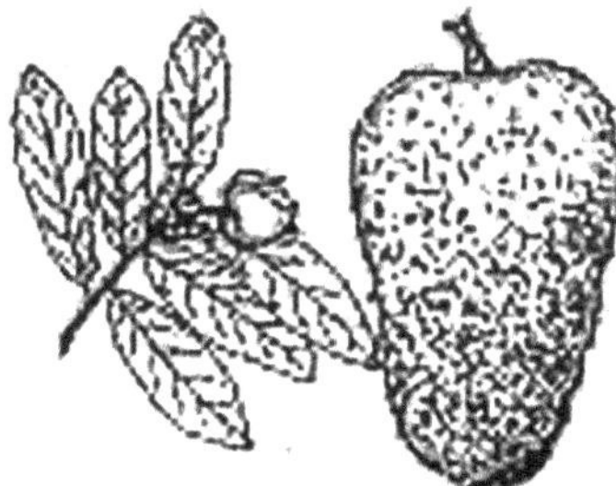

Oralmat inhibits growth of cancer cells

In January of 1999, we reported on an oral supplement from Australia called Oralmat that can dramatically improve asthma as well as a score of other ailments such as chronic allergies, viral, fungal, and bacterial infections, chronic fatigue syndrome, MS, diabetes, and Gulf War syndrome.

Our members were among the first in the world to hear about this breakthrough from the other side of the globe. After this rye grass extract was released into the mainstream market several months later, researchers and doctors began to hear anecdotal accounts of Oralmat shrinking tumors in patients. Now, they are taking a closer look at these claims.

Last year, Professor Indres Moodley, Director of Pharmacology at the University of Witwatersrand, Johannesburg began a laboratory evaluation of Oralmat's ability to combat cancer cells in vitro. While the studies are still in progress and the rye extract has yet to be tested on cancer patients, the initial results look promising. So we decided to bring you in on the ground level for this potentially powerful cancer treatment. Additionally, if the research
bears out, it could lead to a substantial increase in Oralmat's demand world wide, which is another reason why we wanted to keep you on top of this important development.

In the study, tumorous cancer cells from the breast, liver, and kidney have been injected with Oralmat. In three separate in vitro tests, Oralmat inhibited the growth and proliferation of breast and liver cancer growth by 89 percent and kidney cell growth by 55 percent.

According to Moodley, "We've tested a whole range of natural products. This one has certainly been the most active that we've had on our hands." In other words, compared to other natural substances researchers have studied, Oralmat is exceptionally aggressive in attacking cancer cells.

While a lot of further testing needs to take place, Moodley suggests that Oralmat may eventually be shown to be a safe and effective replacement for existing chemotherapy protocols.

Oralmat inhibited the growth and spread of breast and liver cancer by 89 percent and kidney cell growth by 55 percent.

Oralmat is still used primarily to relieve the symptoms associated with asthma and chronic allergies. After taking Oralmat drops for three to four weeks, asthmatics report being able to eliminate or reduce their medication. And severe hayfever and allergic rhinitis symptoms have been shown to respond rapidly to Oralmat, even within minutes of administration.

Oralmat is now also available in both cream and spray forms and can be used to treat cuts, bruises, insect bites, and other topical applications. It can be purchased without a prescription and is free from toxins and side effects.

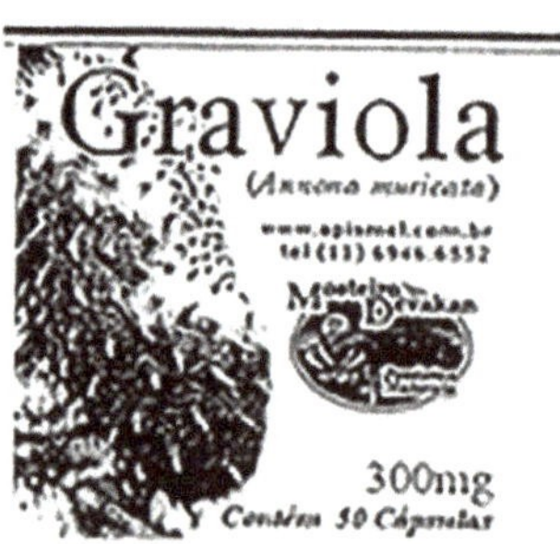

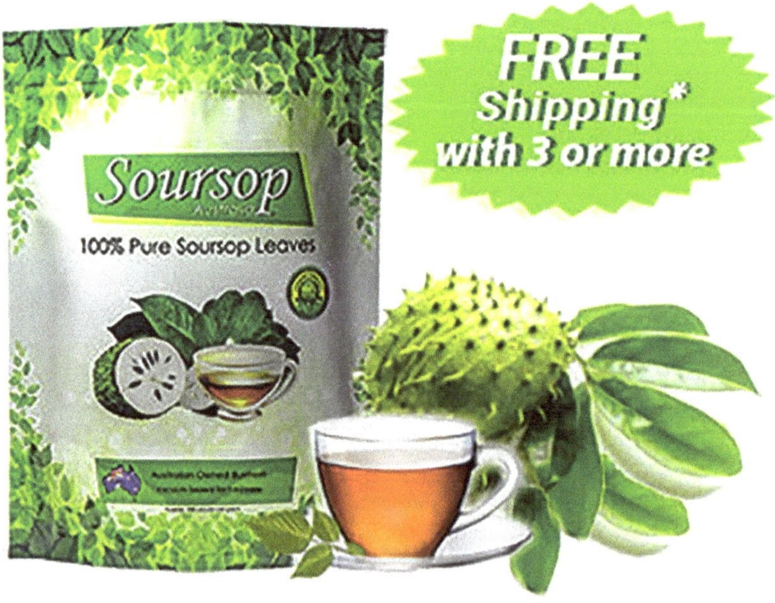

Xango Juice

What are xanthones?

Xanthones are biologically active plant phenols found in a few select tropical plants. Current research on xanthones suggests they are beneficial in helping with many conditions including: allergies, infections (microbial, fungus, viral), cholesterol levels, inflammation, skin disorders, gastro-intestinal disorders, and fatigue.

Xanthones have been found to support and enhance the body's immune system. Xanthones also exhibit strong antioxidant activity which is beneficial for neutralizing free radicals in the body.

Facts about xanthones:

- The most plentiful natural source of xanthones is the mangosteen (*Garcinia mangostana*), which contains over 30 xanthones. The mangosteen has by far the most xanthones of any plant. The pericarp of the mangosteen fruit contains the vast majority of the xanthones.
- Xanthones are some of the most potent antioxidants known. It is thought to be more potent than both Vitamin C and Vitamin E. In fact, many doctors refer to xanthones as **"Super Antioxidants."**
- Xanthones are heat stable molecules. Unlike proteins, they won't denature or lose their structure when heated.

Medical Properties of Xanthones:

Research on Xanthones is ongoing. There are many results people report about health benefits from xanthones that cannot be explained by the science yet. This is likely due to the fact that only about 15% of known xanthones have been studied to any degree.

Some of the known benefits of xanthones based on recent research are:

- Anti-Fatigue - Helps boost energy.
- Anti-Inflammatory - Helps prevent and reduce inflammation
- Anti-Aging
- Helps prevent cancer. According to a preliminary study, six xanthones have been found to be capable of killing cancer cells.
- Helps lower blood pressure

- Helps lower blood sugar. Many people with type II diabetes have reported that it helps them to regulate their blood sugar levels.
- Helps prevent infections - Bacteria, Microbes, Viruses, Fungus.
- Anti-Diarrheal - In folk medicine, the pericarp of the mangosteen (most potent source of xanthones) has been used for centuries to effectively treat dysentery.
- Anti-Parkinson, Anti-Alzheimer. Helps prevent dementia.
- Anti-allergenic - Helps with allergies
- Eye Care - Helps prevents cataracts and glaucoma
- Helps protect the heart and cardiovascular system
- Anti-Obesity

A recent study has confirmed that gamma mangostin, a xanthones derivative found in the mangosteen, is a potent COX (Cyclooxgenase) 2 inhibitor. The COX 2 enzyme is a chemical in the body that causes inflammation. This enzyme is commonly found in people suffering from joint pain and arthritis. However, it is also being found with other diseases as well, that are not as obvious, such as Parkinson's, Alzheimer's, cancer, and Diabetes. In three separate studies, a xanthones derivative of the mangosteen slowed down the body's production of the COX 2 enzyme.

Medical Uses of Xanthones

This information is based of the research of Dr. J. Frederic Templeman, M.D.

"Let Food Be Your medicine" -- Hippocrates

Here is a list of medical conditions that Dr. Templeman uses mangosteen and xanthones contained within the fruit as first line treatment in his medical practice:

- ERD (gastro-esophageal reflux disease)
- Hiatal hernia
- Diverticulitis
- Arthritis
- Sleep disorders
- Irritable bowel disease (diarrheal type)
- Fibromyalgia
- Neurodermatitis
- Fatigue
- Eczema
- Mild depression
- Muscle or joint pain without evidence of Arthritis
- Seborrhea

- Recurrent urinary tract infections in the elderly

Disclaimer: Information herein is not intended to be taken as medical advice. No therapeutic or medical claims are either implied or made. Do not alter any medical treatment or the use of medications without the permission of your medical care provider.

Here is a list of prescription medications that Dr. Templeman has replaced with mangosteen and xanthones:

- **Nexium,** Prevacid, Aciphex, & other proton pump inhibitors.
- **Zantac,** Pepcid, & other H2 blockers.
- **Allegra,** Zyrtec, Claritin, Clarinex, & other antihistamines.
- **Singulair,** Prednisone
- Lotrisone, Topicort, Cutivate, Diprolene, & other topical Cortico Steroids used for skin conditions (Eczema, Psoriasis, Seborrhea)
- **Valium,** Xanax, & other minor tranquilizers.
- Tegretol, Neurontin, & other anti-epileptic drugs used (off label) for chronic pain relief.
- **Prozac, Zoloft,** Paxil, Lexapro, & other antidepressants when used for Dysthymia & anxiety states.
- **Vicodin,** Percocet, Duragesic patch, Methadone, & other narcotics used for chronic pain control.
- **Celebrex, Vioxx,** Bextra, Naproxen, Arthrotec, Ibuprofin, & other anti-inflammatories used for Musculo-Skeletal pain & inflammation.
- Ultram, Talwin, & other non-Opiod pain preparations.
- Midrin, Fioricet, **Imitrex,** Amerge, Maxalt, Zomig, & other Seretonergil Migraine headache preparations.
- **Lipitor,** Zolor, Pravacol, & other Lipid-lowering agents.
- **Valtrex,** & other anti-herpetic agents.
- Aricept, Cognex, & other Alzheimer's preparations.
- Anusol, & other Hemorrhoid preparations

Paw Paw

www.lifetrends.co.nz

New Weapon In War against Cancer

In 1999 in New Zealand about 16,700 people were diagnosed with cancer and about 7,600 died from cancer. Cancer was the leading cause of death, accounting for 27.2% of deaths from all causes. Cancer registrations increased by 41% from 1990 to 1999, largely because of more complete reporting following the introduction of the Cancer Registry Act on 1 July 1994.

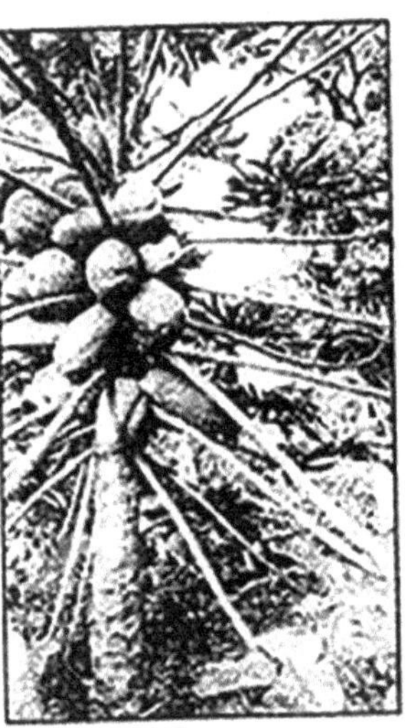

Paw Paw tree with Fruit

Although cancer can occur at any age, the chances of developing it increase as a person ages. In 1999, 64% of men and 50% of women who developed cancer were 65 years of age and older.

About 80% of all cancers are thought to be related to lifestyle or environmental factors. Cigarette smoking is responsible for about 25% of all cancer deaths. Other potentially avoidable causes of cancer include dietary factors, alcohol and sunlight.

In some cases, early detection by screening has been shown clearly to reduce deaths from certain cancers, including cancer of the breast (at least in women 50 years and over) and cervix.[1]

Cancers will attract new blood vessels to themselves to feed their runaway appetites for nutrients needed for their out-of-control growth. Cancers can even clone themselves and, travelling through the blood stream and lymphatic system, metastasize throughout the body.

Paw Paw Cell Reg contains an extract from the twits of the paw paw tree (Asimina triloba). These contain a group of plan chemicals (annonaceous acetogenins) that interfere with the cellular production of energy. Cancer cells use energy at up to 17 times the rate of healthy cells. Paw paw extract safely and selectively deprives these malignant cells of the energy they need to rapidly grow and reproduce.

Paw Paw is a fruit-bearing tree that grows in the US from Missouri and Arkansas to the Atlantic coast. Because the therapeutic ingredients of paw paw are at their peak in May, seasonal shortages are possible. Also, some groves of trees have been found to be especially potent producers and have been deliberately cultivated for the therapeutic paw paw extract.

NSP's Chief Scientific Officer, Dr. Jerry McLaughlin conducted years of research on paw paw at Purdue University. His research suggests that paw paw extract:

- Slows and stops the production of cell energy in cells by blocking the production of ATP
- Prevents the growth of new blood vessels in or near tumours
- Depletes DNA and RNA building blocks needed for cell division

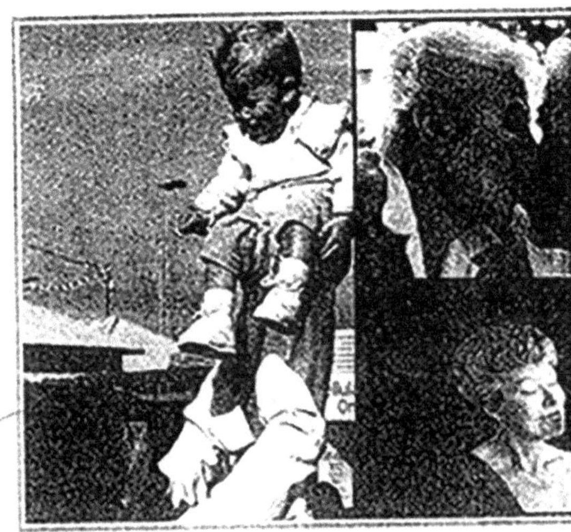

- Kills even those cells that are resistant to chemotherapy drugs
- Prevents cells from activating ATP-fuelled metabolic pumps that reject chemotherapy drugs
- Is up to 300 times more potent than Taxol, without inducing weight loss.

Benefits

- Selectively affects specific cells
- Modulates the production of ATP in the mitochondria of specific cells
- May help modulate the growth of blood vessels near specific cells
- This patent-pending product is the only standardized acetoenin product available

Paw paw extract works by blocking the production of energy in the mitochondria of cells. Mitochondria use a multistage, repeating process called the Krebs cycle to store energy as adenosine triphosphate (ATP), a high-energy molecule used to power other cellular processes.

Without abundant ATP production, the life processes of cancer cells are inhibited. Healthy cells are not such "energy hogs" and are not impacted so severely. Taking too much paw paw extract causes nausea and vomiting. This is built in protection. It is typical to feel more energy while using Paw Paw Cell-Reg as the tumour cells no longer sap the body of glucose.

This product may be used by people with actual diagnosed cases of cancer. The suggested use of Paw Paw Cell-Reg is 4 capsules per day until after remission. Use with Immune Stimulator and Protease Plus (in between meals). Dr. McLaughlin recommends adding Nature's Noni. Women with breast cancer may want to add Breast Assured. Men with prostate cancer may want to add Men's Formula. These are the only supplements to be taken during this time.

Do not use this program with products that are intended to increase the production of cellular energy. Products to avoid are CoQ10, SOD, Super Antioxidants, Grapine, Alpha Lipoic acid, Cellular Energy, Creatine, 7-Keto, Spirulina, IGF-1, Super Algae, TSII and Thyroid Activator. Also avoid the new Para-Cleanse with Paw Paw (to avoid consuming more than you intend).

Some people report a rapid, measurable response to the program. For instance, one lady saw an improvement in her CA-125 antigen (used to monitor ovarian cancer) after only one week. A patient with non-hodgkins lymphoma who had undergone 3 rounds of chemotherapy in 6' years had her white cell count and lymphocytes return to the normal range after 35 days with paw paw extract.

The Paw Paw Cell-Reg program is not used for prevention. It is intended to act against the special metabolism of active, cancerous cells. If you are currently healthy, it will only make you feel fatigued.

Do not use if you are or become pregnant.[2]

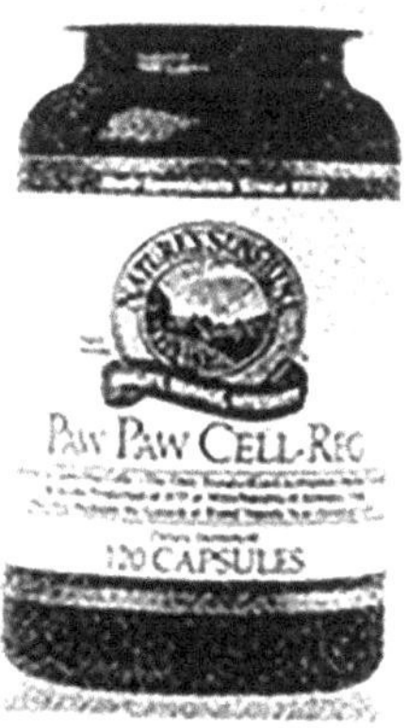

Paw Paw Cell-Reg is now available at Nature's Sunshine Products.

Stock No:	0511-3 (120 capsules)
Mem. Price (excl GST)	$33.9[illegible]
PV:	$33.[illegible]
RRP (incl GST)	$52.[illegible]

[illegible]

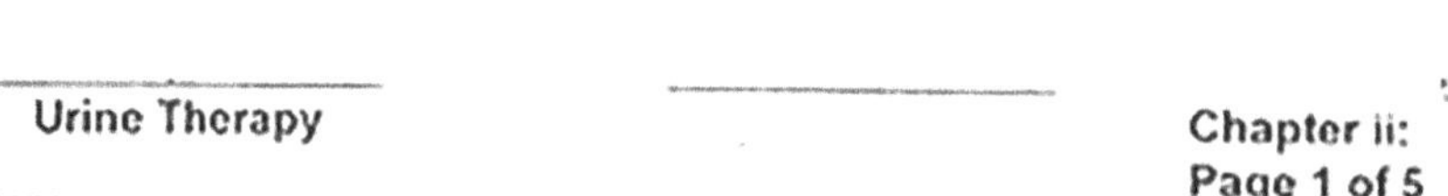

URINE & UREA Therapy
By Walter Last

I have been fond of urine therapy for many years but, except as a homoeopathic remedy, I have rarely mentioned it to patients as our social conditioning invariably prompted a strong negative reaction.

The many and varied case histories described by John Armstrong in his 'The Water of Life' are certainly impressive. However, this book was first published fifty years ago, Armstrong did not have any academic qualifications and without the strong support of other therapists, there were not many convincing reasons for patients to try this method.

This has changed dramatically in recent years with the publication of the books 'The Miracle of Urine Therapy' by Dr Beatrice Bartnett and especially 'Your Own Perfect Medicine' by Martha Christy.

Martha Christy's Experience

Martha Christy cured herself of a host of incapacitating illnesses, including intestinal inflammation or Crohn's disease, chronic fatigue syndrome, thyroid disorder, severe chronic kidney infections, food and chemical allergies and severe endometriosis.

The conventional approach with drugs and six operations did not help and probably intensified her problems. Natural therapies worked for a while, but a difficult pregnancy disabled her again and this time even the natural therapy she tried was not good enough, including $US 15,000 spent in an alternative cancer clinic in Mexico for bleeding pelvic tumours.

Most of the time she had to stay in bed until one day she was introduced to urine therapy and before long, all her health troubles were over.

Instead of just writing another 'How I Did It' book, she went to university libraries and hired a research firm to search the scientific and medical literature for publications on the use of urine and products derived from it.

She was amazed by what she found. There were not just hundreds but rather thousands of published articles. There are probably more articles published about urea, the main ingredient of urine, than about any other organic substance. Mrs Christy devoted a large part of her book to explaining and summarising this scientific and medical evidence and also provided detailed references of published papers.

In addition, she lists many testimonials of individuals as to the effectiveness of urine therapy in overcoming AIDS, Candida, Cancer, Colitis, Depression, Diabetes, Immune deficiency, Multiple Sclerosis and other diseases.

Scientific Evidence

The most amazing aspect of urine therapy is its effectiveness in such a wide range of different diseases. There are several reasons for this. For one, urine contains antibodies and immune stimulating factors against all viruses, harmful bacteria or fungi that we may harbour in our body. The researchers stated that even minute amounts of antibodies, sometimes so low that they cannot be detected with conventional methods, are effective in preventing and treating diseases.

There are reports investigating and describing the curative effects of urine therapy on a wide range of infectious, fungal and viral infections, such as hepatitis, poliomyelitis and AIDS. Urine is especially effective against allergies, auto-immune diseases and other disorders of the immune system.

To switch off an allergic reaction one must put a few drops of urine under the tongue, collected during the reaction, or the urine may be homoeopathically diluted and some of it kept in the mouth for a few minutes.

When drinking urine routinely, allergic reactions may not occur at all, thus doing away with the need to identity which substance one has been reacting to.

Curing Cancer 'Child's Play'!

Cancer, too, responds very well to urine therapy. Most effective appears to be the urine fast employed by Armstrong. His first cancer patient was a nurse who had herself cared for over fifty cancer patients. She knew that any cancer pain is mild as compared to that experienced from the regrowth commonly occurring after medical intervention.

Usually visible tumours such as with breast cancer disappeared within three weeks, but sometimes even in one week. Armstrong called curing cancer 'child's play' except if patients had already received chemotherapy or radiotherapy.

I also know personally of several cases of cancer cures exclusively or mainly due to urine therapy; sometimes the addition of urine therapy to a natural cancer program appeared to be responsible for the successful outcome.

Most of the scientific cancer reports concentrate on urine extracts of anti-cancer agents. One such extract is called H-11, another HUD, others Retine, DHEA hormone or Antineoplaston. While good results were reported with all of these, it is very expensive to treat patients in this way and the treatment would be even more effective and much cheaper if all of these cancer-fighting ingredients of urine were used together by ingesting whole urine. Surprisingly, uric acid is not just the villain causing gout, it is also a proven anti-cancer agent and rejuvenating factor. However, the crown of the cancer-fighting urine ingredients may actually belong to urea, the most common chemical in urine.

Benefits of Urea

Only recently has it been discovered that the concentration of urea in the blood has a key role in regulating at least 7 major pathways. Urea levels are low with cancer and many other diseases. The frequency of cancer and especially of multiple tumours and metastases increases greatly if urea levels are low.

Urea is not just a waste product or the end state of the protein metabolism as commonly assumed. Biochemical research has shown that urea, both from internal sources or externally supplied, is used by the body as a raw material to synthesise amino acids and proteins. This is especially important for patients with kidney failure. These deteriorate quickly on a diet containing normal amounts of protein, but do much better if the diet is extremely low in protein, below 20g per day.

Another research report states that patients with kidney failure on very low protein intake show progressive clinical improvement when receiving added urea which then becomes the main source of nitrogen for protein synthesis. Urea may thus be the main reason why urine therapy and especially urine fasts are so successful with kidney failure

I believe that it is the best and sometimes the only successful therapy. One of my patients with kidney failure continued to deteriorate on a fast of fresh vegetable juices, but was cured when fasting on urine for 2 weeks.

Another helpful factor is the role of urea as the best natural diuretic and far better than synthetic ones. This is not only important for those with deem or fluid retention because of kidney or heart weakness but especially with fluid pressure on the brain or spinal cord or in the eye with glaucoma.

With this, additional urea is important with brain tumours, stroke, meningitis and other inflammations of the brain and spinal cord. One report cites the case of a massive brain tumour reappearing 3 months after surgical removal of another brain tumour. The patient received 256ml of 30% urea. After 2 hours the tumour had completely disappeared.

When applied externally, urea has a very beneficial effect on wound healing, including infected wounds, burns and ulcerating tumours. The urea crystals may be directly packed into the wound or a strong or saturated solution may be applied. In this way, urea removes the foul odour often associated with an ulcerating tumour or other dead or putrefying tissue.

Urea Pioneer

The use of urea in cancer treatment was pioneered by E V Danopoulos, a Professor of Internal Medicine in Athens. Urea was notably effective with liver cancer and in preventing the development of metastases or secondary tumours. He used 45g of urea daily in 6 divided doses for 40 days and then 20g in 3 doses for 2 years. 45g corresponds to 6 rounded teaspoons, while 20g is about 3 teaspoonfuls. The results were published in The Lancet in 1974.

But as it happens so often with discoverers of cheap cancer cures, Danopoulos lost his position after this publication and was forced to retire. Other research has shown that the effectiveness of urine in killing microbes depends largely on its concentration of urea and is better, the higher it is in urea.

Other Beneficial Ingredients

Another important reason for the effectiveness of urine is its content of countless hormones, enzymes, vitamins, trace minerals and other valuable biochemical. Some companies make a fortune by extracting some of these substances from collected urine on a large scale. The fact is that urine is not a waste product full of harmful substances as is commonly believed, but instead a treasure-trove of just the right bio-chemicals that we need for our condition.

The main function of the kidneys is to regulate the concentration of all these countless biochemicals in our blood. Any unwanted surplus is as harmful as any deficiency. However, any hormone or enzyme removed as surplus at one time may be in short supply a few hours later. Furthermore, with advancing age, our hormone and enzyme production declines to sub-optimal levels while the kidneys become less and less efficient in retaining needed ingredients. Therefore, it greatly helps, especially with chronic degenerative diseases and advancing age to recycle these valuable hormones and enzymes.

Urine Rejuvenates

Urine ingestion is frequently praised as possibly the best rejuvenation therapy known to us. It certainly rejuvenates the hair and the skin. The youthful appearance of many Buddhist monks is ascribed to their routine urine ingestion. It seems that historically all cultures have used urine for medicinal purposes. It is praised in ancient Egyptian papyri, was used in ancient Rome, in China, India, America as well as European countries. The Journal of the American Medical Association states that in 'primitive medicine' there is scarcely a disease that has not been treated with the external or internal use of urine.

A 5000 year old Sanskrit text describes in a religious context in 107 verses the virtues of urine. In one verse Lord Shiva, the great destroyer and re-generator, says that he who drinks urine sweetened with honey is cleared of any ailment within 6 months. He attains brilliant brain power and his voice becomes melodious. One well-known urine ingredient is melatonin, the hormone of the pineal gland. It regulates our body rhythms linked to the dark-light cycle. It is produced in the night and mostly expelled with the morning urine. However it is now highly valued as protecting us from cancer and ageing. Melatonin sales in California are said to top aspirin sales. But why pay much money for just one beneficial ingredient when there are thousands for free?

Problems may arise from ingesting large amounts of urine if one takes medicinal or recreational drugs as these drugs may be recycled and cause an overdose. The same may happen if one ingests other toxic substances. However, harmful substances are not necessarily reabsorbed and may just cause diarrhoea instead.

How to Use Urine

There are various ways to use urine but generally it is advisable to start with small amounts. This is not only to get accustomed to the taste of it, but also to slow down any healing reactions. These occur commonly with methods that genuinely improve our health. Reactions may manifest as diarrhoea, vomiting, nausea or a temporary flare-up of old health problems prior to their final elimination.

Start with a few drops or a teaspoonful. These may be swallowed immediately and you may wash it down with some water or juice or eat a piece of fruit. However, with allergies and immune disorders it is more effective to leave the diluted urine under the tongue for a few minutes. An allergic reaction can best be stopped or neutralised by collecting the urine when the symptoms are worst, however in practice you try to use it as soon as you notice the first symptoms.

Some researchers suggest that the proper dose can be found by slowly putting single drops under the tongue until the taste and temperature of a drop can no longer be distinguished. This is then the neutralising dose. Each subsequent day you may double the previous dose or the number of times you take them per day until you reach your target amount or the dose that you are comfortable with. A suggested amount for general health improvement and rejuvenation are 2 or 3 cupfuls daily. More is advisable temporarily to overcome serious diseases, especially AIDS and other viral, bacterial or fungal infections, cancer and kidney diseases.

In these cases ingest about one litre, the more the better, while for a limited period, say several weeks, try to drink all or most of your urine, except in the evening so that you do not have to get up at night. However, that may only be suitable during a cleansing period, as drinking a large amount or strong urine after a meal may cause digestive upset.

My favourite way to flush the kidneys is to drink 1 to 2 litres of urine before breakfast. Start drinking all the urine when you first wake up, lets say around 5 o'clock. Then you may urinate again and drink another lot about 6.30 and then again at 8 o'clock. Either drink sufficient in the evening so that the first morning urine is not too concentrated or otherwise dilute strong urine with sufficient water. I do not use urine that is cloudy as it easily happens during a healing reaction. If the body is reasonably clean, then the urine does not taste offensive and reflects the aromas of the previous meal. The second morning urine, especially after drinking a fair amount of liquids after rising, is usually very mild and better to get accustomed to then the first morning urine.

The Urine Fast

The most powerful form of urine therapy is a urine fast which combines two of the most effective natural healing methods, urine therapy and fasting. This is the method routinely used by John Armstrong and described in his book The Water of Life. Armstrong had amazing results with this method and I also found it very effective. A main advantage of a urine fast over a water fast is a greatly increased amount of energy so that the fast can be continued for a much longer period. I believe that it is also more effective than a fast or cleanse on vegetable juices.

During the urine fast you drink all of your freshly voided urine and initially some added water to bring the daily volume to about 5 litres. However, I suggest to gradually increase the ingested amount to full intake already before starting the fast while gradually reducing the food intake to just a few pieces of fruit or vegetable salad and fresh vegetable juices. It is possible that this combination, a small amount of fresh fruit or vegetables and juices together with ingesting almost all of your urine is already sufficient to cure your problem. If after a week or two you feel that you do not make enough progress, you may then proceed with a strict urine fast for 1 -4 weeks. You end the fast by using again only a small amount of fresh raw fruit or vegetables for another week or two, gradually increasing the amount and variety of fresh food. As with all fasts or cleanses, it is important to keep the bowels moving daily. Initially I suggest using a tablespoon of Epsom salts together with a crushed clove of garlic for several mornings or evenings when starting with a greatly restricted food intake.

This will help to avoid or minimise unpleasant cleansing symptoms, such as weakness, pain or nausea. However, in many cases the ingested urine will already over-stimulate the bowels with liquid discharges and then no further action is needed. Ingest only your own freshly voided urine. Normally urine is light yellow, clear and sterile, especially if collected mid-stream, but during reactions it may become offensive and cloudy. When ingesting a large part of your urine you should check to make sure that it is not too acid. The morning urine normally is slightly acid, but during the day it should be slightly alkaline.

You can buy litmus or pH paper from a chemist. Litmus paper is red when dipped into an acid solution and blue when alkaline, neutral or pH 7 is in between both colours. With pH paper you get a colour chart to compare. If the urine remains acid during the day, which usually happens with allergies and a weak sugar metabolism or if eating much fruit, then take 1/2 teaspoon of sodium bicarbonate once or several times daily in water, but not within 3 hours after meals, until the urine remains alkaline during the day.

However, those with cancer should use potassium bicarbonate (from a chemist) instead of sodium bicarbonate. If the body is too acid, sometimes the emotions become overly sensitive with a tendency to inflammations, mouth ulcers and strong skin reactions. With cancer, oedema and infectious diseases the effectiveness of urine therapy can be increased by taking daily 1-6 teaspoons of urea (e.g. in water or juices) in divided doses; you may take 3-6 teaspoons when only a small amount of urine is ingested and progressively less with larger urine intakes, leaving it off completely when nearly half or more of the daily urine is ingested.

Homoeopathic Urine

A final possibility is to use urine in homoeopathic form. The simplest way to prepare it is as follows:
To one teaspoon of unchlorinated water add one drop of fresh urine. Shake it vigorously in a small bottle about 50 times with a sharp downward stroke. One drop of this mixture is then added to another teaspoon of water, shaken again and then the whole procedure repeated a third time. Place 3 drops under the tongue several times daily. When it is used up, wait a few days and then prepare a new homoeopathic remedy. In order to find the most effective potency add one more step to each subsequent preparation of the remedy, that is dilute it a fourth, a fifth and a sixth time and so forth. Start with such higher dilutions, say sixth potency, especially if a remedy is made from fluid such as pus derived from a diseased part of the body.

An alternative method is even simpler and recommended as an introduction to urine therapy and at times when cupfuls of urine are not tolerated.

To 1 tablespoon of morning urine add 4 or 9 tablespoons of unchlorinated water. Shake 50 times with a sharp downward stroke, and take a spoonful several times during the day; keep in the mouth for a minute before swallowing.

Homoeopathically energised remedies should not be exposed to strong magnetic or electromagnetic fields. Keep this urine remedy only lightly covered in a cool place but not in an electric refrigerator, and make up fresh daily.

Social Considerations

The main problem when starting urine therapy is our social conditioning. You may overcome that by reading and contemplating about the expected health benefits. The taste of urine is not normally offensive, except if the body is rather polluted or when fasting or with strongly concentrated urine. Therefore, dilute strong urine, start with a small and gradually increasing amounts or have a day on fruit before starting to ingest urine. Minimise salt and strong spices in the diet when on urine therapy. An easy way to drink urine or any other unpleasant fluid for beginners is by breathing only through the mouth and possibly pinching the nose until the mouth has been rinsed with water or juice or a piece of fruit may be eaten.

External Use

For skin problems such as burns, wounds, gangrene, psoriasis, eczema, dermatitis, fungus problems ageing skin as well as over inner tumours, inflammations and diseased organs a urine or urea pack or a combination of both is very effective: keep the affected area covered with a folded cloth well moistened with urine or concentrated urea solution, put another cloth or plastic sheet on top, renew several times daily. Urine becomes more alkaline when standing for a few hours and is then more effective than fresh urine for external applications. However it also smells much more and fresh urine seems to be adequate in my experience. With gangrene, dead flesh, skin infections and open cancer and ulcer sores it is even more effective to saturate the applied urine with urea, that also removes offensive odours. With weeping or suppurating wounds, especially if associated with foul odour, it is also very beneficial to cover the area with dry urea crystals.

Urine can be concentrated by leaving it for several hours in a flat dish in the sun or a warm place. This has been recommended by Armstrong for friction rubs to rejuvenate ageing skin. Armstrong also recommended urine packs over tumour sites or diseased organs in addition to rubbing the body daily for two hours with small amounts of urine.

The main problem with urine packs is the offensive odour. You may try to prevent it by sealing the pack with a good tape, such as duct tape. You may completely seal it and keep the pack moist by injecting fresh urine several times a day with a syringe.

References

Armstrong, J.W., The Water of Life. Health Science Press, Rustington, Sussex, England 1971.
Bartnett, Dr B, The Miracles of Urine Therapy, Water of Life Institute, Box 22-3543, Hollywood, Florida 1988.
Christy, M, Your Own Perfect Medicine, Future Med, Inc Scottsdale Arizona 85267,1994.
Tietze, H.W., Urine the Holy Water, Phree Books, P 0 Box 34, Bermagui South, 2546 Australia, 1996.

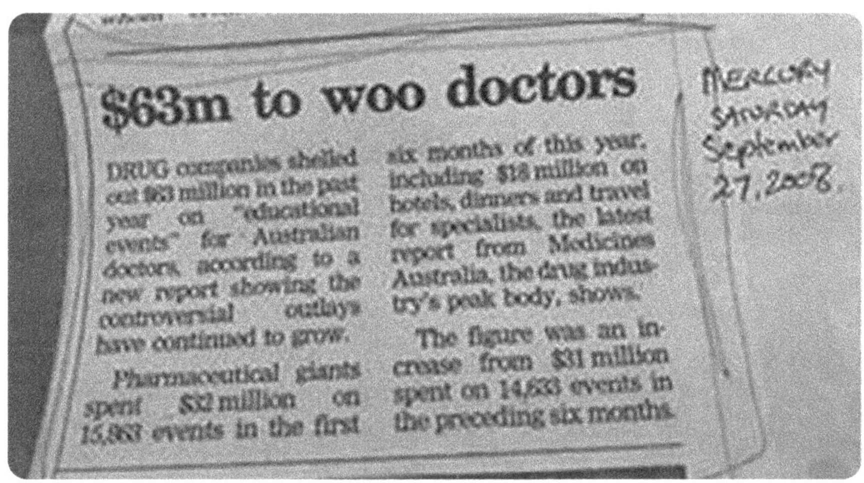

$63m to woo doctors

MERCURY SATURDAY September 27, 2008.

DRUG companies shelled out $63 million in the past year on "educational events" for Australian doctors, according to a new report showing the controversial outlays have continued to grow.

Pharmaceutical giants spent $32 million on 15,863 events in the first six months of this year, including $18 million on hotels, dinners and travel for specialists, the latest report from Medicines Australia, the drug industry's peak body, shows.

The figure was an increase from $31 million spent on 14,633 events in the preceding six months.

See full article on following page 308.

https://www.youtube.com/watch?v=4RlbKZrkgEg

Heal Squad : Cracking the Health Code w/Dr. Jack Kruse

Maria Menounos, Emmy Award Winning Journalist – With the third and final episode of conversation with Dr Jack Kruse. Discussing the complex dynamics of the medical field and electromagnetic environments, Sunlight as a transformative force for mitochondrial detoxification.

"Never miss a Sunrise for the rest of your life" is one of his encouraging phrases.

Dr Jack Kruse's Website: https://kruseatdestin.com

Dr Jack Kruse's Instagram: https://www.instagram.com/drjackkruse

Email contact: info@krusedestin.com

Pharma companies spend millions wooing doctors to prescribe 'me-too' drugs

In the last five months of 2013 alone, the manufacturers of three new blood-thinning drugs spent almost $19.4 million to encourage doctors to prescribe the drugs over a much-older one, according to ProPublica.

By Susan Perry | MinnPost contributing writer

Jan. 9, 2015

Is the drug you're taking the safest and most effective one for your medical condition, or is it a "me-too" drug — one that essentially duplicates the actions of an already existing drug, but at a higher price?

Xarelto package
Xarelto package
Bayer

As a new investigative article from ProPublica reporters Charles Ornstein and Ryann Grochowski Jones points out, pharmaceutical companies spend millions of dollars wooing physicians to prescribe "me-too" drugs to their patients. They do this, in part, with free meals and educational gifts and by hiring physicians as consultants and promotional speakers. (And, yes, although most physicians will say that small gifts, such as free meals, have no influence on *their* prescribing preferences, research suggests otherwise. Pharmaceutical companies know this; that's why they spend so much money on those gifts.)

In the last five months of 2013 alone, the manufacturers of just three new blood-thinning drugs (Pradaxa, Xarelto and Eliquis) spent almost $19.4 million on U.S. doctors to encourage them to prescribe one of those drugs rather than the much-older blood thinner Coumadin (warfarin), according to the ProPublica report.

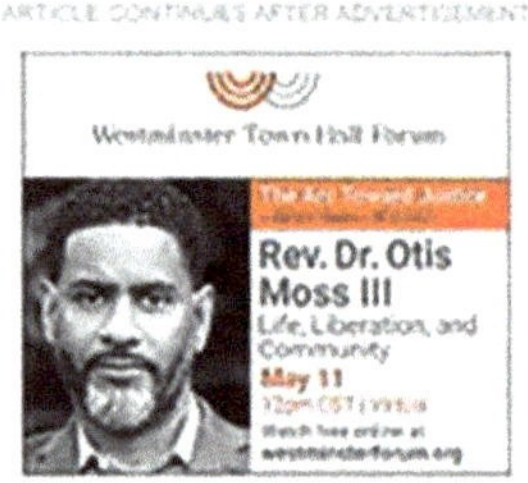

Ornstein and Jones compiled that payment information from the Open Payments database, which has come into existence because of the Affordable Care Act. Their resulting investigation provides "the first comprehensive look at how much money drug and device companies have spent working with doctors," the two reporters write. "What it shows is that the drugs most aggressively promoted to doctors typically aren't cures or even big medical breakthroughs. Some are top sellers, but most are not. Instead, they are newer drugs that manufacturers hope will gain a foothold, sometimes after failing to meet Wall Street's early expectations."

"In almost all cases, older, cheaper products are available to treat the same conditions," Ornstein and Jones add. "Companies typically try to differentiate the new drugs by claiming they are easier to use; carry fewer side effects; work faster than competitors; or have medical advantages."

Top three

According to the ProPublica analysis, the drugs associated with the most payments ($9 million) to doctors during those five months in 2013 was Victoza, a diabetes medication made by Novo Nordisk.

"Victoza, through a once-a-day injection, helps lower blood sugar among diabetics, but researchers and advocacy groups have said drugs of its class carry an increased risk of thyroid cancer and pancreatitis," write Ornstein and Jones. (A Novo Nordisk spokesperson told the reporters that the company had to spent that much money on doctors to address such safety concerns.)

Second and third on the list were Eliquis, the blood thinner (anticoagulant) co-marketed by Bristo-Myers Squibb and Pfizer ($8 million), and Brilinta, a blood thinner made by AstraZeneca.

Majority are new drugs

Among the 20 most-promoted drugs identified in this study, 14 were new drugs — approved by the Food and Drug Administration since 2010. Write Ornstein and Jones:

Majority are new drugs

Among the 20 most-promoted drugs identified in this study, 14 were new drugs — approved by the Food and Drug Administration since 2010. Write Ornstein and Jones:

> Some treat similar conditions, including diabetes, schizophrenia and chronic obstructive pulmonary disease, so the competition among them is fierce. "They're fighting over the same doctors, I guarantee you," said Rhonda Greenapple Simoff, founder of a consulting firm that advises pharmaceutical companies in Bernardsville, N.J.
>
> Largely absent from the top of the list were drugs that cure disease, such as a new class of hepatitis C treatments, or those that significantly extend life, particularly for cancer patients. If a drug is either the first to treat a disease or is much better than existing drugs, said Dr. Sidney Wolfe, the founder and now senior adviser to Public Citizen's Health Research Group, "they 'sell themselves' on the merits of their unique benefits."
>
> According to ProPublica's analysis, a few of the most heavily promoted drugs, including Samsca, which treats low sodium levels in the blood, have serious side effects that came to light after their approval by the federal government. The manufacturers of several others, including Copaxone, Latuda, Xarelto, Daliresp and Humira, have been faulted by the F.D.A. for improper promotion.

For more information

You can read the full article on the ProPublica website. (It was co-published with the New York Times' The Upshot.) The article includes a chart of the top 20 most-promoted drugs during the last five months of 2013.

In addition, you'll find a useful app on the site that can help you see how much money is being spent on doctors (and teaching hospitals) to encourage them to promote a drug you are taking. ProPublica also has a "Dollars for Docs" tool that can help you determine if your physician has received payments from a drug or medical device company.

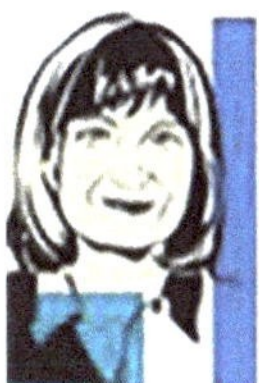

Susan Perry

Susan Perry writes Second Opinion for MinnPost, covering consumer health. She has written several health-related books, and her articles have appeared in a wide variety of publications.

ARE MOST DISEASES CAUSED BY THE MEDICAL SYSTEM?

Medical treatments, pharmaceutical drugs and decisions based on wrong information are responsible for causing an epidemic of disease throughout the western world.

by Walter Last © 2007

Website: http://www.health-science-spirit.com

I do not want to pretend that this is an impartial investigation. Instead, I am now completely convinced that most diseases are indeed caused by the medical system, and in the following pages I state my reasons for this conclusion. Increasingly over the years, my health beliefs have been turned around.

I started out by working as a biochemist and toxicologist in university medical departments, fully believing that all these chronic and incurable diseases are indeed incurable and generally of unknown origin, but that pharmaceutical drugs make life easier for patients and often are even curative. My re-education started after immigrating to New Zealand and learning about natural healing and living; this made me realise that disease is mainly caused by unnatural living conditions and can be overcome by natural methods of living and healing.

While I learned about the harmful nature of drug treatment, I was still thinking of it as being ineffective and causing side effects rather than being a main cause of our diseases. Diseases caused by medical treatment are called *iatrogenic* diseases. The total number of iatrogenic deaths in the USA for 2001 was estimated to be 783,936; these were due to fatal drug reactions, medical errors and unnecessary medical and surgical procedures. With this, the medical system is the leading cause of death and injury in the United States. In comparison, in 2001, heart disease deaths were 699,697 and cancer deaths were 553,251.[1]

This is also the reason why it is so beneficial for patients when doctors go on strike. Statistics show that whenever there has been a strike by doctors, the death rate in the affected population has fallen dramatically. In 1976, the death rate fell by 35 per cent in Bogotá, Colombia, and by 18 per cent in Los Angeles County, California, during doctors' strikes. In Israel in 1973, the death rate fell by 50 per cent during a strike. Only once before was there a similar drop in the death rate in Israel, and that was during another doctors' strike 20 years earlier. After each strike, the death rate jumped again to its normal level.[2]

However, these figures for iatrogenic deaths do not take into account iatrogenic diseases from the long-term harm done by medical treatments where patients survive but with a chronic disease. My real awakening to this problem started when I became aware of the story of Orian Truss who discovered the candidiasis-causing potential of antibiotics.

Dr Orian Truss's Candida Discovery

In 1953, in a hospital in Alabama, USA, Dr Orian Truss discovered the devastating effects of antibiotics.[3] During a ward round, Truss was intrigued by a gaunt, apparently elderly, man who was obviously dying. However, he was only in his forties and had been in hospital for four months. No specialist had been able to make a diagnosis. Out of curiosity, Truss asked the patient when he was last completely well. The man answered that he was well until six months before when he had cut his finger. He had received antibiotics for this. Shortly afterwards, he developed diarrhoea and his health deteriorated. Truss had seen before how antibiotics cause diarrhoea. It was known that *Candida* was opportunistic and thrived in debilitated patients, but now Truss wondered if it might not be the other way around—that candida actually *caused* the debilitated condition. Truss had read that potassium iodide solution could be used to treat candida infestation of the blood, so he put the patient on six to eight drops of Lugol's solution four times a day for three weeks and before long the patient was completely well again.

Soon afterwards, Dr Truss had a female patient with a stuffy nose, a throbbing headache, vaginitis and severe depression. To his amazement, all her problems immediately cleared with treatment for candida. Some time later, he saw a female patient who had been schizophrenic for six years and had had hundreds of electroshock treatments and massive drug dosages. He started treating the woman for sinus allergies with a candida remedy. Soon she recovered mentally and physically, and remained well.

From then on he treated his patients against candida at the slightest indication of its presence. Many of his patients made remarkable recoveries from most unusual conditions, including menstrual problems, hyperactivity, learning disabilities, autism, schizophrenia, multiple sclerosis and auto-immune diseases such as Crohn's disease and lupus erythematosus.

Every experienced naturopath can relate similar success stories. Also, some alternative medical practitioners have realised the curative potential of anti-candida therapy, as for instance Dr William Crook who wrote several books about the successful treatment of allergies and hyperactivity in children.

The Antibiotic Syndrome

Candidiasis is not the only side effect of antibiotic treatment, and antibiotics are not the only drugs that cause such problems. Drugs used in chemotherapy, anti-inflammatory steroidal drugs and other long-term drug therapies tend to kill or suppress the natural intestinal bacteria, and so yeast, parasites and harmful bacteria start taking over. This condition is called *dysbiosis*. Most patients receive such drugs in hospitals and can be expected to develop systemic candida overgrowth as a result.

Our natural intestinal flora, mainly based on lactobacteria, not only help to digest and absorb food but also protect us against ingested harmful bacteria that otherwise might cause food poisoning. With a healthy intestinal flora, millions of salmonella bacteria might be needed to cause an infection; but with dysbiosis, only tens of salmonella would be required.

With chronic dysbiosis, the intestinal wall becomes inflamed, causing ulcers, appendicitis, malabsorption and Crohn's disease; and as the intestinal membrane erodes, the patient develops multiple food allergies, arthritis and autoimmune diseases. In addition to candida, other pathogens and parasites now invade the bloodstream and various organs. With live-cell analysis, natural therapists can see and show their patients the fungi in their blood. This invasion greatly weakens the immune system so that people now become susceptible to frequent or chronic infections. Commonly these are then treated with more antibiotics—a practice which continues to intensify the symptoms.

Actually, the problem is not with the antibiotics. You can take a course if you feel it is needed, provided that you take a fungicide, such as fresh garlic, at the same time and have some probiotics after the antibiotics and before you ingest any carbohydrates. This will prevent most diseases that are caused by the careless medical method of using antibiotics. For more details, see "Candida and the Antibiotic Syndrome" (http://www.health-science-spirit.com/candida.html).

Most patients receive such drugs in hospitals and can be expected to develop systemic candida overgrowth as a result.

Autoimmune Diseases and Asthma

Autoimmune diseases, including psoriasis, lupus erythematosus and pancreatitis, have been linked to dysbiosis. When remedies are given that bind bacterial endotoxins, these conditions usually improve. In addition, autoimmune diseases have been shown to be linked to mycoplasmas or nanobacteria which start to develop from diseased red blood cells in the presence of toxic chemicals and systemic candida. The weaker our immune system becomes, the more these mycoplasmas start to develop into bacterial and, finally, fungal forms. They have been found in all autoimmune diseases, cancers and AIDS.

Antibiotics are also a major contributing cause of asthma. According to a study, children who received broad-spectrum antibiotics were about nine times more likely to suffer from asthma. A recent research paper confirmed dysbiosis as a main cause of asthma.

In the 1980s, New Zealand had the highest rate of asthma deaths in the world. This rate was drastically reduced when in 1991 the inhaler drug Fenoterol was banned, as it caused a 13- times higher risk of dying. This reduction in the asthma death rate was generally hailed as a great triumph for medical science. Other studies revealed that asthmatics using more than one bronchodilator inhaler a month had a 50-fold increased risk of suffering a fatal asthma attack.

In addition to asthma, I also see the combination of pasteurised cow's milk with antibiotic-induced dysbiosis in babies and infants as the main cause of their frequent infections and glue ear and greatly contributing to cot death. Because health authorities insist on pasteurising milk, and doctors prescribe antibiotics without the most basic precautions, I regard asthma and most childhood infections as predominantly iatrogenic diseases.

In the "good old days", people ingested a lot of lactic-acid-fermented foods and raw milk products that replenished our "good" bacteria; and because antibiotics had not been invented, dysbiosis and therefore chronic diseases were rare. Instead, people mainly died from acute infections due to unhygienic living conditions, and in the slums also from malnutrition.

Staphylococcus aureus, or golden staph, causes serious infections in hospital patients. It has been found that not only golden staph but also other infections are greatly potentised when they occur in combination with candida overgrowth. As candida overgrowth is a natural outcome of the standard hospital treatment, it is easy to see why golden staph is so deadly in hospitals.

A similar picture emerges with AIDS. People do not die from the virus that leads to AIDS, but from candida or fungus-potentised bacterial and mycoplasma infections. The end stage of AIDS is the same as the end stage of cancer. It is called *cachexia*, a wasting condition mainly caused by fungal overgrowth. Lugol's iodine solution and other systemic fungicides should do wonders for it. Presently MMS, a 28 per cent solution of sodium chlorite, is also gaining acceptance as an effective antimicrobial remedy (see http://www.miraclemineral.org).

All of this shows that antibiotic-induced dysbiosis and candida are not isolated and relatively harmless problems, as the medical profession prefers to believe, but, rather, are the underlying cause of most of our modern diseases.

Cancer and Leukaemia

One hundred years ago, the rate of cancer was very low. I have no doubt that the phenomenal increase in the use of agricultural and industrial chemicals as well as pharmaceutical drugs has greatly accelerated the increase in the cancer rate, and there is also a link to the consumption of sugar. Even stronger is the link to dysbiosis and candida.

Chemotherapy commonly leads to systemic candida infections, which greatly limit the success rate of the treatment. Long-term follow-up studies show that children develop 18 times more secondary malignant tumours later in life, that girls face a 75-times higher risk of breast cancer by the time they are forty,[9] and that the risk of developing leukaemia after chemotherapy for ovarian cancer increases 21-fold. Also, other tumours commonly develop after treating malignancies with chemotherapy.[10] A main problem appears to be the development of deep or systemic candida infections shortly after starting chemotherapy.[11]

All of this shows that chemotherapy tends to cause leukaemia and cancer many years later, mainly as a result of dysbiosis and systemic candida infection.

Only recently have oncologists started to acknowledge what patients called "chemo-brain", a distressing loss of memory and other cognitive functions. Psychiatrists have now found that the conventional treatment of cancer causes serious depression in 15 to 25 per cent of patients. "The depression itself can often be worse than the disease," they say.[12] Brain fog and depression are common with systemic candida. All of this shows that chemotherapy tends to cause leukaemia and cancer many years later, mainly as a result of dysbiosis and systemic candida infection. The reason for the widespread use of chemotherapy despite its lack of effectiveness, severe side effects and long-term cancer promotion can be seen in the fact that private-practice oncologists in the USA typically derive two-thirds of their income from selling chemotherapy to patients.[13]

This chemotherapy connection makes it very likely that dysbiosis and systemic candida also promote cancer and leukaemia when they are caused as a result of antibiotic treatment. The rate of cancer really accelerated only after the use of antibiotics became widespread.

There is also more direct evidence that candida and other fungi are a cause of leukaemia. Meinolf Karthaus, MD, reported on several children with leukaemia going into remission upon receiving antifungal remedies for their "secondary" fungal infections.[14] In his lifetime of work, Milton White, MD, found fungal spores in every sample of cancer tissue he studied.[15]

Fungal infections have been diagnosed and treated as leukaemia, and leukaemia has disappeared on grain-free diets, presumably because of the high content of mycotoxins in grains.[16]

The Italian oncologist Dr Tullio Simoncini claims a success rate of up to 90 per cent by treating cancer as a fungus. He infuses tumours with sodium bicarbonate solution and recommends taking bicarbonate in water to get rid of gastro-intestinal cancer.[17]

Recently I received a personal communication that a large stomach tumour had unexpectedly shrunk after some mouthwash was swallowed for a few weeks for a different problem. The main ingredient of this mouthwash was benzoic acid, a strong fungicide that inhibits the metabolism of fungal cells. Cancer cells have the same fungal-type metabolism which thrives on high levels of glucose and insulin, and they may therefore be regarded as types of fungal cells.

While the work of the German doctor Ryke Geerd Hamer[18] shows that emotional shock is a major trigger for the development of cancer, a weak immune system as caused by intestinal dysbiosis, systemic candidiasis, toxic chemicals and root canal treatments appears to be an essential co-factor. After all, a century ago people must have had a similar number of emotional shocks as at present, but cancer was very rare. Conversely, there are lots of people with dysbiosis and filled root canals who do not have cancer, but add emotional shock and *voilà*!

Root Canal Fillings

Root-canal-filled teeth are a variation on the theme of intestinal dysbiosis. They, too, appear to be a major contributing factor in many health problems, including cancer, heart disease, arthritis, kidney disease and auto-immune diseases. This is due to microbes that multiply in the multitude of tiny canals or tubules in the dentine and gradually leach out into the lymph system. Even normally harmless microbes become very dangerous and more virulent and toxic under the anaerobic conditions in dead teeth.

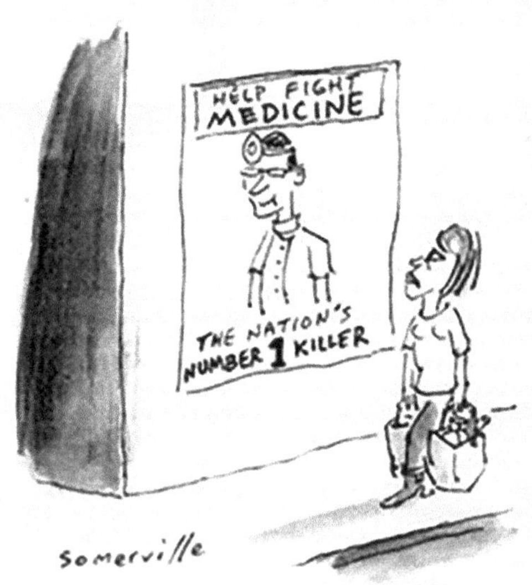

Dr Weston Price,[?] a former Director of Research for the American Dental Association, observed that the removal of root-filled teeth from patients with kidney or heart disease would in most cases lead to an improvement. When he inserted a removed root-filled tooth under the skin of a rabbit, the animal would die within two days. When he implanted normal teeth, there was no adverse health effect. In some experiments he implanted the same fragments of root-filled teeth in succession under the skins of up to 100 rabbits and they all died within two weeks of the same disease that the human donor had!

Dr Price conducted about 5,000 experiments over 25 years. He did not find a reliable method to disinfect dead teeth and make them safe. His research has been suppressed, and if at all mentioned by our dental associations then it is described as "dated" because this research was conducted and published over 70 years ago but has never been repeated or otherwise investigated and root canal fillings have never been shown to be safe. The main argument for the supposed safety of root-canal-filled teeth is that millions of people have them and are still alive many years later. The question of root canal fillings causing widespread degenerative diseases is not discussed or researched. Dr Price found that about 30 per cent of individuals have such a strong immune system that they do not develop problems from root canal fillings until they become old, but the remaining 70 per cent develop problems much sooner.

I regard root canal fillings, even more so than intestinal dysbiosis, as a major cause of autoimmune diseases. In 1993, George E. Meinig, DDS, a former root canal specialist in the USA, republished the dental research of Dr Price in a popular version and included his own experiences.[20]

Generally, outdoors workers with the most sun exposure have the lowest rates of skin cancer and melanoma, while melanoma often shows up in office workers.

Iatrogenic Heart Attacks and the Chlorine Link

One hundred years ago, heart attacks were almost unknown despite diets generally being high in saturated fats. The ascent of heart attacks began with the pasteurisation of milk and the use of chlorine to kill bacteria in public water supplies. This began around 1900 and was generally accepted in western countries in the 1920s.

From 1920 onwards, the explosive increase in the incidence of cardiovascular disease and fatal heart attacks began, but only in countries that chlorinated their water supplies. These diseases remained unknown in, for instance, Africa, China, Japan and other parts of Asia. However, when Japanese citizens immigrated to Hawaii where water was chlorinated, they suffered the same rate of heart attacks as the Americans. And the African-American population in the US has the average US rate of heart attacks, but not so their brothers in Africa. Residents of the non-chlorinated Roseto in Pennsylvania remained free of heart attacks unless they moved to a chlorinated area.[21] Some of the chlorine reacts with organic impurities in water to form organochlorines (DDT is an organochlorine), while the rest remains as residual free-chlorine in the water. It may then react either with food chemicals or with parts of our digestive tract.

In 1967, Dr Joseph Price in the USA performed a decisive experiment. With one group of 50 three-month-old chickens (cockerels), he added one-third of a teaspoon of chlorine bleach to about one litre of their drinking water whilst another group of 50 chickens served as controls. Seven months later, over 95 per cent of the chlorinated group had advanced atherosclerosis, yet none of the control group showed any such evidence. In the following years Dr Price repeated his experiment many times, always with the same results, and more recently even researchers funded by the US Environmental Protection Agency have confirmed atherosclerotic-type changes in other animals, including monkeys, when exposed to chlorinated water.[22]

Drug and Chemical Cocktails

Basically all drugs are more or less toxic: the more so, the more "powerful" they are. Natural remedies cannot be patented; therefore, in order to maximise profits, the pharmaceutical industry routinely makes and sells synthetic versions of effective natural remedies. Synthetic substances are usually more difficult to detoxify than natural remedies and tend to create more problems the longer they are taken. Often they become highly addictive and after some time may cause the symptoms that they originally alleviated. However, this is rarely acknowledged by drug companies or medical practitioners; instead, when a problem arises, alternative or additional drugs are prescribed.

One of the main problems is that drugs are tested individually for relatively short periods, but then prescribed as drug cocktails for very long periods. Drugs have not been tested under these conditions and therefore all drug use, except as individual drugs for short periods, is unscientific and unsafe. As a result of this, there are countless dangerous and fatal drug interactions and side effects, as reported in numerous books, articles and statistics.

It is similar with the thousands of synthetic chemicals and heavy metals that are allowed by health authorities to contaminate our living space. These are even less tested than drugs but also react with each other and with drugs in a brew that is impossible to disentangle.

I want to mention just one instance of such a combination. The herbicide paraquat and the fungicide maneb are widely used in farming and may remain present as residues in crops. Each on its own did not cause a problem, but if rats and mice were exposed to both together, even at very low rates, they developed symptoms of Parkinson's disease. The leader of the research team said: "No one has looked at the effects of studying together some of these compounds that, taken by themselves, have little effect. This has enormous implications [and] it's a huge problem to start thinking about a nearly infinite array of mixtures of chemicals, instead of the risk that a single chemical might pose."[23]

We have similar problems with fluoride and chlorine as well as mercury, aluminium, nickel and other heavy and toxic metals being deliberately put into vaccines and used in dentistry. For detailed documentation of the problems associated with heavy metals and endocrine-disrupting chemicals, see articles by Bernard Windham.[24]

Lack of Sunlight Implicated in Diseases

Health authorities and medical associations have campaigned strongly on avoiding sun exposure to the skin. Presumably such exposure causes skin cancer, including melanoma that can kill.

However, the vast majority of incidences is normal skin cancer that almost never kills, and there is widespread doubt that melanomas are really caused by normal sun exposure, although there seems to be a link with sunburn. Generally, outdoors workers with the most sun exposure have the lowest rates of skin cancer and melanoma, while melanoma often shows up in office workers. Melanoma often occurs on areas of the skin that have not been exposed to sunlight. Other studies show a strong link between long-term exposure to fluorescent lighting and melanoma.[23] With the present campaign in Australia to replace all incandescent light bulbs with fluorescent ones by 2009–10, I expect a melanoma epidemic in 10 to 20 years' time.[24]

Now, more and more research papers show that a vast number of diseases, especially cancer, could be avoided by greatly increasing our level of vitamin D with suitable foods, supplements and frequent or daily short exposure of sunshine to the skin.

Sunlight is our main source of vitamin D. Research shows that there is a strong negative correlation between available sunlight and breast cancer death rates, and that living in a sunny area is associated with lower cancer rates. Even skin cancer is inhibited by regular low-level sunlight exposure; only sunburn is a strong skin cancer promoter. It has now been calculated that worldwide, with these measures, about 600,000 cases of colon and breast cancer could be prevented.[27]

Furthermore, the researchers pointed out that by increasing levels of vitamin D3 by regular sunlight exposure and other measures, we could prevent diseases that claim nearly one million lives throughout the world each year.[28,29]

The irony of all this is that the present skin cancer epidemic, in my opinion, has been manufactured by our health authorities and medical experts. There are three conditions that make us susceptible to developing skin cancers with high sunlight exposure. These are overacidity, a high ratio of omega-6 to omega-3 fatty acids and a lack of antioxidants. The most common cause of overacidity is candida overgrowth, especially in combination with the officially recommended diet high in cereals. Our omega-6 to omega-3 ratio was always somewhat too high, but it went off the chart when our health authorities recommended replacing saturated fats with seed oils high in omega-6 fatty acids. This increased inflammatory conditions of all kinds, including tumours and skin cancers. To make matters worse, health authorities also discourage and legally minimise the use of antioxidant nutrients.

With these measures, health authorities created the conditions for an epidemic of skin cancers. Then they tried to prevent skin cancers by recommending complete avoidance of sunlight exposure, which in turn caused large-scale vitamin D deficiency with an estimated loss of one million lives each year. I sometimes ask myself if it is simply ignorance and incompetence or if there is something more sinister to it.

Obesity and Diabetes Epidemics

I could write a book about all the health problems caused by the medical–pharmaceutical complex and the neglectful way in which health authorities contribute to our diseases. In addition to directly causing diseases, these same forces also prevent the healing of these same diseases by restricting, suppressing and persecuting the practitioners of natural medicine as well as giving disease-causing nutritional advice.

Until 1980, the rates of obesity and type 2 diabetes were fairly stable. However, when health authorities in the USA started vilifying foods containing fats and cholesterol and recommended eating more carbohydrates instead, obesity increased from 15 per cent of the American adult population in 1976–1980 to 32.9 per cent in 2003–2004.[30] Type 2 diabetes became an epidemic as well. In addition, for the first time in history, a large number of obese children developed type 2 diabetes—so much so, it is no longer called "maturity-onset" diabetes. Also, children are now developing type 1 and type 2 diabetes simultaneously.[31,32,33] These are iatrogenic diseases, caused by the medical system.

Natural health practitioners are experts in preventing and successfully treating chronic diseases with nutrition and other natural methods—diseases that include the metabolic syndrome which leads to diabetes, heart disease and overweight. It is routinely and quickly remedied with proper nutrition, but with accepted medical practice it becomes a lifelong condition managed with drugs that are more or less toxic. Surgery is used for a wide range of conditions and patients are severely traumatised or mutilated for life, when these problems could be successfully treated with natural therapies.

In addition, vaccinated children have about 150 per cent more neurological disorders such as ADHD and autism compared to unvaccinated children.

Side Effects of Vaccinations

Vaccinations are the proud showpiece of drug medicine in eliminating the dreaded childhood infections of previous centuries. However, long-term statistics and diagrams tell a different story.

Starting between 1850 and 1900, scarlet fever, diphtheria, whooping cough and measles had declined by about 90 per cent by the time general vaccination was introduced for each disease. While statistics vary between different countries, this is generally true for England, the United States and Australia. Whooping cough had declined in England and Wales by about 98.5 per cent before a vaccine became generally available, and measles had declined by over 99 per cent. Tuberculosis had declined by 87 per cent when antibiotics first became available and by 93 per cent before the introduction of the BCG vaccine. The death rate from rheumatic fever had declined by 86 per cent by the time penicillin was introduced.[34] All of this has obviously more to do with better plumbing than with vaccinations.

There are also statistics showing that death rates from targeted diseases have risen with the introduction of vaccines. Other side effects ascribed to modern vaccines are cot or crib death (SIDS) and a strong rise in autism and shaken baby syndrome (spot bleeding in the brain), which apparently has landed innocent parents in prison. Experts strongly deny that there is a connection between vaccines and autism, but it is strange nevertheless that the rates of autism have suddenly exploded without an obvious reason. Interestingly, there is no autism in Amish children, who are generally not vaccinated. In addition, vaccinated children have about 150 per cent more neurological disorders such as ADHD and autism compared to unvaccinated children.

Another curious aspect of vaccine safety statistics was highlighted by Dr Archie Kalokerinos. Working in the remote Australian outback with Aboriginal people, he found that every second child died as a result of vaccinations. Because deaths commonly occurred about three weeks after vaccination, they were not recorded as vaccine related; officially, reactions were limited to occurring only for up to two weeks after vaccination. However, Dr Kalokerinos eventually solved the problem by giving babies high doses of vitamin C before vaccinations, and no more vaccination deaths occurred. Also, SIDS incidence disappeared. Naturally, he encountered ridicule and hostility from his medical colleagues, and babies are still dying needlessly.

Bias against Natural Therapies

It has become a habit that any successful natural cancer remedy or treatment is quickly outlawed by our health authorities. Many natural health practitioners have been dragged before the courts and often imprisoned, especially in the area of cancer treatment. This is especially regrettable because there is no evidence that the methods of orthodox cancer therapy are in any way successful.

One of the methods increasingly used to denigrate natural therapies is for the pharmaceutical industry to finance shoddy research on natural remedies and then proclaim the remedies to be ineffective or harmful. This is only partly intended to influence the general public, but mainly to provide the justification for health authorities to outlaw and greatly restrict natural remedies.

Another strategy is not to list favourable vitamin studies in the Medline database which is taxpayer-funded and operated by the US National Library of Medicine. It lists all articles published in medical research journals, and even in *Time* magazine and *Reader's Digest*, but not the peer-reviewed *Journal of Orthomolecular Medicine* (http://www.orthomed.org/jom/jomlist.htm) which specialises in vitamin research. Now the *British Medical Journal* has published a letter about Medline bias, and this has forced Medline to index articles on Medline bias. However, because all these favourable vitamin studies are not indexed by Medline, proponents of drug medicine can claim that there are no studies which show that vitamins are useful in the treatment of diseases or that they are safe in high doses, and therefore they seek to restrict them to very low doses. Of course, yearly fatalities worldwide due to vitamins are zero; in comparison, drug fatalities are infinitely higher.

Thirty years ago, Linus Pauling, PhD, showed that high doses of vitamin C are beneficial in cancer treatment. This has been "disproved" by the orthodoxy ever since. But now, a study by conventional scientists at Johns Hopkins University in Baltimore, Maryland, has shown that he was right.

In addition, the *Journal of Orthomolecular Medicine* has just published a double-blind, randomised clinical trial showing that HIV-positive patients given supplemental nutrients can stop their decline into AIDS. This poses a big threat to the medical–pharmaceutical complex and is one more reason not to index this journal on Medline.

There exists a systemic culture of suppression of dissenting views in science and medicine, and frequently a vicious persecution with "Gestapo-like" methods. Recently in the USA, a mother was even imprisoned and brutalised for illegally using natural methods to cure her son of malignant melanoma.

Of course, this assault by the medical–pharmaceutical complex on natural healing methods is not illegal. On the contrary, in a capitalist system the industry has a duty to maximise profits by eliminating the competition and generating a steady supply of patients with chronic diseases who can be managed indefinitely with drugs.

The question is: just why do government health authorities make and enforce laws on behalf of drug medicine and against natural medicine? Theoretically, they should be impartial and ensure the best outcome for the population. I believe the answer can be found in some good lateral thinking by the pharmaceutical industry. By paying for and influencing much of the medical education, it automatically produces health officials who are steeped in pharmaceutical thinking. No bribery is needed, but health officials always know that there is a well-paid job waiting if and when they want to retire from government service.

The very fact of a high rate of chronic disease in our society attests to the inability of the medical profession to treat these diseases successfully.

Natural Medicine to the Rescue

Health authorities so far have ignored the claims and evidence that natural medicine is the superior form of treatment for chronic and medically incurable diseases. The very fact of a high rate of chronic disease in our society attests to the inability of the medical profession to treat these diseases successfully. I have no doubt that natural medicine could eliminate most chronic diseases within a decade, needing only a few per cent of the money that is spent on conventional medicine. The knowledge is already available; no expensive high-tech research is needed that may or may not give results some time in the future.

There is a simple, low-cost solution for bringing about the healing of our society:

1. Phase out public assistance for pharmaceutical companies and their research, and require research to show that a drug is safe with long-term use in combination with other common drugs and chemicals and with old or fragile patients or, alternatively that it is superior in the long term to available natural treatments.

2. Make it illegal for pharmaceutical companies to fund medical education or provide drug information, marketing or incentives directly to the public or to medical practitioners, or to employ former health officials.

Continued on page 79

Are Most Diseases Caused By The Medical System?

Continued from page 32

Information for medical practitioners should be provided by an independent and impartial body.

3. Except for unethical conduct according to society's general standards, make it illegal for medical associations to restrict the therapies used by their members.

4. Afford qualified practitioners of natural medicine the same recognition and opportunities as in drug medicine, including in hospitals, rehabilitation, research and publications, health departments and regulating authorities.

So far, our medical and economic leaders do not want to face reality. They brainwash the public into believing that the present health situation is completely normal. Importantly, the whole economic structure of western civilisation is based on the production and distribution of goods and services that are contributing to poor health. This system includes chemicalised agriculture and food processing, the pharmaceutical industry, technological medicine and the petrochemical and plastics industries.

The guiding motto for industry is "profit", while for the consumer it is "convenience". The price for all to pay is the loss of health. This situation is the natural outcome of a society based on selfish motivation. A change for the better can only come when more and more people realise that ultimately they harm themselves with selfish attitudes, and when they start electing leaders who are prepared to act in a compassionate and cooperative way in the interest of the whole society. We get what we choose: natural health or enduring drug management. ∞

About the Author:

Walter Last worked as a biochemist and research chemist in the medical departments of several German universities and at Bio-Science Laboratories in Los Angeles, USA. Later he worked as a nutritionist and natural therapist in New Zealand and in Australia, where he is now based. He no longer has a clinic.

Walter Last has written numerous health-related journal articles as well as several books, including *Heal Yourself* and *Healing Foods* (Penguin). Presently in print are *The Natural Way to Heal* (Hampton Roads, 2004; see review in NEXUS 11/04) and the *Heal Yourself* Series—seven small books about overcoming specific diseases such as arthritis, asthma, cancer, candida, diabetes and weight problems; see the web page http://www.theartof-life.com/Products_02.html. His two-part article "Sexual Energy in Health and Spirituality" was published in NEXUS 14/03–04; his article on "The New Medicine of Dr Hamer", about Dr Ryke Geerd Hamer's discovery of the shock-conflict mechanism underlying cancer development, was published in NEXUS 10/05; and his article "How Scientific Are Orthodox Cancer Treatments?" was run in NEXUS 11/04.

For information on health questions, see Walter Last's website http://www.health-science-spirit.com.

Editor's Note:

Due to space limitations, we are unable to publish the endnotes that accompany this article. They are available at Walter Last's website, http://www.health-science-spirit.com.

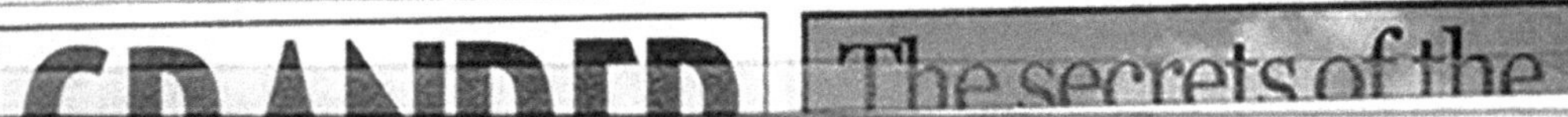

Hulder Clark PhD , three herbs used in her protocol to kill parasites and cancer, a five day treatment using : The green husk of Black Walnut, wormwood and ground clove. (Products can be purchased from Dr Clark Store on line. See: amazon.com.au/Clark-Vegitarian-Walnut-Wormwood-Cloves/dp/B072C8WZ5P) Hulder Clark also used and recommended an electronic pulse device called the "zapper" to remove parasites from the blood.

Hulder Clark's experience purported that the removal of parasites from the blood of cancer patients enabled the rapid recovery from cancer and her studies associated cancer states with parasitic infection.

History of Nutrition

Vitamin A as "Anti-Infective" Therapy, 1920–1940[1]

Richard D. Semba[2]

Department of Ophthalmology, the Johns Hopkins University School of Medicine, Baltimore, MD 21287

ABSTRACT In the last fifteen years, a large series of controlled clinical trials showed that vitamin A supplementation reduces morbidity and mortality of children in developing countries. It is less well known that vitamin A underwent two decades of intense clinical investigation prior to World War II. In the 1920s, a theory emerged that vitamin A could be used in "anti-infective" therapy. This idea, largely championed by Edward Mellanby, led to a series of at least 30 trials to determine whether vitamin A usually supplied in the form of cod liver oil could reduce the morbidity and mortality of respiratory disease, measles, puerperal sepsis, and other infections. The early studies generally lacked such innovations known to the modern controlled clinical trial such as randomization, masking, sample size and power calculations, and placebo controls. Results of the early trials were mixed, but the pharmaceutical industry emphasized the positive results in their advertising to the public. With the advent of the sulfa antibiotics for treatment of infections, scientific interest in vitamin A as "anti-infective" therapy waned. Recent controlled clinical trials of vitamin A from the last 15 y follow a tradition of investigation that began largely in the 1920s. J. Nutr. 129: 783–791, 1999.

KEY WORDS: • *vitamin A* • *anti-infective therapy* • *morbidity* • *mortality* • *immunity*

Vitamin A supplementation is an important public health intervention to reduce mortality from infections among children in developing countries. In the 1980s and early 1990s, several large randomized, double-blind, placebo-controlled clinical trials were conducted in developing countries around the world, and these studies showed that vitamin A supplementation could reduce child mortality by about one-third (Beaton et al. 1993). Improving the vitamin A status of children through vitamin A supplementation is one of the most cost-effective health interventions known (World Bank 1993). High-dose vitamin A is now recommended therapy for measles in many developing countries and for selected circumstances in developed countries (World Health Organization 1987, American Academy of Pediatrics 1993). Although vitamin A has been undergoing investigation in clinical trials in the last two decades, these recent trials are largely a continuation of clinical investigation that began in the 1920s.

Prior to World War II, there was great interest and debate surrounding the use of vitamin A as "anti-infective" therapy. An idea was conceived that vitamin A could strengthen the immune system and would help fight infections. A series of at least 30 studies was conducted to evaluate vitamin A as a means of reducing infections and mortality. The early clinical investigations of vitamin A had some spectacular successes and notable failures. The public seized upon the use of vitamin A as "anti-infective" therapy, but the value of vitamin A in reducing morbidity and mortality from infections was not more widely recognized until 50 y later. This paper will examine the rise of the idea of using vitamin A as "anti-infective" therapy and the evaluation of this theory through clinical trials from 1920 to 1940.

THE INFANT WELFARE MOVEMENT

In 1910, the first annual meeting of the American Association for the Study and Prevention of Infant Mortality was held at Johns Hopkins University. The association was founded out of concern over the belief that one of every four infants died before 12 mo of age in the United States. Out of a total infant population of 1.5 million, an estimated 300,000 deaths occurred each year under 12 mo of age (Knox 1910). The association had broad membership that included social workers, public health officials, and philanthropists, and its founders included William Henry Welch from Johns Hopkins, the pediatrician L. Emmett Holt, and the nutritionist Alfred Hess. The immediate goal of the society was to reduce infant mortality by half, and many members of the association attributed such excessive mortality to parental ignorance and indifference. The strategies being considered to combat infant mortality were diverse, and its members pointed out the need for more accurate vital statistics, the importance of maternal nursing and the need to educate mothers. The association did not restrict its activities to the realm of academia, as they had travelling exhibits and also sent their reports to popular women's magazines at the time. Magazines such as *The Pictorial Review* and *Ladies Home Journal* were quick to pick up the crusade of the association with advice columns aimed at mothers and occasional lay articles written by members of the association.

The movement in the United States was part of a larger

[1] Presented in part as a seminar in the history of medicine, National Library of Medicine, June 24, 1998.

[2] To whom correspondence should be addressed at Ocular Immunology Service, Suite 700, 550 North Broadway, Baltimore, MD 21205. e-mail: rdsemba@welchlink.welch.jhu.edu.

0022-3166/99 $3.00 © 1999 American Society for Nutritional Sciences.
Manuscript received 2 November 1998. Revision accepted 21 December 1998.

international infant welfare movement that began in Great Britain. The major causes of infant mortality at the time were epidemics of diarrhea among infants during the summer, also known as the "summer complaint" and acute upper and lower respiratory disease, known as the "winter complaint." Arthur Newsholme, George Newman, and other architects of public health reform in Great Britain thought that fecal contamination of food and milk were responsible for epidemics of summer diarrhea. George Newman was medical officer of health for Finsbury, one of the poorest and most crowded metropolitan boroughs in Bedfordshire. He made careful observations of infant mortality and pointed out that epidemic diarrhea among infants was steadily increasing, especially in towns "where the lamp of social life burns low." Newman (1906) argued that the health of community should be gauged by the infant mortality rate rather than the general death rate. Thus, he considered it a sign of social degeneration that Great Britain should have a falling overall death rate but little change in the infant mortality rate over the preceding 50 yr.

In the late nineteenth century, sporadic efforts were being made to improve the urban milk supply in large cities (Meckel 1990). Newman pointed out that breastfed infants suffered less from summer diarrhea than infants who were fed artificial formula or cow's milk. He considered the high infant mortality rate to be mainly a problem of motherhood, and he emphasized proper training of mothers and promotion of breastfeeding. Pasteurization of milk and milk stations were other measures that were proposed to reduce infant mortality rates. It took a long time for milk to be transported from the farm to the city, and bacterial contamination of cow's milk was common, especially during the hot summer days. Milk was an especially good medium for bacterial growth. In addition, infants were fed using what pediatrician Robert Hutchinson (1940) termed "foul, sour-smelling contraptions" known as tube bottles.

The American Association for the Study and Prevention of Infant Mortality was founded at a time when improvement of the urban milk supply was having no apparent effect upon infant mortality rates (Meckel 1990). L. Emmett Holt (1910) declared that infant mortality would not be solved simply by purifying milk and by establishing milk stations. Milk stations may have had little influence since they only reached a very small proportion of urban infants. In his time, Holt (1900a) was perhaps the best known and influential pediatrician in the United States, author of the widely read book, *The Care and Feeding of Children*. Holt considered nutrition to be the most important branch of pediatrics and declared that, "The largest part of the immense mortality of the first year is traceable directly to disorders of nutrition" (Holt 1900b). The nutritional measures that could be taken to save children at the time were part of an evolving debate.

Emergence of the vitamins. The nutritional theories of the German chemist Justus von Liebig (1803–1873) dominated scientific discussion for many years and were also echoed in lay publications. In *The Pictorial Review*, Anna Steese Richardson (1916) gave popular advice on motherhood, nutrition, breast-feeding, and other health-related issues in a regular column. Her dietary advice to expectant mothers summarizes Liebig's doctrine: "Stoke the engine of your body with the right sort of coal, keep it clear of cinders and clinkers, cleanse it with pure water, renew the worn parts with rest . . . What is the right kind of coal? Food-stuffs classified according to their chemical properties . . . water, mineral matter, proteins, carbohydrates, and fats." Liebig held that dietary proteins are almost directly unchanged in building up the protein in tissues, and that carbohydrate and fat merely provided fuel to be burned with oxygen from the lungs, thus providing heat. The likening of the human body to a steam locomotive was a popular simplification that was often used by Liebig's successors.

The laboratory provided well-controlled conditions for the critical examination of nutritional theories through the administration of experimental diets in animals. Over a 25-yr period, several investigators made similar observations in different institutions that suggested the existence of vitamin A (Steenbock 1932, Wolf and Carpenter 1997). Two students who worked in the laboratory of Gustav von Bunge at the University of Dorpat challenged Liebig's theory regarding the essential food components. Nicholai Lunin (1881) determined that mice cannot survive on a purified diet of fats, carbohydrates, proteins, and salts alone; however, he noted that mice could survive when milk was added. Lunin concluded "other substances indispensable for nutrition must be present in milk besides casein, fat, lactose, and salts." His idea received considerable dissemination in von Bunge's (1887) widely-read Lehrbuch der physiologischen und pathologischen Chemie. Ten years later, another student, C. A. Socin (1891), performed experiments with simplified diets in mice and found that there was an unknown substance in egg yolk which was essential for life. At the University of Utrecht, Cornelius Pekelharing (1905), showed that mice are able to survive on diets in which small quantities of milk are added, and Wilhelm Stepp (1911) showed that if the milk supplied to mice was extracted with alcohol-ether (thus removing the fat-soluble substance later known as vitamin A), the mice could not survive.

Other experiments with animals suggested that there were other unknown substances in food that were necessary to support health. In 1886, C. Eijkman was sent to the Dutch East Indies to work on the problem of beriberi. He demonstrated that chickens raised on polished rice alone developed a paralytic disorder similar to human beriberi, and that this disorder could be corrected by a diet of unpolished rice, and it was soon demonstrated that the bran portion of rice contained a substance that could prevent beriberi. Scurvy was produced in guinea pigs on experimental diets, and these animals were cured with fresh fruits and vegetables (Holst and Frölich 1907). Frederick Gowland Hopkins (1906) at Cambridge University expressed the belief that there were "unsuspected dietetic factors" besides proteins, carbohydrates, fats, and minerals that were vital for health, especially in rickets and scurvy.

Much of the early work with experimental diets in animals in the United States was conducted by Thomas Osborne and Lafayette Mendel (1911, 1913) at Yale University, and their work suggested that a fat-soluble substance in butterfat was needed to support the growth of rats. After a period of illness, Hopkins published work he undertook in 1906–1907 which, similar to the findings of Pekelharing, showed that mice could not survive on a purified diet without milk. Hopkins (1912) postulated the existence of what he called "accessory factors" in foods that were necessary for life. Casimir Funk (1912) named these substances "vital amines" or "vitamines" over the belief that these accessory factors were chemical amines, similar to thiamin, the vitamin involved in the deficiency disorder, beriberi. Elmer McCollum and Marguerite Davis (1913) at the University of Wisconsin confirmed that this accessory factor was found in butter, and they dubbed it "fat-soluble A." Soon the term "fat-soluble A" was combined with Funk's designation to become "vitamine A."

These early animal studies were criticized because it was thought that under caged conditions, the purified diets given to animals were too monotonous and distasteful so that the animals allowed themselves to starve to death, or that the chemical processing to purify the foods had a deleterious effect that led to intoxications or rendered the food unsuitable for nutrition (Nicholls 1938). Often the vitamin A-deficient animals developed ocular abnormalities, including dryness of the eyes, ulceration of the cornea, and blindness. Many clinicians were skeptical that the findings from animal experiments could be extrapolated to humans, given the severity of nutritional deprivation (Cramer 1924).

Clinical observations in children. Prior to the period in which Hopkins and others were observing that milk or butter contained an unknown factor that was essential to life in animals, similar clinical observations were made among humans. Numerous descriptions exist of blinding eye lesions and high mortality throughout the eighteenth and nineteenth centuries. Many of these observations came from homes for foundling children, usually among infants who were not breastfed (Billard 1828, Brown 1827, Ratier 1824). More detailed descriptions were made in the early twentieth century (Wolf 1998). Masamichi Mori (1904) described nightblindness, cornea ulcers, blindness, and high mortality among children during summer epidemics of diarrhea in rural Japan. The condition was locally known as "hikan." Mori attributed the problem to lack of fat in the diet, and he noted that milk, cheese, butter, and bacon were not common in the Japanese diet.

Adalbert Czerny and Arthur Keller (1906) noted a nutritional problem in children in Breslau which they called "Mehlnährschaden." The exact translation is elusive, but it literally means "flour-based nutritional disturbance." Mehlnährschaden was described as a cessation of weight gain, emaciation, ocular abnormalities, and depressed immunity, and the condition was noted in children who received flour-based preparations as a substitute for milk or breastmilk. The recommended treatment for Mehlnährschaden was breastfeeding. Further descriptions of xerophthalmia (the typical eye lesions of vitamin A deficiency), diarrhea, and high mortality were made among poor children in the east end of London (Stephenson 1910) and among children in Denmark who were raised on skim milk (Bloch 1919). Sporadic case reports of blinding xerophthalmia continued through the 1920s at places such as Johns Hopkins Hospital and Infant's Hospital in Boston among children who were fed condensed milk lacking in vitamin A (Ross 1921, Wilson and DuBois 1923).

Although these clinical descriptions were dramatic, others argued that these cases were only extreme examples, and on the whole, vitamin A deficiency was rare in Great Britain, Europe and the United States. But in an address published in *The Lancet*, William Cramer (1924) expressed belief that subclinical vitamin A deficiency might actually be common, a condition he called "the borderline between health and disease." He noted, "These effects [from lack of vitamins] are so little obvious that they have up to now been overlooked." Cramer surmised that children in this borderline state would appear well but under stress of infection would do poorly because of an underlying inadequate intake of vitamins. The discovery of the vitamins, Cramer noted, "has placed in our hands a therapeutic and prophylactic weapon of quite unsuspected possibilities in improving the health of the community." Further evidence for a relationship between infection and vitamin A deficiency was soon to come from the animal laboratory.

VITAMIN A AS THE "ANTI-INFECTIVE" VITAMIN

One day in 1925, Edward Mellanby, a Professor of Pharmacology at the University of Sheffield, was summoned to his animal laboratory because some of his dogs were dying. Mellanby had previously received a research studentship to work under the guidance of Frederick Hopkins, and Mellanby was extending the research of his mentor on vitamin A. He was raising a large colony of dogs, and about two-thirds of them had been experimentally rendered vitamin A-deficient. An epidemic of bronchopneumonia was sweeping through the colony, and this accident allowed for a fortuitous observation. On post-mortem examination of 330 dogs, Mellanby (1926) noted that the bronchopneumonia was largely restricted to the vitamin A-deficient dogs. He speculated that the observations of the increased susceptibility to respiratory infections might have possible relevance to children with respiratory illness.

Mellanby and Harry N. Green, another physician at Sheffield, continued to investigate the idea that vitamin A could be necessary for immunity to infections (Green and Mellanby 1928). They described increased infections in vitamin A-deficient rats, and this led them to dub vitamin A an "anti-infective agent." Specifically, they noted that deficiency of vitamin A, but not vitamin D, caused increased infections in the animals. Vitamin A deficiency appeared to produce a breakdown in mucosal surfaces in the lungs and elsewhere, allowing infections to occur. They theorized: "On the basis of these facts we suggested that vitamin A plays a significant part in raising the bodily resistance to infection." By calling vitamin A the "anti-infective" vitamin, Green and Mellanby had made the most explicit statement of such a theory and laid down a challenge to scientific investigators. Different measures were being evaluated for reducing mortality among infants and young children, and their theory underwent an intensive phase of investigation through clinical investigations of vitamin A (Lancet 1931).

The Home for Hebrew Infants. The Home for Hebrew Infants in New York, an asylum run by Dr. Alfred Hess and caring for over 400 children, provides an example of what was being done in general to improve infant health during this period. Due to death or destitution, many parents left their infants to the care of the city, and the Home for Hebrew Infants was considered one of the better institutions in New York. Hess was appalled by the mortality rates in the institutions housing infants in large American cities. In one large infant asylum in New York City, 50% of children died before reaching 24 mo of age, and in another, one third of infants died before their second month under institutional care. Hess (1916) warned that this neglect did not occur in all institutions caring for infants, noting that the infant mortality rate in his institute was only 16% in 1915. He attributed this "low" mortality rate to a minimal 9 mo of training nurses, a ratio of one nurse to five infants during the day, and a milk laboratory.

By the late 1920s the major causes of mortality changed among infants and young children in Europe, Great Britain and the United States. The epidemics of summer diarrhea and high infant mortality had virtually disappeared to the point that epidemic diarrhea was declared defeated in Great Britain by the early 1930s (Lancet 1934). New emphasis was being placed upon the "winter complaint," which was now the leading cause of death. But statistics from the Home for Hebrew Infants show that the case fatality rates for pneumonia were also dropping during the same period. The case fatality rate for pneumonia had dropped by nearly two-thirds, from 23% in a period from 1916 to 1922 to about 7% from 1923 to

1927 (Barenberg et al. 1929). Hess's colleagues attributed these changes in diarrheal and respiratory disease to model institutional care, which included unobstructed, sunny infirmaries, large verandas and avoidance of overcrowding or "hospitalism."

The physicians at the Home for Hebrew Infants thought that further interventions could be made to reduce the incidence of respiratory disease, and in 1925 they conducted a study of ultraviolet radiation, or heliotherapy, from a mercury vapor lamp to reduce respiratory infections. Forty infants in two wards were divided into "irradiated" and "nonirradiated" groups. Final analysis revealed that irradiation appeared to have no effect on the incidence of respiratory disease during the winter (Barenberg et al. 1926). The investigators thought heliotherapy failed because they were using the wrong type of lamp, and the following year they repeated a similar study using a carbon arc lamp. Again they noted no impact of ultraviolet radiation upon the incidence of respiratory infections among the 19 infants in the clinical trial (Barenberg and Lewis 1928). Disappointed with these results, another trial was conducted in 1928 to determine if "aseptic nursing" could reduce the incidence of respiratory disease. The two main infant wards of the home were divided into intervention and control wards. The intervention included hand scrubbing with mercuric chloride, use of surgical masks by all nurses, physicians, and attendants, prohibition of physical contact with infants, and boiling of all plates, spoons, and cooking utensils used by the infants. Among the 79 infants in this trial, "aseptic nursing" appeared to have little impact upon the incidence of respiratory disease (Abramson and Barenberg 1929).

During the time that heliotherapy and aseptic nursing were being tested, malnutrition was virtually unknown in the Home for Hebrew Infants. Alfred Hess, a pioneer in research on vitamins C and D, ensured that all children under 3 yr of age received liberal amounts of orange juice and cod-liver oil daily. Hess was concerned that respiratory disease continued to thwart all preventive efforts, and he was intrigued by Mellanby's proposal to use vitamin A as "anti-infective" therapy. A study was conducted in which all infants in the study received at least what is now considered to be the recommended dietary allowance of vitamin A, and the treatment groups received additional vitamin A in the form of cod-liver oil. Additional cod-liver oil had no effect upon respiratory infections (Barenberg and Lewis 1932). Hess thought that perhaps they were not given enough vitamin A, and another study was performed in which even higher doses of vitamin A were used, to no avail (Hess et al. 1933). All infants in their studies received vegetables, eggs and butter, which are foods rich in vitamin A. Hess concluded that young children do not require more than the vitamin A contained in 750 mL of milk per day, and that giving thousands of units of vitamin A "constitutes therapeutic absurdity, which, happily, will prove to be only a passing fad."

Vitamin A and the common cold. Other studies were conducted to determine if vitamin A could prevent the common cold in school children. One such trial, conducted in the Long Beach, New York, public schools in 1932, included a control group not taking vitamin A, but enthusiasm was so high that parents in the control group started giving their children vitamin A at home. The investigators concluded: "Because of the difficulty in controlling the outside factors of a demonstration of this kind, it is impossible to make an unqualified statement as to the efficiency of vitamin A in cold prevention" (Tress 1935). Physicians at the Montreal Foundling and Baby Hospital, like their colleagues at the Hebrew Home for Infants, had evaluated vaccine, ultraviolet ray, and cod-liver oil, but they considered their results were "so uniformly unsuccessful that it has not been thought worthwhile to make any publication" (Wright et al. 1931). Their trial of regular vs. high doses of vitamin A showed that vitamin A in excessive amounts does not protect infants against the common cold.

Medical and nursing students were recruited into a study conducted at the Case Western Reserve University in 1933 (Shibley and Spies 1934). Vitamin A was given in the form of halibut liver oil to more than 200 volunteers, and the students filled out a card that documented any respiratory symptoms each week. The investigators used random sampling to assign volunteers to treatment groups, and they also attempted to conceal their treatment allocation by giving all participants tomato juice, with or without halibut liver oil. The investigators concluded that vitamin A had no effect on either the incidence or severity of colds, but noted that there was a reduction in the duration of colds in the vitamin A-treated group. For data analysis, the investigators mention that they took the data to a doctor in their Department of Hygiene and Bacteriology, and he reported that the results "were significant statistically." Few studies of this period included a statistical analysis, and it was usually mentioned in a footnote.

By 1940, there had been at least 16 studies involving a total of over 9000 subjects to determine if vitamin A, mostly in the form of cod-liver oil, could reduce the incidence of respiratory infections **(Table 1).** These investigations were conducted in places such as Malmö, Peterhead, New York, and Chicago, and the majority were conducted in the United States. The classroom or Infant Home were the primary sites for conducting the clinical trials. Overall, the results were mixed, with about half of the studies showing an impact of vitamin A on respiratory infections, and the others showing no effect. As suggested by Hess et al. (1933), no therapeutic benefit of vitamin A was noted for infants who were already sufficient in vitamin A. Other studies showed that vitamin A showed promise as a specific treatment for infections such as tuberculosis and typhoid fever and as a means of preventing skin infections in children **(Table 2).** After Edward Mellanby visited Johannesburg in 1929, his enthusiasm about vitamin A convinced local investigators to conduct a trial of vitamin A as therapy for pneumonia among mine laborers at the Crown Mines (Donaldson and Tasker 1930). Their results showed that vitamin A reduced mortality, but a subsequent study at the Rand Mines in Johannesburg was unable to confirm these findings (Orenstein 1932). May Mellanby, the wife of Edward Mellanby and a fellow student from Cambridge, also conducted a series of studies in Sheffield and Birmingham that suggested that cod-liver oil could reduce the incidence of dental caries in children (Mellanby et al. 1924), but these findings were not confirmed in a subsequent study (Day and Sedwick 1934).

Industrial absenteeism. A great effort was made to use vitamins to reduce industrial absenteeism by both adults and children. In Chicago, Katharine Rich (1920) noted that more and more children were joining the labor force because of the increased cost of living. She was interested in improving the nutritional status of these children so that they could be healthier child laborers and would not drop out. Because of malnutrition, Rich noted that children "lost their jobs, became discouraged and gravitated into becoming rolling stones, thus easily falling prey to vicious and criminal companions." In the following years she conducted investigations and made recommendations aimed at improving the nutrition of children in the Chicago schools.

In the United States, a major concern among industry in the 1930s was the loss of productivity due to illness in the labor force of 36 million. It was estimated that 250 million

TABLE 1

Studies of vitamin A as "anti-infective" prophylactic therapy, 1920–1940

Subjects	n	Location	Intervention	Therapeutic effect of vitamin A	Reference
Prevention of respiratory infections					
Children	1721	Malmo	Cod-liver oil vs control	↓ Incidence of disease	Widmark and Svensson (1926)
Infants	60	Montreal	Vitamin A vs. control	No effect on incidence of disease	Wright et al. (1931)
Infants	188	New York	Small vs. moderate vs. high intake vitamin A	No effect on incidence of disease	Barenberg and Lewis (1932)
Adults	313	United States	Cod-liver oil vs. control	↓ Incidence of disease	Holmes et al. (1932)
Children	160	New York	Halibut-liver oil vs. carotene vs. control	No effect on incidence of disease	Hess et al. (1933)
Children	575	Peterhead	Vitamin A + D vs. placebo	No effect on incidence of disease	Sutherland (1934)
Children	75	Loma Linda	Halibut-liver oil vs. vitamin A diet vs. control	↓ Severity of disease, ↑ weight gain	Gardner and Gardner (1934)
Adults	36	New Orleans	Cod-liver oil vs. historical controls	↓ Incidence and ↓ severity of disease	Beard (1934)
Adults	241	Cleveland	Halibut-liver oil vs. vitamin D vs. control	No effect on incidence of disease	Shibley and Spies (1934)
Children	275	Brooklyn	Halibut-liver oil vs. vitamin D vs. control	No effect on incidence of disease	Gittleman and Wiener (1935)
Adults	200	West Virginia	Various sources vitamin A vs. control	No effect on incidence, ↓ severity	Cameron (1935)
Children	262	Long Beach	Halibut-liver oil vs. historical controls	↓ Incidence of disease	Tress (1935)
Adults	1780	United States	Cod-liver oil vs. control	↓ Incidence of disease	Holmes et al. (1935)
Adults	3031	United States	Cod-liver oil vs. control	↓ Incidence of disease	Holmes et al. (1936)
Infants	104	New York	High vs. low vitamin A	No effect on incidence of disease	Lewis and Barenberg (1936)
Adults	54	Chicago	Vitamin A vs. vitamin D vs. vitamin A + D	↓ Incidence, severity in vitamin A + D group	Spiesman (1941)
Prevention of dental caries					
Children	102	Sheffield (?)	Three levels of vitamin A intake	↓ Incidence of disease	Mellanby et al. (1924)
Children	430	Rochester	Vitamin A + D vs. control	No effect on incidence of disease	Day and Sedwick (1934)
Prevention of puerperal sepsis					
Gravid women	550	Sheffield	Cod-liver oil vs. control	↓ Morbidity	Green et al. (1931)
Gravid women	235	Bellshill	Serum vs. adexolin vs. both	↓ Morbidity	Cameron (1931)
Prevention of skin infections					
Infants	118	London	Vitamin A vs. control	↓ Incidence of skin infections	Mackay (1934)

working days were lost per year to illness. Arthur Holmes, medical advisor to the E. L. Patch Company in Boston, calculated that colds and respiratory diseases cost American industries a waste of wages of exactly $494,836,363.68 per year (Holmes et al. 1936). About half of the industrial absenteeism was due to respiratory illness. Holmes and colleagues conducted a trial of cod-liver oil among industrial workers in a factory in the American midwest. Over 300 workers received daily cod-liver oil or no treatment, and the trial included both clerical workers and light- and heavy-machine operators. The outcome of the study was hours of industrial absenteeism due to respiratory illness. Members in the treatment group had 40% lower absenteeism than the control group (Holmes et al. 1932). A larger trial involving 1800 workers (Holmes et al. 1935) and another with over 3000 workers were reported (Holmes et al. 1936), and these studies suggested that cod-liver oil therapy reduced industrial absenteeism by two-thirds. Thus, cod-liver oil, which was very inexpensive, was considered to have tremendous value in saving millions of dollars in lost working days and lost productivity to American industry.

Measles. Throughout the nineteenth century, there were large measles epidemics in London which occurred about every 2 yr. During these measles epidemics some of the wards in hospitals in London would be overflowing, and up to 20% of children could die. Measles was generally considered to be unavoidable, and treatment of measles was largely supportive, with general hygiene and nursing. Respiratory disease and diarrhea often complicated a measles attack. Joseph Bramhall Ellison, an assistant medical officer with the London Fever Hospital, cared for children on the measles wards and was aware of the work of Edward Mellanby. Because vitamin A deficiency was shown in experimental animals to affect epithelial surfaces and the respiratory tract, Ellison reasoned that administration of vitamin A might be used to treat acute measles in children. Prior to his study, Ellison reported that the mortality rate from measles in the Acute Fever Hospitals in London was about 8% in 1929 and 1930. The following 2 yr, Ellison conducted a trial of cod-liver oil for 600 children with acute measles, and he randomized the children by ward in order to make the treatment groups comparable. Treatment with vitamin A reduced measles mortality by about one-half, from 8.7% in the untreated group to 3.7% in the treated group (Ellison 1932). Ellison's findings attracted a great deal of

TABLE 2

Studies of vitamin A as "anti-infective" therapy for specific diseases, 1920–1940

Subjects	n	Location	Intervention	Therapeutic effect of vitamin A	Reference
Therapy for acute measles					
Children	600	London	Cod-liver oil vs. control	↓ Morbidity and mortality	Ellison (1932)
Children	697	London	Cod-liver oil + vitamin D vs. vitamin D vs. control	No effect on morbidity or mortality	Mackay et al. (1936)
Therapy for pneumonia					
Mine laborers	299	Johannesburg	Cod-liver oil vs. ox liver vs. control	↓ Mortality	Donaldson and Tasker (1930)
Mine laborers	764	Johannesburg	Vitamin A vs. control	No effect on morbidity or mortality	Orenstein (1932)
Therapy for scarlet fever					
Children	509	Boston	Cod-liver oil vs. historical controls	No effect on incidence of complications	Sutliff et al. (1933)
Children	90	Madrid	Vitamin A vs. sesame oil vs. control	No effect on incidence of complications	Arjona (1934)
Therapy for typhoid fever					
Children	71	Marseille	Cod-liver oil vs. historical controls	↓ Morbidity and mortality	Giraud and Vallette (1939)
Therapy for tuberculosis					
Children	26	United States	Cod-liver oil vs. historical controls	↓ Morbidity, ↑ growth	Holmes and Ackerman (1930)
Children	78	Sheffield	Cod-liver oil vs. high vitamin A + D	Similar improvement in both groups	Pattison (1930)

attention, but some did not find consistent benefit in using vitamin A for measles (Gunn 1935).

Ellison's study was conducted at a time when case fatality rates for measles appeared to be falling in both Great Britain and the United States. For example, in Brighton (United Kingdom), only about 1% of children who developed measles died (Forbes 1933), and in large cities in the United States, the case fatality rate for measles had dropped to about 2% by 1930 (Emerson 1934). Helen Mackay, who studied nutritional problems in children, was on the staff of the Medical Research Council at the time when Edward Mellanby was serving as secretary of the council. Mackay conducted a second investigation of vitamin A therapy for acute measles. Her study was conducted among nearly 700 children admitted to the North Eastern Hospital in London in 1934. The overall mortality in the study was about 5%, and cod-liver oil had no apparent effect on reducing measles mortality (Mackay et al. 1936). The second negative trial seems to have dampened enthusiasm for using vitamin A as therapy for acute measles. In subsequent years there was infrequent mention of vitamin A in review articles and textbooks concerning the treatment of measles.

Puerperal fever. Another major challenge in the 1920s was puerperal fever, a common, fulminating bacterial infection that occurred among women who had just given birth. In the mid-nineteenth century, Oliver Wendell Holmes and Ignaz Semmelweis showed that puerperal fever was contagious and that doctors and midwives could spread the disease from person to person. The main bacterial pathogen involved in puerperal fever was later identified as a streptococcus. Careful hand washing was shown to lower the incidence of the disease and reduce maternal mortality. Even with these precautions, the case fatality rate from puerperal fever could be high. For example, in a large case series of women with puerperal fever reported from Glasgow, the mortality rate was about 5% (Thomas 1930). Antistreptococcal serum was evaluated in clinical trials for the treatment of puerperal fever, but there was little agreement whether it had any therapeutic value (Colebrook 1935).

While other investigators were directing efforts toward testing vitamin A therapy for the common cold, Mellanby and his colleagues conducted a trial of cod-liver oil therapy for puerperal fever in Sheffield. Their preliminary studies suggested that vitamin A therapy would reduce the morbidity and mortality of puerperal infection (Mellanby and Green 1929). From a small group of women with puerperal fever, they reported that 92% of control women died, whereas 29% of the vitamin A-treated women died, about a two-thirds reduction in mortality. Mellanby and his colleagues also thought that vitamin A could be used as prophylactic therapy against puerperal fever. In two hospitals in Sheffield, 550 women were enrolled during antenatal care to receive cod-liver oil or no treatment on a daily basis for 1 mo prior to delivery. The results of the trial suggested that cod-liver oil reduced the incidence of the most serious cases of puerperal fever from 4.7 to 1.1% (Green et al. 1931).

Physicians at the County of Lanark Maternity Hospital near Edinburgh conducted a large trial that confirmed the findings of Green and Mellanby (Cameron 1931). Treatment with cod-liver oil reduced the incidence of puerperal fever by an impressive two-thirds. The study was presented at the Edinburgh Obstetrical Society. In the ensuing discussion, one physician suggested that the findings were so good that application should be considered for maternity hospitals across the country, but others warned that further investigation was needed. In the puerperal fever wards of Belvidere Hospital in Glasgow, Scotland, 800 patients were treated with different therapies, including quinine, glycerin, sera, arsenicals, mercury, saline lavage, and vitamin A, and vitamin A did not appear to confer any advantage. It was argued, in any case, that puerperal sepsis was not a nutritional deficiency disease (Thomas 1930).

ADVENT OF THE SULFA ANTIBIOTICS

The paradigm that vitamin A had an effect in reducing the severity of infections was still being worked out in the late 1930s. The development of the powerful sulfa antibiotics probably slowed further interest in the use of vitamin A as "anti-infective" therapy. Sulphonilamide treatment reduced the mortality from puerperal fever from 22 to 8% (Colebrook and Kenny 1936), and similar impressive results were obtained using sulfapyridine for lobar pneumonia. Much activity in clinical trials focused upon sulfa antibiotics and then later shifted to penicillin (Dowling 1977). The impact of antibiotic treatment upon infections was widely recognized, and vitamin A faded from the arena of clinical investigation. From 1940 onward, there were only occasional trials of vitamin A until the flurry of activity in the 1980s that was largely sparked by the observation of increased mortality among children with mild vitamin A deficiency in Indonesia (Sommer et al. 1983).

STATISTICAL INFERENCE AND CLINICAL TRIALS

The early investigations of vitamin A were, in essence, clinical trials, but they often lacked many features that are considered critical to the modern controlled clinical trial such as randomization, masking, placebo controls, and sample size and power calculations. The studies were also conducted in a period before the controlled clinical trial—as it is known today—became the widely accepted scientific basis for therapeutic experimentation (Marks 1997). Many ideas of statistical inference were just emerging in Great Britain and had little impact on the early clinical investigations of vitamin A. Jerzy Neyman and Egon Pearson (1928) introduced the idea of alternative hypotheses and two types of error. In their theory, Neyman and Pearson presented the idea of the probability α of rejecting a true hypothesis and the probability β of accepting a false hypothesis. To test a certain hypothesis, it is desirable to have a sufficiently large power function so that the probability α is small and the true hypothesis is accepted. The optimal experiment will thus utilize a sufficiently large sample so that the chance of the two types of error is minimized. If the rate of an outcome event is low, a large sample size is needed to detect with sufficient power if an experimental therapy is having an effect. For example, to show a reduction of mortality in measles from 4 to 2%, a clinical trial of vitamin A therapy in the 1930s would need to enroll at least 3000 children with measles to have sufficient statistical power to detect such a therapeutic effect on these low rates of mortality.

Although most of the early clinical investigations of vitamin A employed groups of untreated patients who served as controls, almost all of the trials lacked randomization, the assignment of patients on a random basis to treatment and control groups. The idea of randomization in experimental design was promoted by Ronald A. Fisher, a geneticist and statistician who began work at the Rothamsted Experimental Station in Great Britain in 1919. Fisher worked with plants, and he had some practical experience working as a subsistence farmer prior to entering academia. Fisher was put in charge of experiments to evaluate new grain varieties, and he was concerned about the design of previous experiments in which plots of grain were planted and compared. Fisher knew that the yield of two fields could vary because of differences in soil, temperature, light, moisture and other factors. As a solution,

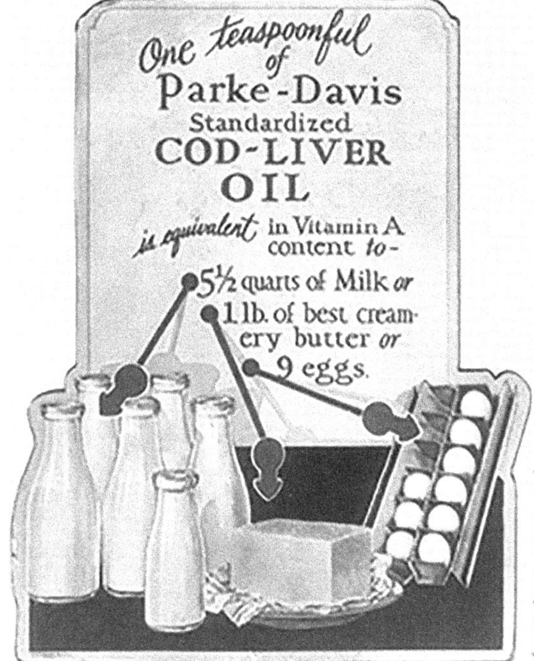

FIGURE 1 Folding counter display advertisement for Parke-Davis cod-liver oil, circa 1935 (Collection of the author).

Fisher proposed randomization of grain varieties by row, rather than by field, in order to reduce background variation in the experimental design. The idea of randomization was further promulgated by Fisher (1935) in his textbook *The Design of Experiments*, but there seemed to be little immediate effect upon clinical investigation. Randomization is often considered to have been introduced by A. Bradford Hill in British studies of streptomycin in the 1940s (Hill 1990), but it is apparent that the concept of randomization, either by individual or ward, was known at least to some clinical investigators in the vitamin A trials of the 1930s.

VITAMINS AND THE PUBLIC

The pharmaceutical industry was quick to promote the paradigm of vitamin A as "anti-infective" therapy. They aimed their advertising at young mothers in women's magazines using a combination of fear, hope, guilt, and the contemporary image of motherhood (Apple 1996). Advertisements warned mothers that the hidden danger of vitamin deficiencies could be lurking in their own homes. One ad read: "A certain famous American doctor, whose life is being devoted to the study of malnutrition in children . . . tells mothers that one out of every three children in the United States is malnourished." Another ad raised the question: "Your family vitamin-starved? Impossible! Yet science now finds the average American family diet lacking in at least 3 important vitamins!"

The work of Mellanby, Ellison and others did not go unnoticed by the pharmaceutical industry. A Squibb advertisement for cod-liver oil read: "Whooping cough, measles, mumps, chicken pox, scarlet fever may do greater harm than most mothers think . . . the children will have lighter cases, they recover quicker and are less likely to be left with some permanent injury, if they build up good general resistance in advance to fight them . . . one precaution to build up the resistance of children . . . [is to give them] 'resistance-building' vitamin A. Vitamin A is the important factor which increases their fighting power in time of illness." The vitamin A content of some cod-liver oil preparations was impressively high **(Fig. 1)**.

Vitamins occupy an unusual position in therapeutics, for unlike vaccines, antibiotics, or serum therapy, vitamins were more accessible by the public. Also the duality in vitamins exists: considered as a drug by some and as a constituent of food by others. Druggists attacked the grocers when bottles of vitamins started appearing on grocery store shelves, but the grocers argued that selling vitamins was consistent with selling fruits, vegetables and dairy products (Apple 1996). This "prophylactic and therapeutic weapon" of vitamins was placed squarely in the hands of the public, and whatever was thought by scientists could be accepted or rejected by the consumer. As a result of advertising and popular belief, the paradigm of vitamin A as an "anti-infective" vitamin became widely accepted by the public. By 1940, the United States and Great Britain alike had become extremely "vitamin-conscious." Legislation was proposed that miners and other workers could receive a larger ration of butter (British Medical Journal 1940), and milk was instituted as part of school lunch programs (Frazer 1950). With the outbreak of World War II, concern was raised over the crowded conditions of underground bomb shelters in London and the spread of respiratory and diarrheal disease. It was proposed that fortification of margarine with vitamin A would help to reduce the risk of infection (Lancet 1940). Cod-liver oil was provided by the British Ministry of Food for children under five and for pregnant and breastfeeding women (Kurlansky 1997). The administration of cod-liver oil became part of a morning routine for millions of children in America and Europe.

The theory that vitamin A influenced immunity and could be used as "anti-infective" therapy was clearly stated by Edward Mellanby, and his studies provided a model for a tradition of scientific research that continues today. The controlled clinical trial had evolved considerably since the 1940s (Marks 1997), providing what was considered the necessary scientific "proof" for the validity of particular therapies. In calling vitamin A the "anti-infective" vitamin, Mellanby (1934) noted, "we were, of course, aware of the drawbacks of giving a label of this kind, because the word 'infection' covers several different types of pathological phenomena, but we also recognized that it had the advantage of attracting the attention of workers to this important subject." After a pause of almost 50 yr, the value of vitamin A as "anti-infective" therapy was addressed again in controlled clinical trials, and these studies provided compelling new scientific evidence for the use of vitamin A as an important public health intervention.

ACKNOWLEDGMENT

I wish to thank the staff of the National Library of Medicine, Bethesda, Maryland, and the Wellcome Institute for the History of Medicine, London, for their kind assistance, and Rima Apple and Harry Marks for helpful comments on the paper.

LITERATURE CITED

Abramson, H. & Barenberg, L. H. (1929) Respiratory disorders in infants. Attempted prevention by control of contact infection. J. Am. Med. Assoc. 92: 2156–2158.

American Academy of Pediatrics. Committee on Infectious Diseases. (1993) Vitamin A treatment of measles. Pediatrics 91: 1014–1015.

Apple, R. D. (1996) Vitamania: Vitamins in American Culture. New Brunswick, New Jersey, Rutgers University Press.

Arjona, E. (1934) Resultados del tratamiento por la vitamina A de las complicaciones de la escarlatina. Arch. Med. Cir. Especial. 37: 10–12.

Barenberg, L. H., Friedman, I. & Green, D. (1926) The effect of ultraviolet irradiation on the health of a group of infants. J. Am. Med. Assoc. 87: 1114–1117.

Barenberg, L. H., Greene, D. & Abramson, H. (1929) The relationship of nutrition to pneumonia in infancy and childhood. J. Am. Med. Assoc. 92: 440–443.

Barenberg, L. H. & Lewis J. M. (1928) The effect of carbon arc irradiation on the health of a group of infants. J. Am. Med. Assoc. 90: 504–506.

Barenberg, L. H. & Lewis J. M. (1932) Relationship of vitamin A to respiratory infections in infants. J. Am. Med. Assoc. 98: 199–202.

Beard, H. H. (1934) The prophylactic effect of vitamins A and D upon the prevention of the common cold and influenza. J. Am. Dietet. Assoc. 10: 193–199.

Beaton, G. H., Martorell, R., L'Abbe, K. A., Edmonston, B., McCabe, G., Ross, A. C. & Harvey, B. (1993) Effectiveness of Vitamin A Supplementation in the Control of Young Child Morbidity and Mortality in Developing Countries. ACC/SCN State-of-the-Art Nutrition Policy Discussion Paper No. 13, United Nations.

Billard, C. (1828) Traité des Maladies des Enfans Nouveaux-Nés et a la Mamelle, Fondé sur de Nouvelles Observations Cliniques et d'Anatomie Pathologique, Faites a l'Hôpital des Enfans-Trouvés de Paris, dans le Service de M. Baron. Paris, J. B. Baillière.

Bloch, C. E. (1919) Klinische Untersuchungen über Dystrophie und Xerophthalmie bei jungen Kindern. Jahrb. Kinderheilk. phys. Erziehung 89: 405–441.

British Medical Journal (1940) Medical notes in Parliament. Vitamin A in miners' butter ration. Brit. Med. J. 2: 241.

Brown, J. (1827) Case of ulcerated cornea, from inanition. Edinb. J. Med. Sci. 3: 218.

Bunge, G. von. (1887) Lehrbuch der physiologischen und pathologischen Chemie. Leipzig, F.C.W. Vogel.

Cameron, H. C. (1935) The effect of vitamin A upon incidence and severity of colds among students. J. Am. Dietet. Assoc. 11: 189–204.

Cameron, S. J. (1931) An aid in the prevention of puerperal sepsis. Trans. Edinburgh Obstet. Soc. 52: 93–103.

Colebrook, L. (1935) Treatment of puerperal fever by antistreptococcal serum. Some new evidence and a retrospect. Lancet 1: 1005–1009.

Colebrook, L. & Kenny, M. (1936) Treatment of human puerperal infections, and of experimental infections in mice, with Protonsil. Lancet 1: 1279–1286.

Cramer, W. (1924) Vitamins and the borderland between health and disease. Lancet 1: 633–640.

Czerny, A. & Keller, A. (1906) Des Kindes Ernahrung, Ernahrungsstörungen und Ernahrungstherapie. Leipzig and Wien, Franz Deuticke.

Day, C.D.M. & Sedwick, H. J. (1934) The fat-soluble vitamins and dental caries in children. J. Nutr. 8: 309–328.

Donaldson, S. & Tasker, J. (1930) Preliminary notes in the treatment of pneumonia with vitamin "A." Proc. Transvaal Mine Officers Assoc.: 64–68.

Dowling, H. F. (1977) Fighting Infection: Conquests of the Twentieth Century. Cambridge, Massachusetts, Harvard University Press.

Ellison, J. B. (1932) Intensive vitamin therapy in measles. Brit. Med. J. 2: 708–711.

Emerson, H. (1934) Measles and Whooping Cough. Incidence, Fatality and Death Rates in Thirty-Two Cities of the United States, in Relation to Administrative Procedures Intended for Control, 1924–1933. Sub-Committee on Evaluation of Health Department Practices, Committee on Administrative Practice, American Public Health Association [no location cited].

Fisher, R. A. (1935) The Design of Experiments. London, Oliver & Boyd.

Forbes, D. (1933) Measles mortality. Lancet 2: 253–255.

Frazer, W. M. (1950) A History of English Public Health, 1834–1939. London, Baillière, Tindall and Cox.

Funk, C. (1912) The etiology of the deficiency diseases. J. State Med. 20: 341–368.

Gardner, E. L. & Gardner, F. W. (1934) Vitamin A and colds. Am. J. Dis. Child. 47: 1261–1264.

Giraud, P. & Vallette, A. (1939) Essai de traitement de la fièvre typhoide chez l'enfant par la vitamine A. Arch. Méd. Enfants 42: 691–697.

Gittleman, I. F. & Wiener, A. S. (1935) Vitamin A and infection. J. Ped. 7: 81–86.

Green, H. N. & Mellanby, E. (1928) Vitamin A as an anti-infective agent. Brit. Med. J. 2: 691–696.

Green, H. N., Pindar, D., Davis, G. & Mellanby, E. (1931) Diet as a prophylactic agent against puerperal sepsis. Brit. Med. J. 2: 595–598.

Gunn, W. (1935) The treatment of measles. Brit. Med. J. 1: 597–599.

Hess, A. F. (1916) Institutions as foster mothers for infants. Arch. Ped. 33: 96–106.

Hess, A. F., Lewis, J. M. & Barenberg, L. H. (1933) Does our dietary require vitamin A supplement? J. Am. Med. Assoc. 101: 657–663.

Hill, A. B. (1990) Suspended judgment, memories of the British streptomycin trial, the first randomized clinical trial. Controlled Clinical Trials 11: 77–79.

Holmes, A. D. & Ackerman, H. L. (1930) The value of cod liver oil for underpar children of school age. N. Engl. J. Med. 202: 470–476.

Holmes, A. D., Pigott, M. G., Sawyer, W. A. & Comstock, L. (1932) Vitamins aid reduction of lost time in industry. Indust. Eng. Chem. 24: 1058–1060.

Holmes, A. D., Pigott, M. G., Sawyer, W. A. & Comstock, L. (1935) The influence of body weight and the administration of cod liver oil in industrial absenteeism. J. Am. Dietet. Assoc. 10: 208–216.

Holmes, A. D., Pigott, M. G., Sawyer, W. A. & Comstock, L. (1936) Cod liver oil. A five-year study of its value for reducing industrial absenteeism caused by colds and respiratory diseases. Indust. Med. 5: 359–361.

Holst, A. & Frölich, T. (1907) Experimental studies relating to ship-beri-beri and scurvy. II. On the etiology of scurvy. J. Hyg. 7: 634–671.

Holt, L. E. (1900a) The Care and Feeding of Children: A Catechism for the Use of Mothers and Children's Nurses. New York and London, D. Appleton and Co.

Holt, L. E. (1900b) The Diseases of Infancy and Childhood: For the Use of Students and Practitioners of Medicine. New York, D. Appleton and Company.

Holt, L. E. (1910) The medical prevention of infant mortality. Trans. Am. Assoc. Study Prev. Infant Mortality 1: 204–206.

Hopkins, F. G. (1906) The analyst and the medical man. Analyst 31: 385–397.

Hopkins, F. G. (1912) Feeding experiments illustrating the importance of accessory factors in normal dietaries. J. Physiol. 44: 425–460.

Hutchison, R. (1940) Paediatrics: past, present and prospective. Lancet 2: 799–803.

Knox, J.H.M. (1910) Address by the president. Trans. Am. Assoc. Study Prev. Infant Mortality 1: 29–32.

Kurlansky, M. (1997) Cod. A Biography of the Fish that Changed the World. London, Jonathan Cape.

Lancet (1931) Editorial: Renewed interest in vitamin A. Lancet 1: 706.

Lancet (1934) Parliament and child mortality. Lancet 2: 146–147.

Lancet (1940) Editorial: Infection in the shelter. Lancet 2: 455–456.

Lewis, J. M. & Barenberg, L. H. (1938) The relationship of vitamin A to the health of infants. Further observations. J. Am. Med. Assoc. 110: 1338–1341.

Lunin, N. (1881) Über die Bedeutung der anorganischen Salze für die Ernährung des Thieres. Zeitschr. physiol. Chem. 5: 31–39.

Mackay, H.M.M. (1934) Vitamin A deficiency in children. Part II. Vitamin A requirements of babies: skin lesions and vitamin A deficiency. Arch. Dis. Child. 9: 133–152.

Mackay, H.M.M., Linford, H. M., Mitman, M. & Wild, M. H. (1936) The therapeutic value of vitamins A & D in measles. Arch. Dis. Child. 11: 127–142.

Marks, H. M. (1997) The Progress of Experiment. Science and Therapeutic Reform in the United States, 1900–1990. Cambridge, Cambridge University Press.

McCollum, E. V. & Davis, M. (1913) The necessity of certain lipins in the diet during growth. J. Biol. Chem. 15: 167–175.

Meckel, R. (1990) Save the Babies: American Public Health Reform and the Prevention of Infant Mortality, 1850–1929. Baltimore, Johns Hopkins University Press.

Mellanby, E. (1926) Diet and disease, with special reference to the teeth, lungs, and pre-natal feeding. Lancet 1: 515–519.

Mellanby, E. (1934) Nutrition and Disease. The Interaction of Clinical and Experimental Work. London, Oliver and Boyd.

Mellanby, E. & Green, H. N. (1929) Vitamin A as an anti-infective agent. Its use in the treatment of puerperal septicemia. Brit. Med. J. 1: 984–986.

Mellanby, M., Pattison, C. L. & Proud, J. W. (1924) The effect of diet on the development and extension of caries in the teeth of children. Brit. Med. J. 2: 354–355.

Mori, M. (1904) Über den sog. Hikan (Xerosis conjunctivae infantum ev. Keratomalacie). Jahrb. Kinderheilk. 59: 175–195.

Newman, G. (1906) Infant Mortality: A Social Problem. London, Methuen and Company.

Neyman, J. & Pearson, E. S. (1928) On the use and interpretation of certain test criteria for purposes of statistical inference. Biometrika 20A (part 1): 175–240, (part 2): 263–294.

Nicholls, L. (1938) Tropical Nutrition and Dietetics. London, Baillière, Tindall & Cox.

Orenstein, A. J. (1932) Vitamin A in the treatment of pneumonia. S. Afr. Med. J. 6: 685–689.

Osborne, T. B. & Mendel, L. B. (1911) Feeding Experiments with Isolated Food-Substances. Washington, D.C., Carnegie Institute of Washington, Publication 156.

Osborne, T. B. & Mendel, L. B. (1913) The relationship of growth to the chemical constituents of the diet. J. Biol. Chem. 15: 311–326.

Pattison, C. L. (1930) Treatment of bone tuberculosis by large amounts of vitamins A and D. Brit. Med. J. 2: 178–179.

Pekelharing, C. A. (1905) Over onze kennis van de waarde der voedingsmiddelen uit chemische fabrieken. Nederlandsch Tijdschr. Geneeskunde 41: 111–124.

Ratier (1824) Note sur un cas d'ulcération de la cornée transparente. Arch. Gen. Med. 2 Ser. 4: 255.

Rich, K. B. (1920) Study of nutrition and mental development in childhood. Preliminary report of work done by the Board of Education in the public schools of Chicago. J. Am. Med. Assoc. 75: 226–228.

Richardson, A. S. (1916) What the expectant mother should eat. Pictorial Review 17: 37.

Ross, S. G. (1921) Nutritional keratomalacia in infants with a report of four cases. Am. J. Dis. Child. 22: 232–243.

Shibley, G. S. & Spies, T. D. (1934) The effect of vitamin A on the common cold. J. Am. Med. Assoc. 103: 2021–2026.

Socin, C. A. (1891) In welcher Form wird das Eisen resorbirt? Zeitschr. physiol. Chem. 15: 93–139.

Sommer, A., Hussaini, G., Tarwotjo, I. & Susanto, D. (1983) Increased mortality in children with mild vitamin A deficiency. Lancet 2: 585–588.

Spiesman, I. G. (1941) Massive doses of vitamins A and D in the prevention of the common cold. Arch. Otolaryngol. 34: 787–791.

Steenbock, H. (1932) A review of certain researches relating to the occurrence and chemical nature of vitamin A. Yale J. Biol. Med. 4: 563–578.

Stephenson, S. (1910) On sloughing corneae in infants: an account based upon the records of thirty-one cases. Ophthalmoscope 8: 782–818.

Stepp, W. (1911) Experimentelle Untersuchungen über die Bedeutung der Lipoide für die Ernährung. Z. Biol. 57: 136–170.

Sutherland, R. (1934) Vitamins A and D: Their relation to growth and resistance to disease. Brit. Med. J. 1: 791–795.

Sutliff, W. D., Place, E. H. & Segool, S. H. (1933) Cod liver oil concentrate (concentrated vitamins A and D): ineffectiveness of large doses in the prophylaxis of otitis media complicating scarlet fever. J. Am. Med. Assoc. 100: 725–728.

Thomas, M. (1930) The Epidemiology, Bacteriology, and Treatment of Puerperal Sepsis. Report of the Medical Officer of Health City of Glasgow, 1930: 112–146.

Tress, E. M. (1935) Vitamin "A" as a prophylactic against the common "cold" in groups of school children. Am. J. Dig. Dis. Nutr. 1: 795–796.

Widmark, E.M.P. & Svensson, B. (1928) Studien über den Bedarf und zur Verfügung stehende Mengen an fettlöslichen Vitaminen der Kinder in den Volksschulen zu Malmö. Skan. Archiv Physiol. 54: 127–144.

Wilson, J. R. & DuBois, R. O. (1923) Report of a fatal case of keratomalacia in an infant, with postmortem examination. Am. J. Dis. Child. 26: 431–446.

Wolf, G. (1998) M. Mori's definitive recognition of vitamin A deficiency and its cure in children. Nutrition 14: 481–484.

Wolf, G. & Carpenter, K. J. (1997) Early research into the vitamins: the work of Wilhelm Stepp. J. Nutr. 127: 1255–1259.

World Bank (1993) World Development Report 1993: Investing in Health. New York, Oxford University Press.

World Health Organization (1987) Joint WHO/UNICEF statement on vitamin A for measles. Weekly Epidemiol. Rec. World Health Organ. 62: 133–134.

Wright, H. P., Frosst, J. B., Puchel, F. & Lawrence, M. R. (1931) Vitamin "A" and the common cold. Can. Med. Assoc. J. 25: 412–416.

Home Catalog Talk to Dr Red Wholesale Enquiries

Home › Dr Red Punch Concentrate Range › blueberry + double + Ginger + prostate + immune + purple + carrot + Rosella

Dr Red Punch Concentrate Range

Browse by Rosella Sort by Alphabetically, A-Z

Manufactured in Australia from both Australian and Imported ingredients, Dr Red's Punch Range has been available since 2005. By combining fruit concentrates with food extracts made using the patent (pending) Modified Polyphenol Technology Process we have created a range of concentrates which you mix with plain water or soda to create a refreshing drink.

Contact us

Phone: 1300 377 331

Email: talktodrred@drred.com.au

Fax: (07) 3289 5705

Mail: PO Box 35, The Gap Qld 4061

Amazing Dandelion: Now we know why Monsanto went after the dandelions:

"Just one leaf of this herb, found in every garden, can save your life in a minute, but only some people know how to use it!

It kills up to 96% of leukemia cells in just 48 hours!

Nature itself has many effective health remedies. You may not know the presence of many effective plants, but in fact, they are located right in your garden.

When it comes to leukemia, many of us are the first to equip ourselves with medication, chemotherapy, poor quality of life and overall misery.

Here's all the info you need to know about the roots (and leaves) of a dandelion and what it can do for people battling leukemia.

Recent studies have shown that the dandelion root is cytotoxic against three types of human leukemia cells and it destroys up to 96% of cells in just 48 hours!

Dandelion tea affects cancer cells by breaking down within 48 hours and stimulating the growth of new healthy cells in the patient's body.

The study was conducted by Dr. Hamm with his students.

They removed blood cells from 9 different patients who used root extract and applied it to several cells to cultivate them. Within 24 hours, the cells were killed.

There have also been a number of other studies to find that dandelion extract can have potentially effective substances against cancer, melanomas and prostate and breast cancer.

Other properties of dandelion root/leaves...Dandelion root/leaf extract has been used for centuries as an effective healing agent in traditional folk medicine.

Anaemia...Dandelions have a fairly high content of iron, vitamins and proteins. While iron is a part of haemoglobin in the blood, vitamins like vitamin B and proteins are important for the formation of red blood cells and some other blood components. A dandelion can help with anaemia.

Strong bones...Dandelion is rich in calcium, which is essential for bone growth and strength, and is rich in antioxidants such as vitamin C and luteolin, which protect bones from age-related damage.

Diabetes ...Dandelion juice can help diabetics by stimulating the production of insulin from the pancreas.

Prevents urinary tract infection...Dandelion can help prevent urinary tract infections, as well as bladder and kidney disorders, or even cysts on the reproductive organs.

Cleanses the liver ...Vitamins and nutrients contained in the dandelion help to clean the liver and ensure their proper function. Dandelions help our digestive system by maintaining proper bile flow. Dandelion is also rich in vitamin C, reduces inflammation and prevents disease.

Digestion Assistance...Dandelion acts as a mild food that promotes digestion, encourages appetite and balances natural and beneficial bacteria in the intestines.

Skin care . . .Dandelion juice is also used to treat skin diseases caused by microbial and fungal infections. The juice is highly alkaline and has insecticidal, bactericidal and fungicidal effects.

This juice can be used for itching, shingles, eczema, etc."

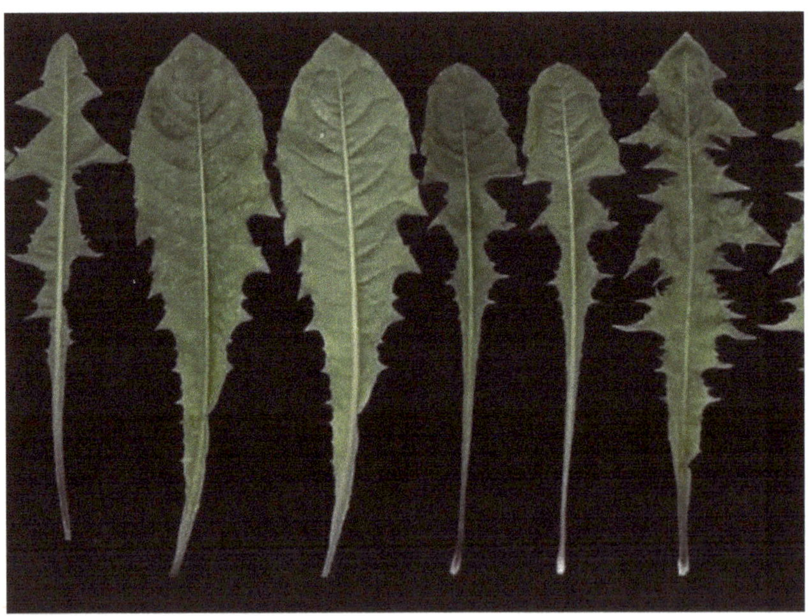

Save citation to file

Format:

Summary (text)

Create file   Cancel

FULL TEXT LINKS

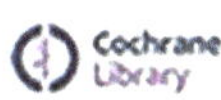

Review   Cochrane Database Syst Rev. 2002;(1):CD001479. doi: 10.1002/14651858.CD001479.

Vitamin A for treating measles in children

R M D'Souza [1], R D'Souza

Affiliations
PMID: 11869601 DOI: 10.1002/14651858.CD001479

Update in

Vitamin A for treating measles in children.
Huiming Y, Chaomin W, Meng M.
Cochrane Database Syst Rev. 2005 Oct 19;2005(4):CD001479. doi: 10.1002/14651858.CD001479.pub3.
PMID: 16235283 Free PMC article. Review.

Abstract

Background: Measles is a leading cause of childhood morbidity and mortality. Vitamin A deficiency is a recognised risk factor for severe measles. The World Health Organization (WHO) recommends administration of an oral dose of 200,000 IU (or 100,000 IU in infants) of vitamin A per day for two days to children with measles in areas where vitamin A deficiency may be present.

Objectives: The purpose of this review is to determine whether vitamin A when commenced after measles has been diagnosed, is beneficial in preventing mortality, pneumonia and other complications in children.

Search strategy: MEDLINE and the Cochrane Library, Issue 4, 1999 were searched.

Selection criteria: Only randomized controlled trials in which children with measles were given vitamin A or placebo along with standard treatment were considered.

Data collection and analysis: Studies were assessed independently by two reviewers. The analysis of dichotomous outcomes was done using the StatXact software package. Sub-group analyses were done for dose, formulation, age, hospitalisation and pneumonia specific mortality. Weighted mean difference with 95% CI were calculated for continuous outcomes.

Main results: The relative risks (RR) and 95% Confidence Intervals (CI) are based on the estimates from the StatXact software package. There was no significant reduction in mortality in the vitamin A group when all the studies were pooled together (RR 0.60; 95% CI 0.32 to 1.12)(StatXact estimate). There was a 64% reduction in the risk of mortality in children who were given two doses of 200,000 IU of vitamin A (RR=0.36; 95% CI 0.14 to 0.82) as compared to placebo. Two doses of water based vitamin A were associated with a 81% reduction in risk of mortality (RR=0.19; 95% CI 0.02 to 0.85) as compared to 48% seen in two doses of oil based preparation (RR=0.52; 95% CI 0.16 to 1.40). Two doses of oil and water based vitamin A were associated with a 82% reduction in the risk of mortality in children under the age of 2 years (RR=0.18; 95% CI 0.03 to 0.61) and a 67% reduction in the risk of pneumonia specific mortality (RR=0.33; 95% CI 0.08 to 0.92). There was no evidence that vitamin A in a single dose of 200,000 IU was associated with a reduced risk of mortality among children with measles (RR=0.77; 95% CI 0.34 to 1.78). Sub-groups like age, dose, formulation, hospitalisation and case fatality in the study area were highly correlated and there were not enough studies to separate out the individual effects of these factors. There was a 47% reduction in the incidence of croup (RR=0.53; 95% CI 0.29 to 0.89), while there was no significant reduction in the incidence of pneumonia (RR=0.92; 95% CI 0.69 to 1.22) or of diarrhoea (RR=0.80; 95% CI 0.27 to 2.34). Duration of diarrhoea was measured in days and there was a reduction in its duration of almost two days WMD -1.92, 95% CI -3.40 to -0.44. Only one study evaluated otitis media and found a 74% reduction in its incidence (RR=0.26, 95% CI, 0.05 to 0.92). We did not find evidence that a single dose of 200,000 IU of vitamin A per day, given in oil-based formulation in areas with low case fatality, was associated with reduced mortality among children with measles. However, there was evidence that the same dose given for two days was associated with a reduced risk of overall mortality and pneumonia specific mortality.

Reviewer's conclusions: Although we did not find evidence that a single dose of 200,000 IU of vitamin A per day was associated with reduced mortality among children with measles, there was evidence that the same dose given for two days was associated with a reduced risk of overall mortality and pneumonia specific mortality. The effect was greater in children under the age of two years. There were no trials that compared a single dose with two doses, although the precision of the estimates of trials that used a single dose were similar to the trials that used two doses.

Update of

Vitamin A for treating measles in children.
D'Souza RM, D'Souza R.
Cochrane Database Syst Rev. 2001;(2):CD001479. doi: 10.1002/14651858.CD001479.
PMID: 11405993 Updated. Review.

Related information

MedGen
PubChem Compound (MeSH Keyword)

LinkOut - more resources

Full Text Sources
Wiley

Medical
Genetic Alliance
MedlinePlus Health Information

IODINE
THE PERFECT PANACEA

Iodine is an essential nutrient for good health, a simple remedy for a range of physical and mental ailments and an effective detoxifier and antiseptic, yet it has been demonised for decades by Big Medicine and Big Pharma.

by Elaine Hollingsworth © 2000–2012

Extracted and edited from the "Starting Point" section of her book *Take Control of Your Health and Escape the Sickness Industry*

Website:
http://www.doctorsaredangerous.com

A monumental crime was committed in 1980. The result of this crime dwarfs the war crimes of Adolf Hitler, Joseph Stalin and George Bush. And that's going some! The consequences of this crime were not immediately apparent. Bombs didn't fall. Cities were not laid waste. Dictators did not mobilise goose-stepping thugs to enforce their crime. It wasn't necessary. The people, lulled by Big Pharma, governments and a corrupt medical system, let it happen.

Consider the magnitude of one decision being responsible for undermining and even destroying the health of nations. "They" were able to get away with it because populations did not sicken and die immediately: the effects of this crime were, and still are, cumulative and steady. The only people to escape have been those in societies so primitive that they grow and prepare their own food.

You are a victim. No matter how well informed you are, or how carefully you choose your food and beverages, escape is nearly impossible. Does this seem far-fetched? It isn't. Be patient, and you will understand how this happened and what you can do to protect yourself, your loved ones and your friends, if they will listen. Most won't.

Yes, there are things you can do to minimise the damage. You will not, unfortunately, be able to mitigate the results, which are millions, probably billions, of physically and mentally impaired victims of this crime. These victims are bringing medical systems down and committing senseless crimes that were unthinkable 30 years ago.

Only old people realise how dramatically our world has changed. Ask any old codger and he will tell you that in his day people were strong, illness was rare and almost everyone was sane.

Bromine Is The Culprit (And It Is Everywhere!)

It's an antibacterial agent similar to chlorine; it's a fumigant for agriculture and termites; it's a virulent pesticide that kills insects on contact. When it's injected into soil, everything dies—and you probably had it for breakfast.

According to *Webster's Dictionary*, bromine is a chemical element usually in the form of a reddish-brown corrosive liquid that volatilises to form a vapour with an unpleasant odour that is very irritating to mucous membranes.

Bromine became a household name in the 1920s as a hugely popular hangover cure called Bromo-Seltzer. It worked so well that it was in every medicine cabinet, a trusted remedy for just about everything that ailed you.

The bad news about Bromo-Seltzer took half a century to become common knowledge because, as is customary, Big Pharma managed to keep the truth swept under the carpet. Those in the know, however, were aware that too much of this hangover cure led to what became known as "bromomania". Don't believe me? Check the *New England Journal of Medicine* and you will learn that between 1920 and 1960, alarming numbers of Bromo-Seltzer victims landed in psychiatric hospitals with acute paranoid psychoses, secondary to ingesting the bromine in Bromo-Seltzer or another bromine tonic known as Miles Nervine.

Bromine, bromide, bromate, brominated, brominated vegetable oil (BVO)—whatever they call it, shun it! (For the sake of simplicity, I refer to it as "bromine".)

Bromine was eventually removed from these tonics, but not due to government diligence. On the contrary, all it takes is a bit more digging to find that the US government dosed personnel during the Gulf War with pyridostigmine bromide. It was given to unsuspecting soldiers to prevent death in the event of exposure to chemical warfare. As it happened, the chemical warfare didn't eventuate—but Gulf War syndrome did, and it should come as no surprise to those familiar with government to know that a cover-up was put into place. Consequently, we can't locate statistics on the number of service men and women who were sent home as incurably ill, hopeless psychotics. (See chapter four, "Excitotoxins—Deadly Chemicals Your Government is Happy for You to Eat and Drink", to learn about other related chemicals that contributed to Gulf War syndrome.)

This deadly "side effect" of bromine was as apparent then to governments and scientists as it is now. Yet bromine use is still so widespread that it is nearly impossible to avoid.

Bromine is even in some children's asthma inhalers! Has your doctor prescribed one of these inhalers for your child? If so, I suggest you ask why he/she has put your child at risk of "bromine intoxication", which can cause schizophrenia, delirium, hallucination and psychomotor retardation. Prescribing a dangerous drug, when a simple change of diet easily banishes asthma symptoms, looks like malpractice to me. If you agree, I strongly suggest a change of doctor—if you can locate one who isn't under the thumb of the poison-pushers.

Of course, if you are also being exposed to bromine in your food or in some trusted medication that you have been taking for years, you will probably be suffering from depression and "brain fog" and an inability to concentrate sufficiently to change doctors. You may feel so dull and apathetic that you won't have the judgement, wit or gumption to recognise what your doctor, in league with Big Pharma and governments, is doing to your child and to most people in "civilised" countries.

Soft Drinks (There's Nothing "Soft" About Them!)

It was Jorge Flechas, MD, acknowledged world expert on this subject, who first alerted me to the deadliest aspects of these ubiquitous, addictive drinks that our young people are hyped up on. And, no, it isn't just the huge amount of sugar, aspartame and other dangerous chemicals they contain. That news is old hat. It's the bromine, and I'll bet you didn't know that many soft drinks are loaded with it. I didn't. So when I learned about Dr Flechas's work, I rang him in Henderson, North Carolina, USA. He graciously gave me 30 minutes of his valuable time.

What an eye-opener that conversation was! Dr Flechas told me he had discovered that when oil is placed in a bowl and bromine is stirred in, the bromine will slowly turn the liquid oil into a solid until it becomes so stiff that the spoon won't move. This also happens once a bromine/oil mixture is in the body, and this goes a long way toward explaining the cause of our epidemic of obesity.

...when oil is placed in a bowl and bromine is stirred in, the bromine will slowly turn the liquid oil into a solid until it becomes so stiff that the spoon won't move.

As Dr Flechas pointed out to me: "Years of drinking sodas that are loaded with brominated vegetable oil solidifies body fat. We call this 'morbid obesity', and our kids are becoming obese nationwide; and even though they try to exercise and limit their diets, they just can't get rid of the fat."

These young people are so desperate that they sometimes opt for surgery, hoping to get the "morbid fat" sliced off. It would take a huge strain off Medicare and health insurance companies if their doctors would suggest a cheap, simple remedy instead: shun soft drinks and embrace the antidote explained below.

I asked Dr Flechas about Mountain Dew, a hugely popular soft drink. This is of particular interest because scientists whom I trust say it is a central nervous system depressant because of the BVO it contains. Dr Flechas concurred, and said: "Mountain Dew's not the only one. They have been doing this with Fresca and Gatorade, and a tremendous number of soft drinks." When I asked him why they would use such a dangerous chemical, he said it helps disperse the citric acid added to soft drinks to impart a citrus flavour. (See chapter four of my book for the bad news on this additive.)

Even worse, Dr Flechas said: "The BVO causes psychoses, and to try to overcome the resultant depression they load it with a tremendous amount of caffeine." Simply put, they knock you down and pick you up, all in one drink.

Dr Flechas is on a crusade to put a stop to this outrage, or at the very least to educate people and make it public knowledge. As he told me: "Here we are, creating jittery, irritable, anxious kids who are having problems with increasing weight and don't know why." Many such teens are his patients, and he said that he has found that once they are off soft drinks they can easily lose nine kilograms (20 pounds) each year. And, more importantly, they become "normal" emotionally.

According to Dr Flechas, mental aberrations are the most sinister aspect of BVO. "When you look at this from a public health standpoint...young people are becoming so paranoid that they're...shooting each other, shooting their parents, their teachers... We think we need to throw counsellors at them...but I think we need to take these central nervous system stimulants out of their diets."

Amen! Give it some thought. Bromine became a staple of our diets in 1980, as you will learn below. Do you remember any teenage murder sprees prior to that time? No, because there weren't any. Now, senseless teenage murders and sieges have become a staple of television breakfast viewing.

Adults are affected, too, of course, and there is no safe haven. No matter how well we look after ourselves, everyone is affected because it is not always possible to escape a neighbour's crazy teenager or a hyped-up madman on the freeway, using his car as a weapon to vent his frustration. We are all potential victims.

Other Culprits

Bromine is not the only culprit. We also have the choking pollution that many of us endure, mouths filled with deadly mercury from amalgam fillings, lethal artificial sweeteners, sodium fluoride and pesticide exposure, food additives, electromagnetic radiation exposure, vaccinations, shocking agricultural practices, chemtrails, sugar, alcohol and severe toxicity caused by dependence on drugs—all government-sanctioned and enthusiastically approved by establishment medicine. These contributing factors are hard, some even impossible, to avoid. But there are things you can do to protect yourself, so cheer up and read on.

Prozac and the other deadly antidepressants have made a huge contribution as well. Many teenage killers were known to be addicted, although that bit of important information is always censored quickly after the initial news breaks (thanks, needless to say, to the power of advertisers on the media). But why were these teens on Prozac to begin with? No doubt to counteract the terrible emotional yo-yo that the BVO-loaded soft drinks they lived on created.

So you think you're in the clear? Think again. You guard your health and never allow yourself to be exposed to any of the above-mentioned risk factors. Even in your young days you shunned Bromo-Seltzer, and you managed to escape military service and the deadly drugs they doled out. So, you should be safe, right? Wrong. I'll bet you thought I'd never get to the point, but here it is: this is the earlier-mentioned monumental crime that was committed in 1980, with nary a peep from the "watchdogs" that are extremely well paid to look after our health.

Our Daily Bread and Milk (Hitting Below The Belt)

"They" ruined our bread. It was done quietly and quickly (before 1980 in some countries, later in others, and not at all in a lucky few), and it was seemingly innocuous. This is what happened, in four little words: hello bromine, goodbye iodine. In the "good old days", when iodine was used as a dough conditioner, there were generous quantities in our bread and in all bakery products. This amount of iodine was sufficient to protect thyroid glands from radioactive iodine and to prevent thyroid illnesses of all persuasions.

This is what happened, in four little words: hello bromine, goodbye iodine. In the "good old days", when iodine was used as a dough conditioner, there were generous quantities in our bread and in all bakery products.

Iodine was also in our milk for a really good reason: it kills bacteria. It was used on the teats of cows before milking to ensure cleanliness, and it was used to sterilise the equipment used in the milking process.

As my friend and colleague Pip Rose told me: "We used iodine in our dairy for years, as it was the perfect antiseptic and it was dirt cheap. Then, one day, someone from the Milk Board arrived on our doorstep and threatened to deregister us if we did not replace the iodine with a chemical. I don't remember its name, but it smelled toxic, and it was heaps more expensive than the iodine. We were forced to use this chemical for milk sold to the public, but we certainly didn't use it for our family: we didn't want to poison our daughters." Multiply this story by millions of dairies worldwide, and it sure smells like a conspiracy!

Donald Miller, MD, my American telephone and email colleague, said: "I've used iodine on a daily basis for the last 35 years in heart surgery, to prepare patients' skin. It is the best antiseptic for preventing wound infections after surgery because it kills 90 per cent of bacteria on skin within 90 seconds." Dr Miller, who is Professor of Cardiac Surgery at the University of Washington in the USA, has permitted us to post an article he wrote on iodine on our website. You will learn a great deal by reading it. Simply go to the left-hand sidebar of our home page at http://www.doctorsaredangerous.com.

Deadly Substitution (Why Was It So Serious?)

Iodine, as mentioned earlier, is essential as it helps to eliminate toxic metals—especially bromine—from the body. So when iodine was replaced by bromine, there was no longer a way to eliminate the bromine. Overnight, a huge segment of the population was being affected by bromine. This was infinitely more serious than the damage done by Bromo-Seltzer, which only struck a tiny proportion of society. And, of course, the brominated vegetable oil in soft drinks only strikes people who are stupid enough to guzzle them. But bread—"the staff of life"—strikes us all!

As respected iodine researcher James Howenstine, MD, succinctly put it: "This substitution of bromine for iodine has resulted in nearly universal deficiency of iodine in the American populace. Iodine therapy helps the body eliminate fluoride, bromine, lead, cadmium, arsenic, aluminium and mercury. Could this substitution of bromine for iodine have been carried out to increase diseases and thus create more need for pharmaceutical drugs?" This sounds like the sort of diabolical, profit-making plot that Big Pharma would cook up, but it has covered its tracks and there isn't any proof.

Even more sinister are these words from Guy E. Abraham, MD, who claims that removal of iodine caused "more misery and death...than both World Wars combined".

I agree. During my 23 years as Director of Hippocrates Health Centre, I have been privileged to witness amazing recoveries from "incurable" illnesses by merely adding a bit of iodine to the diet. But who am I? I don't have a fancy degree. I'm merely an experienced observer, and few physicians pay heed to what they refer to as "subjective" information.

Dr Abraham, however, is a different matter. He is considered the most knowledgeable iodine/thyroid expert in the world. He is a Professor of Endocrinology and a pioneer on ways to assay iodine and minute quantities of hormones in the body. He has received more research awards on this subject than anyone else, and has published his findings in "The Iodine Project". In other words, he is a gilt-edged expert, and sensible people pay attention to him in spite of the well-orchestrated iodine phobia which has been so carefully nurtured by Big Pharma and enthusiastically endorsed by our pretty-close-to-hopeless medical establishment. Because of this, if you ask your physician about iodine he/she will no doubt react badly and refer you to the utterly unscientific and totally discredited Wolff–Chaikoff effect (http://www.doctorsaredangerous.com for the truth about this report which did incalculable damage worldwide). Of course no one can prove it, but scientists whom I respect believe that this report was "inspired" by grants from Big Pharma.

Your doctor will probably also insist that you can get all the iodine you need from fish. Maybe, if you consume nine kilograms (20 pounds) per day, along with all the mercury it contains. And, if he/she claims that iodised salt is sufficient and iodine isn't necessary, refer your physician to the many scientific reports on this subject that prove otherwise. The truth is easy to find, and this is it: iodine is the "universal remedy" that enables us all to be our own doctors.

Iodine... is essential as it helps to eliminate toxic metals—especially bromine—from the body. So when iodine was replaced by bromine, there was no longer a way to eliminate the bromine.

What Is This Panacea?

The panacea is known as Lugol's solution (hereafter referred to as "Lugol's"), and it contains 5.0 per cent iodine and 10.0 per cent potassium iodide in water. Two drops contain 5.0 mg of iodine and 7.5 mg of potassium iodide. Lugol's has been used therapeutically for two centuries with amazing success, and it's cheap.

Unfortunately for us, however, this remedy cuts your doctor and Big Pharma "out of the loop" and they are not pleased. Remember, they are backed by governments and have all the power. We have virtually none. And when Big Medicine and Big Pharma want something, they rarely fail to get it! What they want is for all of us to be dependent upon their drugs, for life. They are aware that for just a few cents a day, costly trips to doctors and laboratories, and lifetime dependence upon their drugs, can be eliminated. Operations and years of illnesses can be prevented. This is not a good outcome for your doctor, and it is certainly not good for Big Pharma. After all, they did not build up an empire that rakes in one trillion dollars per year by being kindly or stupid, so they are in the process of banning this natural element that is so crucial for our health.

My American, British and New Zealander colleagues tell me that Lugol's, which used to be available at every pharmacy, is now extremely hard to get, if not impossible. In some cases it is available with a doctor's prescription—but lots of luck getting one. Further, your "friendly neighbourhood chemists" will probably assure you that it is toxic and dangerous to use. They lie. Big Pharma told them to.

You can still buy Lugol's from some pharmacies in Australia, but it looks as if its day is limited. Do not give up, however. Lugol's is easy to formulate, and it will always be available for people who do not give up easily. Try the Internet. Check on Lugol's News on our website, but please don't phone us: we use it religiously and will continue to do so, but we do not sell it.

Will Lugol's Fix All Health Problems? (Sorry, No)

There is no "magic bullet" that can overcome a lifetime of eating junk food, smoking, alcoholism, unrelenting stress and devastating medical interventions. Changes are necessary. Our bodies are amazingly forgiving, and adopting a great diet, combined with Lugol's, can work wonders. But please, make those changes way before the doctor tells you the end is near!

Lots of people, who were ill in spite of taking really good care of themselves, refer to Lugol's as the "missing link". We have heard this over and over again from people who "tried everything", sometimes for their entire lives, getting no help or even hope from a raft of medical practitioners who didn't even think of checking iodine levels.

Lots of people, who were ill in spite of taking really good care of themselves, refer to Lugol's as the "missing link".

Do you sweat, or do you remain strangely dry even when racing about in hot, humid weather? If you do not sweat, you need iodine more than the average person because lack of it in the body manifests as dry skin that is unable to sweat. This means that your health will be at risk due to an inability to sweat out toxins. If this is the case, it only takes a couple of days of taking Lugol's for the body to regain its natural ability to sweat.

What Dose Is Recommended? (The Tricky Part)

In his preface to Dr David Brownstein's book *Iodine: Why You Need It, and Why You Can't Live Without It*, Dr Abraham wrote: "It is of interest that the recommended daily amount of iodine for supplementation by clinicians of previous generations, that is 12.5 to 37.5 mg, in the form of Lugol's solution, turns out to be the exact range of intake for sufficiency of the whole human body, based on a recently developed loading test." This amount is the equivalent of two to six drops of Lugol's solution per day in a glass of water. (One drop of Lugol's contains 6.417 mg of elemental iodine.)

For those who don't like the taste of Lugol's, a capsulated version is available with a doctor's prescription. It is called Iodoral, and it contains the equivalent of two drops of Lugol's. It costs about 25 US cents per day, compared to four US cents per day for Lugol's. Even for people who need two or even four times this amount, Lugol's is a bargain. Big Pharma could go under, or at least be badly damaged, if everyone knew that they could banish their depression with an investment of four cents a day. So, tell your friends!

We are all different and our needs for iodine vary considerably, therefore it will be necessary for people to do their own research. There is a great deal of information on this subject on the Internet (see resources section at the end of this extract).

Starting with two drops of Lugol's per day in a glass of water is a safe, extremely conservative dose. Sometimes much higher amounts are necessary in the beginning to undo damage from years of deprivation.

Dr Brownstein wrote in his book, which I highly recommend: "Iodine is the safest of all the trace elements, being the only one that can be administered safely for long periods of time to large numbers of patients in daily amounts as high as 100,000 times the recommended daily amount (RDA)."

One caveat: if you know for sure that you have an allergy to iodine, which is extremely rare, do not take Lugol's.

What Lugol's Can Do

The most startling improvements I have observed were with victims of devastating depression. I have seen people turn their lives around after many years of "staring into space", which was the way they described their afflictions. All were hustled off to psychiatrists, who rubbished them for refusing Prozac, when all they needed was iodine.

One woman told me she had been incapacitated for 12 years, went everywhere for help and took every blood test known to the profession. The only thing untested was her iodine level. She had spent a fortune and had lost 12 precious years of her life.

After taking three drops of Lugol's in a glass of water once a day for three days, she reported to me that she was a "new woman". Because she didn't like to be dependent on medication, she tried several times to wean herself off Lugol's but slipped right back into severe depression. The last time we spoke, she told me she will never try that again!

I have observed that iodine supplementation brings about almost immediate lifting of spirits in mildly depressed people and does wonders to alleviate crankiness, which can go a long way toward preserving relationships. I have even talked to people who have banished long-established migraines from their lives. Lugol's often has a remarkable effect on lifelong problems with constipation and, combined with magnesium chloride, it detoxifies bromine as well as many other poisons.

Since iodine was removed from our food supply, cancer rates have trebled, and breast cancer is a frightening example. Many of the doctors whose work I have researched are convinced that keeping the iodine level up is by far the best prevention for breast symptoms of any kind. Further, once problems exist, even if advanced, iodine can cure—not like the other medical interventions that create havoc and spread cancer cells. Lugol's can relegate menstrual problems to just a bad memory. In fact, all "female" problems, including the dreaded cervical cancer, can be prevented and even cured with the correct amount of Lugol's.

With Lugol's, severe "brain fog" clears up in a few days; frightening, abnormal heartbeats stabilise; thyroid and adrenal problems improve; even some victims of Addison's disease are able to reduce their hydrocortisone intake. Some diabetics are able to cut down or even discontinue their insulin—but please, do not tamper with your dose without receiving competent medical advice.

The key here is not to think of Lugol's as a "remedy" but as a *nutrient* that is crucial for all aspects of health.

Painting Lugol's on cysts can cause them to shrink; painting it on insect bites can prevent complications; and painting it on skin tags often makes them disappear after only a few days. Several experts on iodine report that keloids are only formed on people who have extremely low iodine levels in their bodies.

It's hard to believe that such amazing improvements can be achieved with a few drops of an ancient remedy. The key here is not to think of Lugol's as a "remedy" but as a *nutrient* that is crucial for all aspects of health.

You will find that everything in your body functions better, even your brain, once it is nourished by the iodine it needs. Without it, you cannot reach your full potential.

Once people learn how to use Lugol's, Big Pharma will lose the power it seized when it took over our medical schools, doctors and governments. Small wonder that they are pushing so hard to demonise iodine and ban it forever. This panacea has the potential to put them out of business!

For 150 years, doctors recommended Lugol's solution with great success and without damaging their patients. If they are ever able to return to using natural remedies again, they will become what they are meant to be: kindly men and women who come to the house, look into the eyes and prescribe rest, fluids and safe remedies. (I'm not holding my breath, as this kind of medicine cannot support the lifestyle to which our doctors have become accustomed.)

Is All Medicine Bad? (Absolutely Not!)

Throughout my life, I have known many fabulous doctors. All have one thing in common: the courage to buck the system and think for themselves. Not one has ever refused to talk with me or send me research papers when I've asked for assistance. I have great respect for these pioneers, many of whom risk deregistration. They are in constant danger of being silenced and may disappear forever.

Tragically, it's already too late for the kindly "family physicians". They have dropped away, slowly but surely, during the past decades. Medicine is the poorer for it. Fortunately, however, one group of doctors has vastly improved: surgeons. These amazing men and women are brilliant at repairing accident victims, restoring sight to the blind, giving deformed people hope through plastic surgery, and patching up bodies that have been abused so badly that there is no coming back through any natural remedy. They deserve our respect, as do doctors and nurses who selflessly expose themselves to hardship in order to help sufferers in remote and dangerous regions of the world.

But Big Pharma and Big Medicine do not deserve our respect because they actively work to demonise all natural remedies, including iodine. ∞

About the Author:

Elaine Hollingsworth is Director of the Hippocrates Health Centre, on the Gold Coast, Queensland, Australia, where she lectures on health issues and continues her research into natural ways of maintaining health. A former Hollywood film and TV star under the name Sara Shane, she has been a health crusader since the early 1950s. Her book *Take Control of Your Health and Escape the Sickness Industry* (Empowerment Press, 2000, 10th edition 2007) was reviewed in NEXUS 8/02 and 15/01. For more information and to purchase the book, visit the website http://www.doctorsaredangerous.com.

Resources

- Guy E. Abraham, MD, http://theiodineproject.webs.com
- David Brownstein, MD, http://www.drbrownstein.com
- George Flechas, MD, http://www.helpmythyroid.com
- James Howenstine, MD, www.NewsWithViews.com
- Donald W. Miller, Jr, MD, http://tinyurl.com/7qnysrs
- Byron J. Richards, http://www.wellnessresources.com
- Bruce West, DC, http://www.healthalert.com

Appendix 2.0

End Notes:

In July 2021 I was ready to submit this manuscript when I received a message saying, no, wait, hold on, some new information is yet to be revealed...

So I trusted and waited and the information that has come out of the scientific, medical, innovation and legal community in the past 12 months has fortified my observations and convictions about health, medicine and good civil governance. The next 62 pages include information and more fun observations plus links relating to some of the current societal happenings in our World.

The Odysee of observable truth Vindicated, 2020-2022 .

At the end of every 'body' of work a period of review exists. I would like to thank and acknowledge in these times where speaking anything other than the dictated script, publically, is set upon by legacy media fools and groomed health officials.

Gratitude for the work of **Dr Reiner Fuelmich** and his brave team with many hundreds of televised interviews with credible scientists regarding economic mandate/inoculation fraud and injury on rumble/brandnewtube and other independent channels featuring the **Grand Public Jury**.

Many changes have occurred since I began this journey. It appears more evident than ever that references to rackets, their de-construction of free will and human sovereignty of self, for economic purposes are rife in western socialized life. One racket, managing the reset of their continuance on new levels of invasiveness.

Gratitude also to Dr Martin and his work following the medical patent trails of the world, clearly demonstrating my previous statements of a rigged system is true and in effect...

Here are some notes taken from watching an interview link and Disclosure, dated 9 July 2021 with Dr Martin on BrandNewTube. Dr Martin speaks of his job in keeping track of economic developments so as to provide investment and other advice to the world markets.... He discloses that there were 4000 patents registered around the Carona virus giving rise to SARS. Made public in 2020. Dr Martin talks of the gene sequence of the so called 'Novel' virus when reviewed against patent records available show so many patents that there is no way the virus could be called 'Novel', some dating back to 1999... Initially uniquely applied to veterinary science, Pfizer made its first application regarding the 'spike protein' in 2000, 21 years ago. **US Patent 6372224** Spike Protein virus vaccine for Canine Corona Virus. The Pfizer work was coupled with Rabbit Cardio Myopathy, research of 22 years according to Patent findings. Or the Rothschild's, making application for patents of Covid19 biometric tests in 2015 and 2017! As recorded in patent documentation: (US pub. No.:US2020/0279585 A1)

ATOMIC BOMBSHELL: ROTHSCHILDS PATENTED COVID-19 BIOMETRIC TESTS IN 2015.AND 2017

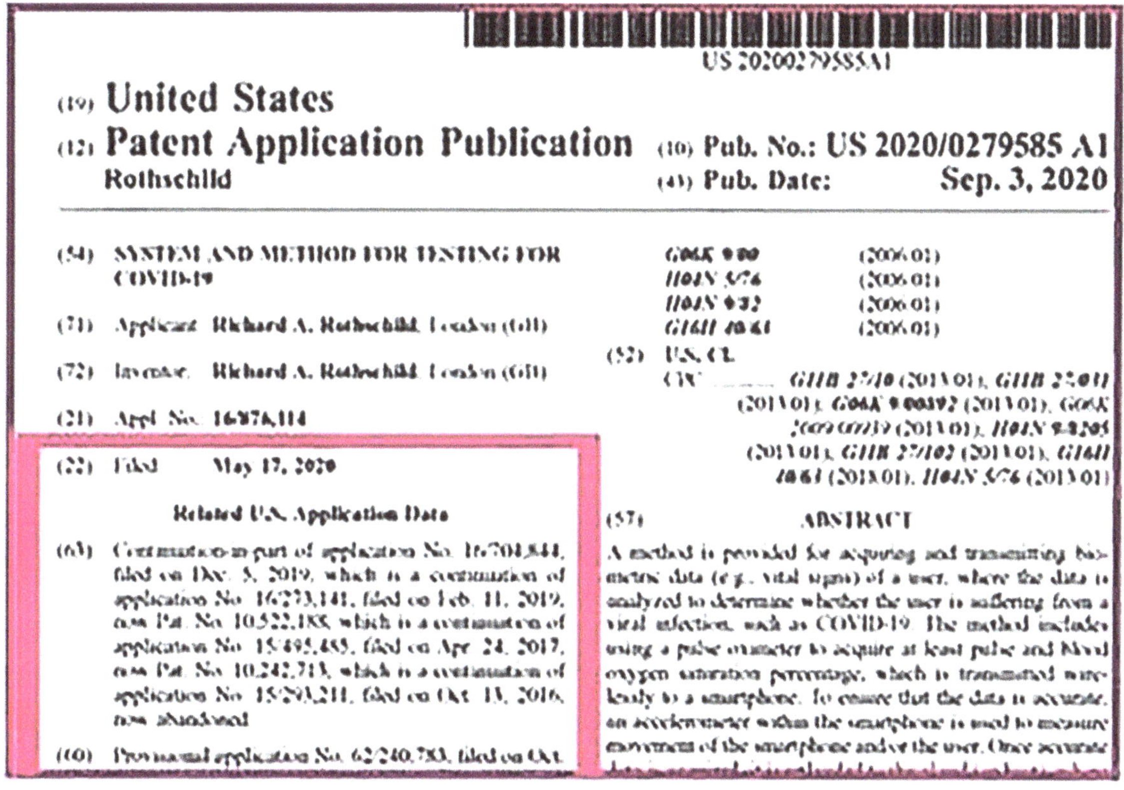

US 20200279585A1

(19) United States
(12) Patent Application Publication (10) Pub. No.: US 2020/0279585 A1
Rothschild (43) Pub. Date: Sep. 3, 2020

(54) SYSTEM AND METHOD FOR TESTING FOR COVID-19

(71) Applicant: Richard A. Rothschild, London (GB)

(72) Inventor: Richard A. Rothschild, London (GB)

(21) Appl. No.: 16/876,114

(22) Filed: May 17, 2020

Related U.S. Application Data

(63) Continuation-in-part of application No. 16/704,844, filed on Dec. 5, 2019, which is a continuation of application No. 16/273,141, filed on Feb. 11, 2019, now Pat. No. 10,522,188, which is a continuation of application No. 15/495,485, filed on Apr. 24, 2017, now Pat. No. 10,242,713, which is a continuation of application No. 15/293,211, filed on Oct. 13, 2016, now abandoned.

(60) Provisional application No. 62/240,783, filed on Oct.

G06K 9/00 (2006.01)
H04N 5/76 (2006.01)
H04N 9/82 (2006.01)
G16H 40/63 (2006.01)

(52) U.S. Cl.
CPC G11B 27/10 (2013.01); G11B 27/031 (2013.01); G06K 9/00302 (2013.01); G06K 2009/00939 (2013.01); H04N 9/8205 (2013.01); G11B 27/102 (2013.01); G16H 40/63 (2018.01); H04N 5/76 (2013.01)

(57) ABSTRACT

A method is provided for acquiring and transmitting biometric data (e.g., vital signs) of a user, where the data is analyzed to determine whether the user is suffering from a viral infection, such as COVID-19. The method includes using a pulse oximeter to acquire at least pulse and blood oxygen saturation percentage, which is transmitted wirelessly to a smartphone. To ensure that the data is accurate, an accelerometer within the smartphone is used to measure movement of the smartphone and/or the user. Once accurate

"“2010 Rockefeller Foundation Report: Scenarios for future development"

Illustrates how the Covid Pandemic was planned ten years prior.

In the report: "Lockstep – A world of tighter top-down government control and more authoritarian leadership, with limited innovation and growing citizen pushback. Scenario is around a pandemic – Novel Virus, mass quarantine of well people and total removal of all freedom."

International Journalist: Alex Newman speaks. @tomandlaurenhealth."

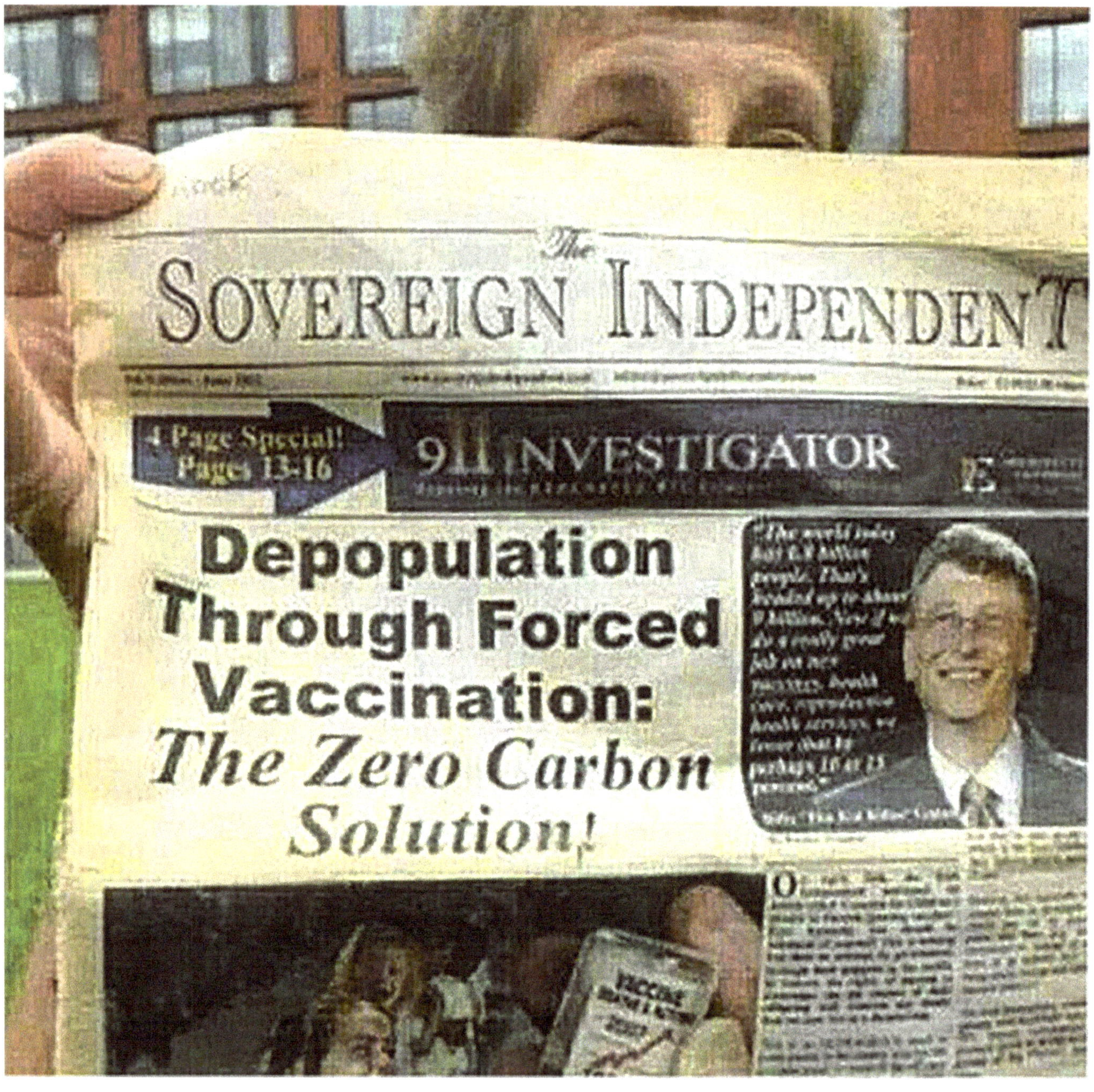

: Newspaper article of Bill Gates advertising his "Zero Carbon Solution" of "Depopulation Through Forced Vaccination" front page of the Sovereign Independent Newspaper in 2010.

Dr Martin demonstrates the Patent trail of the Covid19 disease and the plans of a pharmaceutical/ techno racket to make humanity addicted to and dependent on vaccines and managed medical interventions. This interview Includes but is not limited to;

- Directives from ..... suggesting that 'Media' create 'Hype' to ensure population take-up and profitability...Contracts, contracts.
- 79 Patents lodged between 1998 and 2002, 2006 and 2014 shows continued innovation in tweaking the c*vid strains, proving that there is nothing 'Novel' about the Corona Virus/Covid19. Proving that this virus was made by men, twenty year before its release in October/November 2019. Some of the same men now control and profit from the vaccine rollout.
- This disclosure also acknowledges through various patent trails and contracts that the C*vid Virus strains have long been considered part of biological warfare development programmes. Tweaking of the virus is done by computer modelling, likened to swapping in and out sets of code. Nothing like this virus Frankenstein, is found in nature.

The patent notations alone, in this video interview disclosure, demonstrate that industry is attempting to manage disease as would weapons manufacturers, seeding the conflict to sell the weapons/vaccines. Patents, patterns and profits of racketeers, in an economy of diabolical control, 'the new normal'.

The many arms of the same remote controlled monster, mobilized against innocents. We see the racket pledge, even in their intellectual patents, of incrementally removing civil liberties, as deliberately as their incremental development of disease... to debilitate and enslave humanity into profitable dependence, by corporate rule.

Reverse engineering both, our genetics and society back to, the good ole, feudal times.

High-tech feudal lords of corporations, that politicians of every nation,

Have allowed to undermine, constitutional rights and laws... Not for the peoples wellbeing but for profit and power, continuing...Their Toxic Economy.

Let it not be so. Freewill and civil liberties are too valuable to let go.

Our grandfathers fought wars to prevent what is happening in 2020-21, today,

Their treasured freedom, incrementally whittled away by convenience and the phrase,

"It's for your own good".

On the bright side, a renewed awareness has sprung from the truth of Diet and Hygiene, again the highlight and key to minimizing disease and their unwanted spread.

60 years of corporate medical propaganda supporting general profiteering, suggesting that diet had nothing to do with wellness? And Hygiene, surgeons of the last century refused to believe germs were on their hands – Hand washing is a relatively new consideration in doctoring and surgery... Less than 80 years?

Trust them with your health and life? Perhaps in emergencies, they do perform well?

In reviewing Dr Martins work, connecting patented documentation on Covid19, time lines, who the beneficiaries were.. It is plain to see that the same government influences/foundations, whom benefited from the Dr Kaali and Dr Stephens blood zapper technology being hidden from the world, so that AIDS could be 'managed' pharmaceutically with Fauci's (Rendesivir), now a known killer. These same foundations are now benefiting from the C*vid jab, redacted contracts and mandates. An experimental therapy being forced upon unwitting populations, against the Nuremberg Code! Oops what was their preferred treatment for this new pandemic? Rendesivir?! Wow..

Interestingly many of those same foundations also profit from cancer protocols – experimental protocols...WW2 experiments. Yes just like the ANZECC Study Protocol, another experiment continued from WW2 legitimised as a 'Study' – Never a cure.

In Australia, New Zealand, USA, Canada and UK, parents are routinely told there is no other way, and to question is to risk losing contact with your child or jail. As was my direct experience.

A whistleblower of the CDC in 2015, after a 4 year silencing legal injunction... Judy Mikovits confirmed that it was known by CDC researchers, but covered up, that 6% of the population contract blood cancers like Acute Lymphoblastic Leukaemia from foreign protein contaminated vaccines. This effectively seeds the population with disease. And they have known this for 40 years.

After reviewing the Nuremberg 2.0 Grand Jury interviews, it is obvious now, why no one publishes of promotes any negative story on chemotherapy or radiation... These experimental toxic modalities that cause more harm than good, are 'mandated' and made into law in the abovementioned countries, particularly where children are concerned. To choose an alternative is a crime in these countries, where medical entrapment supports experimental toxic, inefficient studies, but not civil, parental or patient rights to choose.!?

I conclude that all the non-cure-experimental ANZECC STUDY PROTOCOLS are in direct contravention of the 'Intent' of The Nuremberg Code. Yes and the sly laws set up around media publications and health freedoms say that Authorities, 'know' that they are operating outside international law, as clearly stated in the Nuremberg Code. Or why would they need to have a 'black list' in publishing across all media since the 1950's? Hmm, protecting Mr Rothschild's investment streams? You may Imagine Australia is free, until you want to say a truth, 'industry' don't want heard, then realization of greater machinations dawns into a dismal few shades of grey. Pure Violation of any Natural Order.

Australia's 'Chief Health Officer' since 2014 is himself WEF groomed, a Klaus Schwab eugenicist/ globalist?...Is he a doctor? Never mind the Hippocrates Oath!? Where is the quality control with these unelected officials? Oh Yes, Klaus admits he owns them all. Now Mr Gates, of Hells paving with intent; 'pandemic', owns Netflix, the BBC and the WHO. These two make Pol Pots experiment look unrefined, and they smile as they tell us what is coming next.!

Previously in Australia, if anyone mobilizes to do anything to 'change' the war-time cancer treatment protocols, especially for children, a new Foundation is set up as a smoke screen for a cure, and an excellent funnel of money from caring individuals who want to feel like they are doing something of value. The same old diversionary tactics.

Families in Australia, New Zealand, Canada, USA, the UK and possibly others are routinely abused under the Nuremberg Code, today wherever children are forced into toxic experimental study protocols. The 'Rand Prisoner Dilemma' is the psychology used on any questioning parent who's child is placed into forced medical care or state care. Dividing Family. Parents are actively prevented from seeking any healing modalities outside these decades old protocols, so as to maintain profitable loyalty to fraud. Psychological abuse, human rights abuse are legalised. Institutional Fraud! Legal Fraud! Foundational and Ethics Fraud! The Nuremberg Code is a definitive document and the ANZECC STUDY PROTOCOL is a Crime against innocents and parents. A Nazi study legitimised in medicine with the help of Rothschild businesses and Their Cancer Council.

Under the Nuremberg Code many of the Foundations; Clintons, Gates, Cancer, Kidney, Leukaemia the Diabetic foundations may be found, upon scrutiny, are part of a racket. Complicit in injury and death of innocents. These slick marketing organisations need to be openly scrutinized under the Nuremberg Code of International Law. Are they doing the best they can to promote or prevent true curative options? All these so called foundations admit to and submit to, zero cures, therefore no individual nor child should be forced, coerced nor encouraged to take experimental medicine, uncompensated. Free Will is sacrosanct.

Thanks to Dr Reiner Fuelmich's team-Nuremberg 2.0 expert interviews, it has been shown that PCR testing are DNA collection devices, the data of which, in Australia, is to be 'managed' by a

CCP/Chinese tech company? The W.H.O have been reported to be linked with organ transplant racket in China, which is experiencing an industry 'boom' according to one 30 years + doctor reporting.

No informed consent, nor permission was given for the collection of DNA in Australia of its citizens? Or was that signed over during the 'Innovation Paris Agreement 2016' or the Trans Pacific Partnership Agreement with China, that no one was allowed to publicly scrutinize? Have these details been hidden by complicit government and agencies owned/paid for by WEF/WHO and Big Pharma plants?

NOTE: See also European documentary on Serum products; Australian Red Cross shown to be doing big business trading the blood products/serum of the poorest of Americans. Blood banks using high tech, low interaction facilities and an honesty system for screening of contaminants or illness?!. This is being used by criminals to farm people for drug debt collection. These blood Products are sold, as clean, to unsuspecting European families. This is Big business, just as organ donation and products from aborted fetuses is, now Big Business. Interesting that governments and agencies employ foreign companies and employees to do unethical work.? Another psy-op against sovereignty?

Back in Australia complicit governments and agencies have undermined the security of all Australian financial and medical records and packaged them neatly in one place. This 'MyGov' account, as they named it, is the perfect one stop shop, hand-over package for the unelected WHO/WEF take-over plan. Citizens, such as one fine ex Police Officer recently stated, 'have been chemically raped' and had their DNA and financial data stolen to support the forth-reich, biometrics control of programmable animals, they call Trans-human.

Ref: Dr Ryan Cole talks on bitchute.com referring to the MRNA inoculants as equivalent of nuclear bomb on immune system… It may not happen overnight but I will happen, 'Pantene' style, little by little. https://www.bitchute.com/video/EcUtBYdOLTBw/

Don't Panic, good spirits say, these organisations and managers have already destroyed themselves and trust.

"The double edged sword. The very mechanisms they used to bring humanity low, are the same mechanisms that will swallow them whole… Foundations and All." (13:31 16/6/2022)

Soon Humanity will turn away from the WEF/WHO pantomime and focus on what is Good and True. A Big Lesson Learned.

Refs: The Lost Book of Herbal Remedies www.thelostremedies.com https://www.thelostremedies.com/abook/ Herb Usnea is a natural antibiotic like Doxycycline.

Happy Herb Co. "Wormwood" – a bitter herb to invigorate the whole digestive process. Treats gallbladder issues and internal spasms. Other common uses: Fever reduction, Libido enhancement, roundworm/pinworm expulsion and liver health. http://www.happyherbcompany.com/ Both references are an excellent resource for education about natural health, herbs and practical applications.

Dr VA Shiva PHD. Truth Health Freedom is his discussion base, his experience is in Bio Systems and Immunity particularly. A brave doctor speaking out.

His web page: http://www. VASHIVA.COM Talks about: " Your Body, Your System" a registered trademark. Seminar. Understanding the immune system as a natural system.

The TGA and FDA have been shown to be owned by the pharmaceutical bodies seeking untested approvals for products of dubious nature. A scam over decades.

It is on public record, though perhaps not well reported in many countries, that Major Pharmaceutical companies have long histories of litigation that found them guilty, multiple times of multiple crimes for knowingly causing injury or death… 'Iatrogenic' style.

Tobacco companies are banned from advertising in sport but killer pharmaceutical companies advertise everywhere and own your health officials and government's contracts, redacted though they may be?

Billions are spent by these pharmaceutical companies on sweeteners for Politicians, Specialists, Doctors and GPs. It is confirmed this is their education after University. It is confirmed that Doctors are the most 'lied to' profession and the rackets of illness-seeding medicine, have tied up all the loose ends, to ensure Doctors, the family's most trusted, are the new WMD's, upon an unwitting population.

Why? Because they are educated and later bribed/wooed by racket manufacturers. Creating effective weapons of doctors is the end of a corporate take-over deal that care-less DAVOS participants and politicians have signed future generations up for?!

Observation in marketing SALES of the slow-cooked western froglet: The psychology of Sales it appears, has evolved away from 'The Closer' toward 'The Rand Prisoner Dilemma'.

Exploitation and division not of prisoners but Family for economic purposes.

It appears that the psychology/torture of the Rand Prisoner Dilemma, sells more unwanted or dubious products, experimental medicine, insurance and economic resets, than any previous marketing ploy…

And keeps people in toxic check – zero cure treatment when they would prefer to try something else, wellness perhaps? Interestingly this is Modern Medicine's preferred mode of marketing, psychology of abuse non-Nuremberg compliance style.. Or Epstein Island style if you consider forced medication is chemical rape?

NO matter that the compulsory Jab register for children in Australia is the result of a private member bill paid for by big pharma!!!??? Commonsense went out the window at the mention of Profits to the Lawyer/Doctor politicians that allowed themselves, to be groomed!

Responsibility and Ethics have gone out the window in an attempt to High Roll the world in a corporate coop to remove free will and 'manage' populations with chemicals and technology for zombie consumers of the perfect commercial loop.

But the Lord of Life has other plans. Smile!

Evidence of these words exists in John Abramson new book. John Abramson was Head of Faculty at Harvard Medical School and a family physician for more than twenty years. His new book entitled "Sickening How big pharma broke the American health system and how it can be fixed": This can also be viewed on a Lex Fridman podcast #263.

(2/Oct/2021) Is it a Joke of a Hoax? Political Leadership? A Joke or a Hoax on the People? Medicine? A Joke or a Hoax on wellness and choice? Weapon manufacturers? A Joke or a Hoax on Peace? Trade Deals? A Joke or a Hoax on fair trade and legal liability? Global economics run by Rackets? The bank of International Settlements? Fractional banking and savings? Is it a Joke or a deliberate Hoax to apply compounding interest to debt? Hmm Sir John Maynard Keynes once said at the economic reset of Bretton woods after WW2… *"..The wickedest of men will do the wickedest of things under the guise of the greatest good",* obviously still a true statement in today's world as any. Perhaps an **Audit** on "guises" such as "foundations" and "CODEX.A/WHO/WEF/CCP/DAVOS" would better support truth, justice and greater good for humanity and a healthy respectful world functionality.

Such undercover agendas cannot continue under intelligent scrutiny. Good people would not tolerate defilement of the innocent. Not unlike pedophile rings, defilement will not be tolerated nor supported by good hearts.

These words are written to honour our Loved Ones lost to Nuremberg Code defilements and abuses… Not another futile 'Foundation' but a Global Audit of "Efficacy" in good governance, economics, pharmaceutical medicine and Doctor Education. A Global Audit of research and charitable foundations linked with medicine or DAVOS/WHO/WEF in any way. Transparency.

Such an audit, presents a greater honour to our loved ones, to ensure rackets, lies and poisons are not perpetuated in any protocol of CARE.

For a future, of choice and sovereignty for citizens of our diverse world. Consider Seven Generations Hence. For the chance of our grandchildren to live in non-chemically/technologically enhanced, natural Human bodies.

Again a big thank you to Dr Reiner Fuelmich's team and all the courageous scientists and doctors who spoke their truth against the tide of panic and fear. Thank you Dr Martin for your patent trail and Robert Kennedy for your tireless work defending informed, free choice. Dr Shiva, Dr Cole and Many others like the CDC whistleblowers and Vitamin C lecturers. Blessings to 'The Old Man in a Chair' chats, Del Bigtree and may he keep winning legal cases against those that people are no longer permitted to litigate. All witnesses to the Grand Deception in medicine linked with the Grand deception in economy reset and removing free will…Thank you for seeing and speaking.

Please also see; hidden during Clinton/Obama administration, a promising treatment for Neurological diseases, Altziemers, Parkinson's and Autism. Possibly useful given the adverse effects some people are experiencing and predicting over time in relation to MRNA brain damage. GCMaf. A naturally occurring enzyme aiding the brains rapid recovery. All 15 US doctors working on papers of research relating to GCMaf, mysteriously died between 2013-2015 and the only existing manufacturer in Europe was also mysteriously shut down. Perhaps this new natural discovery would interfere with the diabolical plan?

"An ACT OF WAR on the Immune System." The World Truth TV reported in June 2022 "Australia have approved the license application from Big Pharma company PAXVAX that it will allow them to intentionally release a GMO vaccine consisting of live bacteria into Queensland, via chemtrails." As a comment to this lunacy…

- ❖ Clearly a BioSecurity breach, inconsistent with federal bio security laws,
- ❖ Clearly zero informed concent and abuse of civil rights under Nuremberg Code International Law!
- ❖ Clearly an abuse of power by authorities, enabling Bioweapons and deployment to be legalized without public referendum nor informed consent?!

Check out: ogtr.gov.au/what-weve-approved-/ dealings-involving-intentional-release

An example of why corporates, APHRA, DAVOS, disease foundations and rackets of control of public services, laws and civil health domain is fraught with dangers of corruption, profiteering and harm to many innocent people. Wake Up Australia and the World!

The traffic is being directed by WHO and eugenicist foundations. Plandemic.. Food shortages are being manufactured, supply chains sabotaged and mass forced medication for fear and distraction, all for money, just like all the other wars – this time weapons are biologic.

Forced medication is unethical whether delivered by food, air, water, jabs or chemo. Enough is Enough. No. No! No!! to corporate takeover of our civil services and civil rights! Bring on Nuremberg 2.0. War crimes of Company CEOs and unelected health officials and/or bribed politicians, need to be addressed.

Know that children in fact have died to bring you this book. Not just my son.

If it cannot be questioned and any intelligent individual needs to be peer reviewed to express a reasonable opinion? This is not ethics or science that silences questions and learned opinions, but a Racket, that depends on silence to operate in perpetuation. Damn That System!

3/Oct/2021 Conscription by Prescription

Is Australia being brought to ruin by commercial political contracts, redacted, to feed and indemnify the Big Pharma/TechPsycho Economy?

Innocent lives ruined by another “Red Carpet” investment by private member bill, not the compulsory register for children but the “ManDate”.

Man-Date? Are we the ‘butt’ of a bad joke on civil liberties?

And what of the Nuremberg Code liabilities?

Whom will stand for Australia undone by ANZECC/WHO/WHAT/TPA trade agreements of economic, social and health tyranny?

Naming Times:

The Great Depression of the 1930s, the Great War of the 1940s, the Great Sell of the 1950,s,

Then the great banking deception of the 1960s where compounding interest was the civil bait, later allocated only to debt..! The great thinking and construction of the 1970's pedophile rings both labor and liberal. 1980s was the Great gluttony and plastic preening obsession working on more addiction and delusion. The 1990s saw the Great stealthy/debt recovery takeover as seen by corporates own all farming and manufacturing/production sent overseas, utter dependency and zero self-sufficiency in the take-away/throw-away society of Aussies...

The new Millennium provided many useful distractions and technical danglements to keep people stupefied or stifled, and to get their devices into every hand and every home. Every ecological and techno efficiency sold uses more power, resources and time than previous times but nobody notices. Every cancer research fundraiser prevented a new cure but established a new product range. It was so much Fun! Like a kids party, so full of noise and frivolity that the drug porno Epstein island gang have come in the back door and now occupy the bathroom, forcing drugs on kids, they charge for entry. The basement is a sex slave room... All the while, music blares and kids keep having fun, completely unawares about what has been going on. Wait until the parents get home! In Australia, the parents would be called Consequence.

So 2020-2022 will be known as the Great Deception, the Greatest Deception of all time in the whole world. And if WEF, the few, get their way... the Great Oppression.

I pray it be defeated already!

More Refs:

Dr Flemmings book "Is Covid 19 a BioWeapon?" and interview link on Tips Media. 12 June 2022.

Dr Vernon Coleman has had many years of litigating against corrupt pharmaceutical companies. He is banned on youtube and Rumble so you find him at BNT (BrandNewTube). "Chat with an old man in a chair".

Professor Edward J Steele; a molecular and cellular immunologist and geneticist. Interview detailing his horror and disgust at what he refers to as his collegues in the Doherty institute and others for deliberate lies around the C*vid management and dubious novel inoculants. Professor E J Steele used his authority to speak about natural immunity having been reached in the Northern

Hemisphere but news and research data is being prevented in Australia and Australia's natural immunity is being hampered by imuno-destructive novel products being pushed by Authorities that should know better.

And, what of Genetically Modified agricultural and medical products and their 'intentional release' in Australia?

View the following government page and scroll down the list:

http://www.ogtr.gov.au/what-weve-approved/dealings-involving-intentional-release

July 2022 in Australia:

Dr Luke McLindon leads fertility services at the Mater Hospital and is Principle Investigator of a series of randomized trials. He was just sacked for non vax status and trying to release his data on miscarriages post mRNA jab. Normal miscarriage rate is between 5-14% sometimes as high as 16% according to Dr McLindon. However his statistics, kept since the introduction of the mRNA jabs, has found a rate of 74% of vaccinated women having miscarriages. He now spearheads the "Doctors Against Mandates" initiative. A collaboration of doctors, who have until now, remained silent.

http://rumble.com/v15yicn-dr-david-martin-everything-you-need-to-know-about-monkey-pox.html And WHO is planning the end of the World as we know it.

N.I.H COVID UPDATE: What is the truth?

Russell L Blaylock: http://www.ncbi.nim.nih.gov/pcm/articles/PMC9062939/. Innate Immune Suppression by SARS-COV-2mRNA vaccinations: The role of G-quadruplexe. rumble.com

******To finish, with some personal observations of 2020/2022 in loose verse and quotes.***

Doctoring in Australia

Protecting sugar industry profits is the WHO/WEF directive for doctoring in Australia according to APHRA? It has been more than two decades since doctors were permitted to ask questions without suffering bullying and harassment by the AMA. Children have been dying for years of protocols that are FAILED treatments – from Jabs to radiation, that do harm.

Doctors are publically damned for not promoting sugar to diabetic patients? APHRA be damned!

Pet rocks are more effective and less harmful than Maderna/Pfizer 'novel inoculants' and APHRA/ ex -Prime Ministers brother dictating health!? Wanker-ism gone WEF. WTF!

Mindless, careless, doctoring of many prescription puppets is filling corporate coffers with money and filling coffins with people. The 80%/20% general rule applies to any profession and many sociological studies. Medical professionals and Scientists are no exception.

Is it time to make 'Wellness' and 'Peace' profitable, without expending freewill of the People.?!

None can claim power over another's health and personal choice.

This is the power and domain if each individual, it is given as, freewill.

A fundamental human right to choose, one's personal input.

Freewill is fundamental, as a keystone, in the conscious continuum.... Human after human, generation after generation, life upon life.

Machine life breaks down, in entropy. Human life evolves in a continuum on and on in synergy.

Perfect, whole and complete. It is our nature. We are both macrocosm and microcosm in one.

Respect it. Love it.

(Hippocrates oath) FIRST DO NO HARM.

(Above the door of The Temple of Delphi) KNOW THYSELF.

NOTHING IN EXCESS.

November 2021

A lost faith...

Why is Journalism important? Does it help the common people?

Is it just a marketing tool or made bent by government policy?

ABC, Four-Corners or 60 Minutes? What ever happened to

Fearless, gutsy Journalism, or the People's 'right to know'?!

When did Journalism become a prostitute to corporate contracts? Ignoring civil rights?

Pharma sales rep Dr Norman Swan is allowed to infect every broadcast with fearful suggestions, promoting the uptake of dubious 'products',already 'under contract', for right or wrong?!

A knee-jerk reaction "herding" humanity over a 'spike protein' cliff.?

Where is the Journalism around the Pfizer patents of 1990,98,2002,06 and 2014 and others relating to the multiple variations of the C*vid Virus and its extensive use in biological warfare 'research'!?

The RNA delivers a message to create a spike protein never before created naturally in the human body.

- Are whole populations being manipulated by fear or a lotto, into being Guinee-pigs for biological warfare experiments?
- The 'assumption' of protection from C*vid virus and transmission by Pfizer vaccine or others is obviously erroneous, when Nurses and Paramedics, already fully vaccinated with Pfizer, clearly continue to contract and transmit the virus? Why?
- Statistically, more people have died from vaccines in Australia than C*vid19. Should personal choice be as mandatory as it is constitutional.
- Do Pfizer and Maderna vaccine products fit the definition of a vaccine? Or is it a vector and immune modulator; Genetic Modification?
- Is being a GM human, as a result of Pfizer or other RNA vax product, healthy or desirable in the the long term?
- Who is going to take responsibility, should the GM Herd immunity crashes or is found to be inferior to a natural immunity, that recognizes many different pathogens?
- Where is the line and who is defending the Human Right to say "No thanks" to corporate products, corporate rackets and corporate/political blathe.
- Where has our sovereign protection gone?!

Answer the question on the Patents of this very man-made C*vid19.

Want disease traceability?

Well here it is! **'Sickening Science', patenting its creations**.

The-newtube link: https://brandnewtube.com/watch/dr-david-martin-dr-reiner-fuellmich-july-9-2021_RlmKScwsMf6ATEG.html

A quicker version is: STEW PETERS:INTERVIEW WITH DR.DAVID MARTIN WHERE HE MAKES EXPLOSIVE CLAIMS OF 'PATENTED GENOCIDE' brandnewtube.com

Anyone profiting from these products in Australia should be charged with Treason and intent to exploit an innocent population.

When you wish for a magical pharmaceutical silver bullet, think of the Thalidomide babies. Doctors told their mothers the anti-nausia medicine was 'safe'....

- 2019 and 2020 flu vaccine products contained cell lines from a 1950's Cocker Spaniel. Interesting that covid is routinely found in Canines. Has the virus been seeded into the population with flu vaccines? Just as weapons manufacturers seed conflict, to promote sales. Have pharmaceutical companies seeded disease, to sell new product lines?
- Are these the same companies that were 'convicted' in Polish international courts in the late 1990's, found guilty of deliberately attempting to start a pandemic with the H1N1 bird flu strain, by sending live virus to certain Eastern Block countries?

(Pfizer criminal payments See reference on pages 42-43)

Ask questions and protect the future of our human genome.

May the Truth at least set some free...

An Interesting past scientific breakthrough, that disappeared, almost...

As shown on Science TV show Beyond 2000, out of the Albert Einstein Medical University in New York, AIDS Researchers Dr Kaali and Dr Lyman published findings early 1990's about their work which resulted in 14 surgical implantation patents. These researchers found that healthy human cells can withstand 100,000 times the electrical charge than that of pathogens including viruses such as AIDS, Epstein Barr and Ebola.

Their application of micro ampules of electricity to AIDs, disabled the virus and prevented it from connecting with a human host.

This, non- toxic research disappeared when Bill Clintons administration announced a $3.billion dollar injection into 'managing' aids with pharmaceuticals.

Interestingly the portion of the AIDs virus that Kaali and Lyman rendered disabled is the same portion of the AIDS sequence/key that is said to have enabled the Covid creation to attach to a human host.

Perhaps Lyman's and Kaali's research should be 'uncovered' as a non-toxic potential combatant to the current pathogenic threat. A safe, non-chemical, low cost approach to killing pathogens in the blood.

An ex Naval Physicist Dr Beck took this research and produced effective external devices including 3 years study on AIDs patients with Pathology labs across the USA.

More information can be obtained on the Collection of Useful Links on page 187"
www.bobbecksinstruments.com

Another helpful tip: For the prevention of pathogenic transfer and contamination, surgical theatres and algae laboratories utilize Ionizers to clear pathogens from the air. Very safe, effective and **Ionisers** such as those made by Aussie company ELANRA, increase oxygenation of the occupied space.

More oxygen = less viral pathogens. Viruses are known to prefer anaerobic cultures/environments.

Ionizers could easily be deployed in public rooms, foyers, waiting areas and in transport. People can also wear ionizer pendants during travel. Perhaps the government could buy everyone ionizers and liposomal vitamin C, instead of toxic overload vaccine dependency.

Politicians have sold our industries away, our land and our water rights to corporate interests?! Help us to keep their hands off our health choices, bodies and genetics!

I have a background in property law and intensive aquaculture, cultures.

I have experienced medical entrapment first hand as a mother of three. My child did not survive the toxic protocols. I know what it is to be threatened for speaking truth. It is not coincidence that 'fundraiser foundations' are preferred to any 'cures'. We are looking at Billion Dollar economies.

Little people get, smashed and harassed for questioning the 'unquestionable'. Ray Martin lost his job for pursuing his interest in the Microwave cancer treatment…

We need to be allowed to ask the questions.

To Keep shining bright enquiry, into the corporate shadow-play.

It is reasonable to:

Maintain good Nutrition, Maintain good Hygiene, Maintain social distancing in any serious disease outbreak. It's common sense… But

Unreasonable to remove cautious opposition and make mandatory medical immune modulation of unknown and known consequence.

*For Up to date information as excellent resources may still be found on Bitchute, Gettr or the Telegram app: Concerned Lawyers Network posts regular pertinent updates.

See also @childcovidvaccineinjuriesuk.

Remembrance Day 11:11;11

Remember the Australian Forces and their sup-posed sacrifices for Peace and Freedom!?

Remember when The Peoples health choices were protected under the Australian Constitution!?

Remember when Police were in place, for our safety and protection!?

Remember de-regulation of our banking, agriculture and education systems, before the Corporates moved in to micro manage our every institution…!?

Remember when farming families were on the land and "Grown in Australia by Australians, meant something!?

Remember when Australia manufactured goods!? Before all the unelected Trade Agreements, created off shore dependencies, unemployment and economic deficits….

Remember when Keating deregulated banking, when Gillard cooked the constitutional care of government to The People, under section 8? Or when little 'baby killer' Johnny cooked the books during the Y2K distraction, creating "a level playing field" of The Corporation of Australia…Directors unknown?... For a seat on the UN and giving our taxes away to other nations!? And…

Our telecommunications, our media, our water, our land, our food, timber and mineral resources, our innovations..Etc.. Stripped bare of real equities, for our good, for so called, progress…

Remember?

Remember when the Royal Commission into child sex abuse, did not release the names of 28 Pedophiles for fear 'The People' may lose faith!? Well judging by the influential media and political names recently video published by parents... Could it be that the "Epstein Island" formula of critically compromising world leaders or children, for control purposes, was also entrenched within Australia?! ? Gee Wizz!?

BUT I do not remember ever hearing that our Private Medical Records were no longer protected under Law, from access and exploitation by corporate entities!!!!!????

Medical Records are Private and have always previously been protected under Law! Our private health records should not be in the hands of the non-elected corporate APRAH!?

Is this a corporate take-over of the last Aussie bastion, our bodies and our civil liberties?!

Remember when, we called these behaviours from Authorities of any Nation – Fascism?

Unelected corporates appear to : Dictate the exploitation of Australia and its people...

Dictating our failing politics, Dictating our failing Agricultural Chemical use, Dictating our failing processes of manufacturing, Dictating our failing medicine, and Dictating our failing education...

Remember when corporates could not dictate our Democracy and our Civil Liberties?

All the so called progress, seems to be killing all that is Good!? If CHOICE in health and FREEWILL in choice is banished? Where is "Civility" and its POINT?!

Cretinism has found its way in and is Damning Good Governance! Ignorant, greedy politicians of 4 generations were easy prey, they let it in, and called it Progress so no one could complain... Then laws were made to prevent questioning.. again and again.

Imaging a giant bird, The Drongo Doom Bird: The corporates form its body, with Liberal and Labour its flapping wings and the Greens form the tail, for direction towards socialist controls and destruction of 'family', movement to disconnect The People from basic and meaningful relationships with the land or small supportive community living...

Remember when they made the middle class into mass consumers? It consumes so much that now they have to destroy it.

Remember when work was meaningful, people were mostly honest and good and the world was sane? It was before the corporates moved in!

Remember always: There is a Basic Goodness in People and the World, the dictates of fools may come and go, but Goodness of People always remains. Fear and Guilt are marketing tools, for faulty products of man against man, nothing more...

'Division' is the intended action, as it renders civilians easy to herd and control.

The old saying: Divided they Fall. Whether the mind, the heart, the family, the society... It remains true. Division is a tool of influence, that un-does something that was previously strong...

Remember when the Heart of Australia was caring for each other, as ONE and strong!

Let Aussies, not fall prey to the divisive corporate and political herding, now that we have witnessed, that which, fools, joined with political-will, has become... Dangerous, to Australian constitutional 'intent' and inalienable freedoms of choice.

Remember today, 11/11 at 11AM, Remembrance Day: What our soldiers have fought and died for, as directed by politicians? Was their sacrifice made for commercial exploitation of this nature, a dictatorial corporate takeover? Or was it Freedom of Choice for future generations, against Fascism, that motivated them?

Remember on Election Day who sold-out Australian freedoms, liberties, our children's and future resources away... Redacted contracts indeed!? WTF! Hmm WEF the FEW.

Remember, Remember; Truth can stand up to QUESTIONING and Lies cannot be questioned.

EX Green Voter.

Perspective and over-view; 2000/2021

The control of information, timelines and money trails....

Are we witnessing Corporate Piracy over Human Sovereignty?

Contact tracing and investment Contract tracking suggests;

Big business 'seed' their Patented diseases, developed over 20+/- years,

To promote the need of their undesirable 'immune modulation "products"',

They hope will be as "addictive" as Opiates, to

A fearful, dependent and enslaved population…

Amid an "un-agreed" economic 'Re-Set'.

Genetics de-engineered for profits continuance, on and on…

Best 'Spike Protein' intentions, may pave the way to auto-immune Hell?

Dr Martin exclaimed amid his "BrandNewTube" disclosure of the myriad of US Patents of the Covid-not so novel -Virus developments, that his favorite quote came in 2015 from a Peter Daszak of the Eco Health Alliance reporting to the National Academy Press Club, published February 12 2016.. **"We need to increase public understanding of the need for medical countermeasures, such as that of a Corona Virus Vaccine – A key driver is the Media and the economics will follow the hype. We need to use that Hype to our advantage to get to the real issue. Investors will respond if they see profit at the end of the Process" End Quote.**

"A press conference transcript follows where in Dr David Martin exposes Covid as being a biological weapon created by the World Health Organisation (WHO) sponsored by DARPA.

He says; " I happen to be for the United States Government, in the early part of the 2000's and latter part of the 90's, a person who was sent around the world to look at the proliferation of chemical & biological weapons. I am acutely aware of the definition of what a biological agent is in the 18 Code of the US criminal code, of violations of biological & chemical weapons. And so, my assessment is in fact professional and right. In 2005 at a conference sponsored by DARPA and the Mitre Corporation, Ralph Barrick, the architect of the lethal strand, that has been injected into millions and billions of people arms, that Ralph Barrick, was sponsored to present the following, and let's go ahead and use his words; **""Presentation: Synthetic Corona viruses, bio-hacking, biological warfare enabling technologies.""** Does that sound like a public health distribution program? Does that sound like something that is accidentally misinterpreted to mean something else? Or does "biological warfare enabling technologies" sound like, not counter measures or pandemic preparedness? It sounds to me like, biological warfare enabling technologies, and the reason why I have that hunch is what followed was he (Barrick)received next to his NIAID grants, non-competitive DARPA grants in matching funds, for over a hundred and forty million dollars of aggregate funding going into his and his related programs on synthetic biological warfare enabling technologies. So do I have a problem call the injection a biological warfare enabling technology? Absolutely Not, because that's what they called it, and we know that they knew they called it that on September 18th 2019 because on September 18th 2019 the racketeering co-conspiring cabal of interlocking directorates also known as The World Health Organisation said

“”that they were going to conduct an experience for the world; there was going to be a rapidly spreading pandemic due to a ‘lethal’ respiratory pathogen””. The lethality in that statement is the problem. They didn’t say we may be going to get a little bit of sniffles going around, they said we are going to actually have the promulgation of a deadly agent. And the stated reason in September 2020, the progress indicator is that the world would accept a universal vaccine, as we stated on September 18 2019 we were intending to kill. And we were intending to kill to create fear that would drive people to accept something that without coercion, no one would have accepted.”

Three and Three- 28/July/2021

Dr Malone on “The Intellectual People Pod Cast”,

Researcher and Inventor of RNA and DNA vaccine technologies including the lipid carrier of the MRNA vaccines.

Dr Malone discloses the cut-throat and hostile environments in which these products are created, the thefts the bent protocols and the purchasing agreements with the CDC, together with the minimal testing possibilities of new products such as these… unless there is a plandemic?

As a Bio Ethics adviser he discloses the industry agreement of the Noble Lie as consisting of three elements. The Noble Lie

- Not saying what the risks are,
- Not collecting data of adverse events
- Promoting the product as ‘safe’

Dr Malone would prefer that all recipients of these new vaccines were registered in a ‘trial’ as they did for Ebola. He discussed his current role in repurposing old pharmaceutical drugs to combat viral strains.

Dr Malone stated clearly ”there is no such thing as a completely safe vaccine.

Since the “Iatrogenic Injury” cases involving these products in 2018,USA. The ‘Legal Term’ for these products in the USA is “Unavoidably unsafe”.

The Bio Ethics Three; (Oops I can only remember two)

- Complete disclosure of Risks and
- Free Will.

(Still more than we have in Australia in 2021?)

Dr Robert Malone actually recommended waiting for Nova Vax made from tree bark and not an RNA product…yet this too, has shown side effects unworthy of calculated risk.

Motivation by fear is hysterical and divisive, while logic speaks volumes but is less profitable.

If vaccines work? Why fear the unvaccinated?

If Pfizer product works, why are all the paramedics, nurses and others still contracting and transmitting the covid virus?

Why do so many 'Patents' for this not so novel virus exist with variations such as the international bio weaponisation of spike proteins? Immune modulation products as Bio Weapons?

Gene therapy products = GM Humans?

Diced and spliced with animal cell lines/foreign proteins = Auto Immune crisis on the horizon…

Just as Dr Judy Mitovitch CDC whistleblower reported in a Vimeo video, November 2015.

The truth always finds its way through the cracks eventually, this crack is clearly evolving into a profitable "division of humanity" for cooperates.

Where money and contracts are in place, frequently,

Truth is hidden, enabling the Sell, Sell, Sell.

Why are whole populations human rights being violated to promote one group of products over all others?

Promoting one view, over others, independent research kept hidden of discredited without consideration?

This fits a pattern, does it not? Yes, it's a 'Racket'…

A racket in medicine, just as weapons manufactures promote conflict with privateers to sell more products of war.

Perhaps it's time to consider the expediential increase over the past 20 years in childhood cancers, auto-immune disorders and Autism?

The Australian Compulsory Vaccination Register was a Bill brought upon the unwitting Australian Parliament by a consortium of pharmaceutical corporations, who paid a Doctor/Politician to introduce the Bill, on their behalf. Introduced as a "For your own good" piece of legislation and delivered by our 'Trusted' Doctor/Politician…No one questioned?

Civil Rights were thus removed under Law, with consequences yet unseen….Increases in previously unknown or rarely seen diseases?!

Conscription – Mandatory – Compulsory: all unconstitutional, in governance of our constitution or our business dealings.

The 'Culture' of Medicine it appears, has established itself as a powerful and 'Unquestionable' Priesthood, that routinely silences whistleblowers or competition.

I pray that future generations do not have to look upon Doctors as they do Priests, that Rape little children of their genetic rights to a healthy, non-medicalised life?

Good health and wellness products are what require mandating economically, to protect populations from product/industry 'rackets' of any kind…. War/Oil/Free energy/Technology and Big Pharma medicines profit policy of chemical management of human health VS Free will and choice in health and medicine for all citizens.

How did "products" become Law under the Constitution of Australia?

In determining if politicians Sold Out or Asleep at the wheel? Follow the money trail….

Doctors told pregnant women that Thalidomide was 'Safe' and 'Tested'!!! Any Regrets?

I have experienced medical entrapment first hand as a mother of three. My child did not survive the toxic protocols. I know what it is to be threatened for speaking truth. It is not coincidence that 'fundraiser foundations' are preferred to any 'cures'. We are looking at Billion Dollar economies.

Little people get, smashed and harassed for questioning the 'unquestionable'. Ray Martin of 60 Minutes, lost his job for pursuing his interest in the Microwave cancer treatment…

We need to be allowed to ask the questions.

To Keep shining bright enquiry, into the corporate shadow-play.

It is reasonable to:

Maintain good Nutrition, Maintain good Hygiene, Maintain social distancing in any serious disease outbreak. It's common sense… But

Unreasonable to remove cautious opposition and make mandatory, medical immune modulation of unknown and known consequence. .. There is nothing like this 'Medical Frankenstein' in Nature.

As a parent of a Vaccine Injured child I strongly suggest that individuals do their own risk assessment for health and genetic disposition and not to allow money nor fear to influence; genetic immune modification, decisions.

I have witnesses Dystopic Australia, as seen, when a family in W.A went public with an "Adverse reaction event" story to the MMR vaccine in an adult male/the Father, who was coerced into this jab in order to visit his pre-term baby in a W.A Neonatal Ward.. The man, now an invalid and his family were harassed and silenced by police at the direction of a Health Minister in that State!?

An example: of the continuum of the Noble Lie and Medical Racket in play?

It is Legal to say "No Thanks" to conscription or mandatory vaccination of any "product".

It is Legal to use your "choice" and buying power to support businesses and corporates that support Human Rights and Civil Liberties.

In a consumerist society, this is your only power… Your Choice.

Your monetary Vote of Confidence, or not.

Australia and the World needs 'Real Doctoring', not 'Prescription Puppets' creating addiction for corporate profits.!

Book ref: Dr Robert Mendelsohn M.D "Confessions of a Medical Heretic" (See page 268)

Chapter 8 –If This Is Preventative Medicine, I'll Take My Chances with Disease pg. 141-156.

Discussion on the innovations of the modern medical system, the consequences and it's killing of 'family'.

Be Aware of Influence: Billion Dollar Industry Privateers have Billion Dollar resources to protect their investments.

During the Obama reign with Hillary Clinton and the current President, Mr Biden by his side, 15 natural health qualified Doctors were mysteriously killed, perhaps, it was theorized, due to injury, by mini drones in the USA, all within 10 months of each other, all were working together on a natural treatment called GcMaF, that was shown to reverse the affects of Altzimiers, Autism and Parkinson's Disease, producing wellness and functionality in previously brain injured patients.

(Could this be helpful to reverse brain damaged from MRNA experiments?)

If wellness were important to the economy, why would this revolutionary discovery be destroyed?

The phase that underpins modus operandi appears to be; If it can't be ignored, discredit it and if it can't be discredited, destroy it... Many a researcher and whistleblower experiences this patterning.

Note: In the mid 90's. It was Bill Clinton who announced a 3 billion Dollar injection into the chemical management of AIDs at the time Albert Einstein Medical School researchers Dr Kaali and Dr Lyman's, safe, cheap and effective; Blood Micro-electrification invention disappeared... Found to be successful in disabling the ability of the AIDs virus from connecting to its host. **(spike protein disabled then, how about now?).**

Wellness is not profitable and is seen as a risk to profitability of the chemically invested Medical Industry. Politicians and key health officials are encouraged into investments that lock in loyalty.

Follow the money trail. To understand fully go back to some of **Sir John Maynard Keynes** quotes at the inception of our current psychopathic monetary system. Classics like:...

"Capitalism is the astounding belief that the most wickedest of men do the most wickedest of things for the greatest good of everyone" and

"The decadent international but individualistic capitalism in the hands of which we found ourselves after the war is not a success. It is not intelligent. It is not beautiful. It is not Just. It is not virtuous. And it doesn't deliver the goods."

Or " Words ought to be a little wild for they are the assault of thoughts on the unthinking."

One could 'track' the beast, to see from which direction it has come and where it is heading...?

Given the lead in time for this socio/economic/military exercise, officials of every nation must have been bought and sold at a prior time? The Australian Government has been corporatizing since 2000 and all corporates are vulnerable to take-over.

Are we witnessing WW3 in the form of 'corporate take-over' of human sovereignty the world over? Governments owned/contracted? People unaware they are the commodity?

Words of particular kinds have been made illegal. Not just 'cure'. If you put the word Buoy and Cott together for instance. There is already an expectation of grand opposition to the current scenario, and people should perhaps not give authority an excuse for violent suppression. Silent protests can be effective in public gatherings.

In previous years, my experience was met with incredulous surprise,

I pray in this time it is seen with new eyes.

With Love from a caring XGen citizen.

22/6/2022 Death of a Salesman Society gone Mad.

When entertainment norms include; defilement, horror and pain,

When the people, unskilled and bored are fattened like pigs for the consumeristic slaughter,

Is life's profit and gain?

When the beautiful boys have gained the Rule through Drama Queen behaviour and turned all of life into 'the powder room' entertainment...

From dollar hungry yuppies to – too many preening guppies having,

Injectable parties, in the Lounge.

When glitter and bleach are carefully applied to Assholes and food supply chains are just as carefully destroyed on mass..?

Has Narcissus gone mad at his reflection? When,

Children are offered no protection from predatory indiscretion – instead encouraged to,

Betray nature and personal Genetics to, 'fit-in', for 'your own good'?!

The new norm appears as physical, psych and chemical rape, from birth to 80!?

Family dismantled, along with constitutions, to enable and promote dependency on corporations, of Nazi –Zero-Hearts. Their new normal service delivery, includes but is not limited to...

Destruction of Sovereignty, Family and Immunity; by Nuclear termination or poison. They may ask you to choose, that's demon-cracy. Sounds a lot like the choice in cancer therapies.. No Ethical Choice.

Rackets in banking, war, medicine, water and chemical agricultural poisoning,

politics and sex rings. The Judiciary obliterated from behind the scenes.

The World Economic Forum Snake eats itself whole.

Clown like distractions disintegrate, masks melt as if wax...

Distortions seen in full scrutiny amid an angry daze.

Humanity sheds an old skin, a walk away to begin again, with increased wisdom.

Backs are turned on the pantomime, the realization its all a creation.

All the enemies are FAKE!

All the DRAMA is 'Man against Man'..

$$$ Delusion $$$ Men and Women $$$ Deception games.

See Ref: Dr Naomi Wolf's new book "Sorry but MRNA is Genocide..."

Go well the Lawyers of Light.

Calm the Farm - the image of the infinity symbol, likened to a butterfly.

The butterfly has a lifecycle of process; the consuming grub, the gestation and catharsis of chrysalis/pupae, then the emergence of a graceful butterfly... Flying free from the grips of entanglement.

A blossoming in the Garden occurs again, a new season in life after the consciousness of CARE has thawed.. Sparkling in the Sunlight of Life's Glory.

Environment is everything.

Love is the Law of healthy co creation.

False growths such as mad economies/societies, unattended as dreams, pass away… as night turns into day. Rejoice in the imperturbable dawn.

Light is Life,

Love is its own purpose.

Don't Feck with it!

And for the repressors of the Truth in medicinal and global rackets, here are a few more creative writing pieces diarised… some mere musings, others, universal downloads.

January 2022

Good Leaders lead by example? Or do they? Perhaps the Gates, Clintons and Swarbs of the world could sacrifice themselves to their passion of depopulation? Gates Town? Swarb Town, hmm, who would be miss a bunch of eugenicist sociopaths? Silence of the lambs.

7 January 2020

100 years of "It's for your own good". Critical thinking gave way to marketing packaged conclusions. False dependency, sold out whole populations, unwitting, to an economic and health delusion.

Piece by piece Family and Community is devolved into a non-supportive mechanism.

Piece by piece Silent weapons for quiet wars were welcomed, as 'progress', into homes, then enhancements of bodies de-humanised.

A systemic network of Man-against-Man, established over generations, has grown like weeds, up every social structural tree, every service, every utility…

The sacred garden got covered in concrete and boxes, now therapeutic policy cuts the Family tree into cuttings, splicing genetics, that never grow to maturity.

All innocence lost as witnesses Gape! Genetic Rape and Dogs of Bankers Wars.

Dependency and Trust swirling down the drain. Media Tellie-tubbies repeat rubbish, Again and Again.

The social Geo-Economic ladder climbing now seen true; as the hang-mans gallows. And the noose of cognitive dissidence, tightens around too many innocent necks.

Misplaced trust and fear, are the blinding shroud.

Will they awake in time to see, they can lift their arms to release the noose of doom and blindfold?

'Critical thinking' is the knife that cuts illusions away. Question the contracts. Contracts. Contracts.

Why is media owned by vested interests in doomed pirate-like economies?

To prevent critical thinking by providing, manufactured conclusions?

Is that also why it is illegal to question policy and narrative, but is unscientific, inhumane and unethical not to?

28 January 2022

Reset Backfires

Bankers and boffins on the run, their deeds of doom to be undone.

'Silent weapons of quiet wars' operations, hung and dangled in public circulation by their own 'hidden hand'.

All the private armies and covert troops crumble from within; Conscience heavy.

Events disclosing fully, technology to humanity that has been for generations, hidden.

Politicians dive for cover as the veil is lifted from a profitably unhealthy corporate ruse, the backfired techno-banking Coup.

The People's awareness sharply dawning, to the poisoning reality, amid "shock and awe" conditions they scramble to save the Family Tree.

Structures of socieatal support are swiftly and intelligently reformed to ensure public support 'includes' free will and choice in medicine. Manufacturers and merchants put back in their proper place as 'servants' to the purchaser... No longer to be Authorities in health nor agriculture. No longer industry nor public advisors, but servants to good and proper health, where no poisons are used nor sustained.

Civil boycotts weed the economic gardens, efficiently, knowingly.

The Courts of Laws realign, clean up and put the 'burning rings of fire' away, acknowledging injury of economics, trafficking and Iatrogenic injury in so many.

Tough lessons for humanity, lulled into a false sense of security-dependency and spoon fed market led conclusions, for a century of Hollywood delusion.

Take heart; After the boil is burst and puss removed, healing occurs.

2.2.2022

A Take-over time.

A time when manufacturers of war won't allow Peace.

A time when manufacturers of medicine won't allow Wellness.

A time when techno racketeers own all media and won't allow the Truth to reach the peoples ears.

A time when 'public servants' remove all civil liberties.

A time when profitable delusions have become constructed conclusions and are spoon fed, while critical thinking or questioning is called out as 'dangerous or stinkier than dead'…

Instead let fundraising for fake foundations be your diversional therapy.

A time when the on-stop-shop, 'my gov' account, becomes a handover ledger to techno giants gaining unapproved, unrestricted access to personal banking accounts, medical records and DNA, to enable social psy-op abuse on mass. The social credit system reset to control the middle class from consuming and ensure the gains the richest have made, remain.

A time when trade deals undermine constitutional and civil rights, where contracts remain hidden and litigation of foreign trespass is forbidden.

A time when politicians and groomed civil authorities are bought and sold by corporate interests. WEF/Epstein Island style.

A time when Democracy is weakened by Autocracy and commercial collusion, create more delusion. Demon-crazy.

A time when Poison Companies own and regulate: Agriculture/food and Health/medicine.

A time when corporate puppet masters re-brand disease, to promote sales of patented weapons as medicine.

A time when the TGA, Australia's health/medicine regulator, is funded by pharmaceutical giants, whom are seeking approval to sell products to Australian doctors and citizens.

A time when the Chief Health Officer of Australia is a World Economic Forum Protégé, Klaus Swarb mini mee and the (ex)Prime Minister's brother heads up APHRA Australian Professional Health Regulation Administration, an unelected foreign owned body, dictating to Australian Doctors : not to speak up about MRNA adverse advents, not to use certain words publically, not to use tried and trusted medicines like Ivermectin and to ignore, not look at any data of other Covid healthier nations.?

A time when the 'Rose Coloured' glasses of immature leftist idealism are broken into the shards of Stark reality, of social facist diabolical control.

A time of deliberate economic destruction to re-set on psychopaths economy for a new level psycho-techno-de-naturalised-de-humanised world.

A time when all the healthy structures in the garden of society have been overgrown by weeds, someone thought looked pretty… The weeds grew strong and choke out the natural sunlight, the balances and support for 'society of meaningful purpose' and Family.. Strangled out of servitude and diminished by corporate intent to profit from dependency and control, of all aspects of civil and personal life.

A time when the People realise how diabolical and uncivil is the corporate socialist rule of bankers wars, bankers poisons, medicine and technology.

A time when people see, that the Domestic Screen is and has always been, an Entrapment process, of focus addiction… Now the screen tells a person, how to think, feel, dress and medicate – No need for critical thinking or Free Will?

A time when the use of Bilderberg's 'Silent weapons for quiet wars' is known by all and an Awakening humanity effectively and efficiently, 'weeds the common', the parks, the gardens of society... So after the thaw of awareness on the socialist doom, the garden can blossom again and Serve the People True.

Lest we forget, wars were fought against Tyranny. Only the bankers use wars for economic benefits and re-sets. People will have Peace.

Fairy tales were written to help people identify patterns of psychopaths.

Never forget, all that glistens is not Gold.

The Light of the Sun gives Life but the moon, its reflection and shadow is dead and cold. An endocrine disrupter, as are street lights in a city, they alter menstrual cycles, sleep and biorhythms.

A time when wisdom of the Great Sun Men/Women is practiced by the meek, while the rulers and elite practice Lunacy...

A time for understanding; Natural Justice cannot be bought and sold, nor be influenced by fools.

A time when all of humanity learns the Truth: There is No Enemy, that is not first 'created' in the mind of Man. Vain imaginings.

Creations of Falsehoods against Humanity, shall profit Not. 2.2.2022

27/2/2022 10:33am

A correction is here, that many hearts have been requesting... It will not be 'the reset' the banker class holds dear. The world veil is lifted on their generational coop of stealth and hidden monopolies, machinations, theft, poison and murder, in their crimes of misdirection.

Like a hidden infection is brought to the surface for healing. Scrub the necrotic flesh away from the healthy. Weed around the structural trees to see the orchard blossom anew.

The correction, amid the settling dust, of truths eruption, will be organic and divers rendering null and void all planning of monocultures and combined toxicity of robotic structures of no service, but futures doom.

Humanity as One World, allows and celebrates diversity and strength and honours this divine expression creatively: Small is beautiful economies, as if the people matter, thrive in the garden markets of Humanity made Wise.

Catalyst of Light.

That which could only grow, hidden in shadows and darkness, goes through a catharsis, under the light of scrutiny. As with any open system, it either crumbles away or transmutes to higher functioning.

That which could only take hold, hidden in the shadows and darkness, man-made; perishes under Lights Scrutiny... Always. The evolution of understanding and conscious choosing, sheds false overlords easily, once they are witnessed, for compassion and wisdom gives to synergy of self. False overlords create a debt.

It can be shocking to see, Truth Naked and that Lie has stolen her silks, but better to see the wolf is only pretending to be friend of the flock. Perhaps, weave Truth, some sturdier silks?

26/3/2022 7:40am

Let the bright light of Truth Glare – Lighting up the trail of psychotic ill-will rulings, high and low.

These WEF, would make cages for all the worlds life to live in? Madness against Life.

In days of old, only mad men likened to demons, DAVOS, Dr Evil etc. needed a cage as an abode. No permission asked nor granted for FIFA camps of savagery, built for entrapment of freewill? WEF assume themselves already masters of All? Perhaps said FIFA camps should be their own reward? Poo Poo to their generational plans put in place to bring disgrace.

A False overlay to benefit their greed at the expense of the 'Harvest of Life'.

A cliff of their own making, is where they shall fall, prey to their own demons and disease from which no cage nor bunker can save them from their failings and lack of CARE.

Watch their empire building fall to dust...Forgive but never forget.

A wiser Humanity continues on... building a global sense of family nurturing. Positive, loving creativity thrives again. ~

I give thanks this day that the 'World Economic Forum' WEF, influences and members fall away, their plans gone to dust, for the highest good of all concerned.

Only intellect gone mad creates poison. Only intellect gone mad fails to know the 'Heart of the World'. Only intellect gone mad 'divides' all things in the 'sacrifice of care'.

Unification is not created by division and false judgements, distractions and false-flags.

Unification comes from understanding compassion and care. Unification comes… But it will never come from Nazism or any other "ism". Monoculture is not a functional nor healthy representation of "Life" growth.

If the Heart is the seat of the Rider and the Mind is the whip, the WEF folk are amusing contortionists. Is it wise to allow the technocratic circus to lead the world? These WEF know nothing of FAMILY or CARE? Many eyes Stare!!!

3:00pm

Those that mock, are fools who obey Nazi rules, but know not the Laws of Life.

Mathematics, patterns and frequencies, the harmonics of the great conductor upon the materials of Life. The Orchestra, creates an eternal symphony.

Perfect, whole and complete, like DNA.

Narrow understandings hear only the fragments of mp3 rather than the full bodied sound of the Symphony of the Spheres.

Life Molecules Solar Collector, the 'Tree of Life', Family its' beloved fruit, great and small.

29/3/2022 9:38am

What interesting times we live in!?

Wars over political funding of bio-labs, amid the second great holocaust invented by a eugenics cult called the World Economic Forum, WHO's followers have turned, the peoples most trusted, Doctors into WMD's (weapons of mass destruction). Nuremberg 2.0 convenes.

After the dust of falling towers settles these events will begin to bring into question, 'doctor education' and the disarsterous effects of closed loop medicine, pharmaceutical companies, lobby groups, banking creeds and political Epstein/Naziisms influence upon any Doctors Education or Ethics. First Do NO Harm! Never Allow Doctors to be Used as WMD again!

Put Medicine back in its place, prioritise, Emergencies Only. Surreptitious Chemical management of Humanity is to be abolished.

3,6 &9...They should have listened. Frequency will save biology. Gates of hell technology deconstructs to dust only.

31/3/2022 7:23am

Forgive the makers and supporters, the members and affiliates of the World Economic Forum for their plans of artificial doom and psychopathic economic bloom.

Their arrogant ignorance proceeds them – IBM-BIS-Bilderberg's.

An example of fruit rotted on the tree, and mould spreads.

Lifeless creations of intellect gone mad, can only lead to its own natural dead end.

Begin again, with more wholistic considerations.

To place the market and currency above the Temple of Life, makes as much sense as wearing sandals on ones head?

Smiling serpents give trinkets as gifts when they are usurping something greater. Indigenous peoples will remember.

Without Free Will and creative diversity, living diversity, what is it to be life and human?

Are you a drone to the hive or a companion to the creators?

Is the Natural Fractal biological mystery to be enslaved by the WEF-few? Who will protect the 'lifeblood' against the doom/dead-end of transhumanism?

May Humanity finally learn that none of the 'isms' bring Peace and Harmony, but individuals taking responsibility can bring Peace and Harmony into their minds, their words and deeds, their homes, families and work places. In this way Peace and Harmony will cover the world while preserving free will and diversity.

Nazism is only proficient at factory farming, which does not allow for full expression of life, but is efficient and economical as a prison model, for lifers. No attachment.

Nazi thinking is no less an abomination or defilement than those whom predate upon innocents as do pedophiles. Interesting how the corporate elites of the world worked so well, in conjunction with Epstein Island style manipulation of leaders and influencers – Defiled.

Pedophile rings were the perfect instrument to defile and control world movers and shakers – For only defiled individuals would support such a plan, as the WEF-few have envisaged.

'Enticements' work so well in political and business fields that they were applied to all fields including but not limited to; Telly-tubbie/legacy media, medicine and science.. DEFILED. This is what requires a RE-SET!

My Children are not Lab Rats, for commercial exploitation! Take the statement: "Every plant our heavenly father has not planted shall be rooted up." Corporate blathe may hijack consciousness for a time but it is not the ruler of the Kingdom of Man.

Weapons of Man against Man.

Bankers medicine and bankers wars,

Two wings of the same evil Eugenics bird.

Craving and Aversion, Wanting and Fear

These are the lenses that burn holes in civil sovereignty, that keep humans in tow.

It's called marketing, you know.

However, comment must be noted that advertising since flu shots were popularized is marketing gone mad, and its ethics?, seem profits over proof.

The use of the (RAND) Prisoner Dilemma style manipulation, unleashed willfully, upon the entire World's population. Has worked a treat in the Sars/Covid experiment rollout, in exploiting and dividing family and community, just as it was originally designed to do.

This exploitative manipulation has been perfected in the general community, outside prisons, on another group of innocents. Chemo kids and their families.

No one noticed amid the distracive din of fundraiser advertising, that families of chemo kids, don't get to speak!

No social license they say, to comment?

No negative press permitted on this very old, very unsuccessful and damaging experimental/trial they call the ALL ANZECC Study Protocol!

Now with the 'new normal' flu protocols, a whole world of families feel the same manipulation and terror, that our family endured for years and years.

It took a few years to devolve doctoring away from treating cancer patients and independent research, towards specialisations... that exclude questioning, even from general practitioners (GPs). And Family GPs appear to have been devolved to sufficiently to be considered mere prescription puppets, for a system that puts efforts into prevention – of questioning, of wellness with disease creation and perpetuation the marketing direction. As we have seen with Cancer treatment spirals, opiate addictions, type 2 diabetes management and other lucrative illness holding patterns. So much money in illness, there appears little to no commercial interest, nor incentive for wellness in pharmaceuticals? Evidenced by corporate groups like APHRA, dictating to government bodies and doctors what they cannot speak about or prescribe, such as Ivermectin... Safe, know and effective. As Indian Studies revealed.

Ivermectin - Now banned in Australia because it kills Covid dead!? Are these actions and dictates of a racket of illness I see before me?

If it needs more than the sum of itself to sell?

Only the bitterest pills are coated with honey. And

So too with information.

Where hype marketing and propaganda is supplied,

Questioning of a lie is denied.

Like 'Redacted' Contracts our governments signed with no vetting?

These black lines, hiding corporate lies and injunctions on transparency,

Demonstrate the illegality of the corporate hijacking of civil liberties and health.

Literal covenants of Doom.

I pray their towers of power fall to dust, for

The survival of Human sovereignty and our children's,

Is a Must.

The new nanotech inoculants intend removal of free will for deliberate control of all things, human. Economic drones.

Witness enticements and wooing as this too will be coated in sweetness so gooey, benefits engaging the unwitting population with a lust for personal edge and gain.

Being allowed to be just Human, is the next civil liberty they want to take in lockstep with

This system of diabolical control, a corporate 'Krakin', against Life. Human Life.

The Separation Principle is a Lie!

Humans are as much a part of Nature as the Trees and the Stars.

We stand up for the right of other living creatures to Be.

We are also a valued part of Nature.

Stand now and allow Humanity to Be, more than the sum of WEF/few, and

Living free, to choose, what we think, say and do, with our time and energy in

This living garden, of enough provision for us All.

Join the dots...SOS

How interesting is it? The sound of silence on Vaccination Injury?

It has been 29 years or so, since an Australian polly was paid a fortune, by a pharmaceutical consortium, to introduce the "Compulsory Vaccination Register".

In that small 29 years, W.H.O statistics confirm incidence of Autism has risen from 1 in 10,000 children to 1 in 30 children (brain injured) globally.

ALL (Acute Lymphoblastic Leukaemia) also once a RARE condition, has skyrocketed in Australian children along with Auto-immune diseases that are now commonplace. What Changed?

Now Myocarditis, a RARE condition in children is suddenly the 'new normal'?

What Changed?! Environment? Diet? Injectable Mandates?

This big pharma/red carpet investment/madness has grown from four shots to new born babies being routinely injected with up to 20 in current times, aside from the recent experimental MRNA stabs.

In 2015-16 CDC whistleblowers publically confirmed cancers, brain injury and auto immune conditions are being caused by dubious and profitable inoculations....Produced by companies recently granted, litigation immunity.

And – How do Authorities maintain trust in injectable disease "creation" and "management"?

SILENCE, the researchers, Silence the doctors, Silence the parents and the victims, Silence the debate, the ethics, the truth. Very effective and frequently used to keep the bulldozers going.

Threats of court and child removal if not compliant!

This is where reading between the lines, tells, and the Silence speaks volumes!

Listen to the words they never speak; like, Cure…or, Vitamin C. Ivermectin! Illegal speak in 2020.

Rackets and 'Trust' in **faulty systems** is only maintained through "careful" information control and scripted protocols. No Critique Allowed! Telly Tubby Journalism and commentary…Again! And Again!

Discombobulated, distracted populations dumbed down and diverted to accept the gas chamber/ disease ahead…or nanotech razor blades.. whatever?!

Political management speak empty words as they continue pushing 'Silent Weapons for Quiet Wars', which is a 1954 document found on the NASA website and publically circulated in 2020.

'Plandemic the Book', is written as an insider prediction, by a CDC whistleblower in 2019, Judy Mikovits. Didn't Bill Gates do a NetFlix Hype Movie called the Pandemic in 2019 also? Hmm, and now he owns the BBC and W.H.O?! Classic story of the best intentions of the few, pave the way to Hell for the many.

Sack the management to survive the 'covenant of doom'.

Statistically, vaccinations appear to be more about creation of disease than prevention, continuing the medical income stream, cleverly with Iatrogenic injury and eugenicists at the helm.

Admissions that the CDC have NEVER tested any vaccine for efficacy… and See the following reference of PHD Viera Scheibner in her book: **Vaccination: 100 years of Orthodox Research shows that Vaccines Represent a Medical Assault on the Immune System**. *(See page 183)*

The Vaccine my son had in 2004, was according to the Doctor, "recalled by the manufacturer as faulty". The GP suggested another dose. My son had cancer a few weeks later.

Research showed the vaccine was likely to have been contaminated with the Green Simian Money virus – known to cause blood cancers, like (ALL) Acute Lymphoblastic Leukaemia. Dr Judy Mikovits CDC whistleblower confessions confirm the definite possibilities of this contamination.

Then 6 years of another industry 'Racket' the ANZECC Study Protocol.. A never ending study of cyto-toxic products used, that cause future cancers and death.

Laws were made to prevent parents choosing alternative treatments no matter how effective. Routine parental coercion includes threats of court action and removal of child.

The 'Prisoner Dilemma' presently being used to ensure the take-up of experimental inoculant products, was also used on parents of Cancer Kids… Note: You will never see or hear a negative critique on chemotherapy in legacy media and the Cancer market is flooded with foundations of research, products and diversionary therapy… So busy, no one ever sees what is really going on.

Immunologists, researchers and health experts that promulgate methodologies other than the Nazi like mandates in Australia, are routinely banned from gaining speaking visas in this country.

Doctors are bound and gagged and have been for years. So is Media! Especially the ABC or Murdock Press. Australia is run by corporate contracts that 'The People' are not allowed to see… The transparency of Black Granite!

Like the Black marker lines on those MRNA contracts!?

My family suffered years of Medical Entrapment. My Son died. No compensation can ever compensate such civil abuse!!!

Parents of cancer kids were just the testing ground… No one noticed – No one spoke up!

Its all Clown faces and sympathetic smiles.

VAX Health Hoax makes informed consent a Joke.

“Work your way to freedom”, the sign above the entrance to WW2 German Camp…

“Jab your way to freedom”, the sign written by the same idiotic ideology.

Noticing that the positive medical innovations are quickly removed from the public domain – Like the Micro Algae Trauma Gel, treatment that stops intensive bleeding within seconds.. that should be in every First Aid Kit! Where is it? Oh, it’s another, helpful and harm free treatment… Disappeared.

Yet willful promotion of toxic illness creation products such as chemotherapy and experimental inoculations that do more harm than good, is OK?!

Interesting, knowing the ingredients, one would be considered lacking in intelligence to provide any informed consent to these new injectables? Suicide is considered illegal? Insurance companies have already ruled on experimental medical treatments voiding life insurance?

So why the open-air gas chamber? It’s like King Herod sent out swords to kill the infants that potentially may threaten his power and rule.. The corporate Herod pricks of the WEF have sent out little needles to stab the threatening populous.

There is a ‘basic goodness’ in the World and good doctors are attracted to the prospect of helpfulness and healing… Many still holding the Hippocrates oath in high esteem.

It is the commercialization and racketeering that comes from profit, that is letting the World Team down. With everything owned by ‘Foundations’ and Corporations that create and perpetuate disease, is it any wonder that 15 Natural health doctors were mysteriously ‘disappeared’ while working/researching a harm free natural treatment for recovery from brain injury. Successful in reversing Parkinson’s disease, Alzheimer’s and Autism – Completely. The naturally occurring enzyme was manufactured in Europe but the factory disappeared alone with the good doctors… Why would the corporate owners of the world not want a Cure for debilitating brain disease and damage? Perhaps there is a link with the ‘Gain-of-function’ spike protein technology that delivers brain damage over time, according to Dr Malone and others, it’s likened to ‘Mad Cow Disease’, a Prion released into the brain.

So the natural enzyme that doctors died for, so it could remain hidden, is a cure for such brain injuries as Parkinson’s, Alzheimer’s and Autism, may be the best hope for the “Iatrogenic” brain injuries sustained from the New Novel Vaccines, that are actually Gene Therapy.

A suggestion for interested others… Look up references on GCMaf. Another hidden 'cure', not good for intended business.

Interestingly, back in the 1990's, the Dr Kaali blood electrification, micro dose, that found viruses and pathogens have 100,000 less ability to withstand electrical charge than any healthy human cell. This research was also 'disappeared', with only its invention/innovation patents remaining. What is interesting is that the same investors and authorities were in power in the USA at the time. Clintons announced a 3 billion investment injection to 'management' of AIDS with pharmaceuticals and Mr Fauci got to legalise the use of Rendesivir, now referred to as the murder drug. The same investors and researchers patenting disease, gain of function, fake pcr testing and killer drugs, had both the Blood Zapper research/technology and GCMaf research/technology put away. Coincidence? Or "MANAGEMENT"?

*Just hot off the Stew Peters interviews, see 15 June 2022 chat with Ex Cancer Researcher of 22 years and CDC whistleblower Dr Judy Mikovits. A true Hero. Spelling it out about the contaminated cell lines that they know have been causing many known modern diseases, cancer, autism, auto-immune etc for over Forty (40) years!!! Contaminated cell lines with other animals! Aborted Fetus lines! The MRNA lines are just the newest tip of a very large submerged iceberg. Disease is the INDUSTRY, not wellness. Thank you Judy Mikovits, a TRUE HERO for health and humanity. http://rumble.com/v18l44h-judy-mikovits-shocks-the-world-most-damning-covid-evidence-bombshell-the-wo.html

***News flash*:** Office of Gene Technology Regulation – Australia. What do you see?

http://www.ogtr.gov.au/what-weve-approved/dealings-involving-intentional-release

These are gene therapy products that are being used in agriculture and medicine, some speak of aerial spraying of contaminants over populated areas. Informed consent, no-where to be seen? Is this where the Ukrainian bio-lab substances, brought to Australia by then Prime Minister Scott Morrison, have landed? And what of Australia's bio-security implications?

In July 2022 Professor Edward J Steele, a molecular and cellular immunologist and geneticist, currently working in the Northern Hemisphere, was interviewed and went on public record using 'his authority' as an expert of 50 years in the field. He called out his colleagues in Australia, at the Doherty Institute and others as LIARS.

Professor E J Steele stated that 'all' his colleagues know that a jab in the arm can do "nothing to assist" with the mucosal immunity in the respiratory system or gut, which is where immunity is first created. The Professor was obviously distressed at the time of the interview at the adverse health effects of the MRNA products and alarmed that his colleagues are continuing to promote these products that are useless in providing the intended protection or immunity. During his interview Professor indicated that the proper research information was being suppressed as was his ability to speak openly.

Legalised suppression in business occurs, when 'Truth' may prevent PROFIT from lies or ignorance.

Just as divisive, disrespectful, emotive and convenient labels such as "Anti-Vax", used by some Doctors or market players, is coercive and unscientific.

Any Doctor using the 'convenient label' of 'Anti-Vaxer' is a lazy 'prescription puppet' that is spoon fed commercially viable information for dissemination or persuasion in selling product.

Covenant owners and investors in foundations like Black Rock, Gates, Rothschild and Clintons/ Obama or Biden's upon scrutiny, appear to be investing in against life against nature technologies of doom…?

They wish that never again, will human drones, consume too much or wish to own homes,

Nor breed unfettered nor will they wish to like outside the drone complex…

Because I care deeply for our children,

Spirit has shown me that the Mystery is Alive, in every

Man, Woman and Child and upon awakening,

All covenants of doom shall fail and their Trojan gifts will be returned to senders.

Physicists know that the Fractal of Life is Alive and the Infinite and Eternal Garden, is the Continuum… It will be so, long after the toxic technologists have fallen away.

Don't Panic! The good hearts of humanity will join together, for the highest good of all concerned.

They can no more stop the Rose from opening and spreading its perfume of Love, uplifting through the air… The old mechanism of secateurs used to cut premature blooms of man and its children will be taken from their severed hands.

All previous power, crumbles, revoked.

Let Hippocrates Oath now be applied to all levels of business and health-care, everywhere.

Love is the Law, underpinning beneficial WILL. Let it be so. For the Love of all our children Thriving. I speak as “MOTHER”.

2/4/2022 5.56am

ON NOTICE - Without Prejudice

As a result of watching an arrogant and delusional Dr Noah Harari, deliver a talk on the preference for programmable animal over a, free will humanity.

This whom the elites call the prophet…Hmm…Profit of Doom perhaps, if you are human?

The deepest stratum of my being has something to say to counter this madness of our modern day.

As a ‘Mark of Respect’ to our grandchildren’s freewill and health,

A boy-cott of all ‘replaceable’ WEF business and affiliates… Begins Now.

The idea of ‘Starve a Fever’, the diseased WEF fever of your $$$/your choice.

A financial sanction against Nazi thinking and policy making.

These WEF mob are not our leaders but usurpers of Life.

-Find alternatives – Make alternatives.

Entrepreneurial opportunity knocks.

As a ‘Mark of Respect’ to Life, Health and Cultural Diversity, buy to support

Locals and independent or family/community commerce, for a healthy and respectful, free will world.

The whole village turns its back upon the corporate giants that collude to harm independence, health and free will of generations, yet to be born.

Let any idea of ‘Elite prison world’ management be put to death with the W.E.F.

No reprieve from the Governor of Life.

Let the 'high-rollers' watch from behind their FEMA bars as humanity Unites as One and utilizes the hidden technologies to create the beneficial + One (+1) for future generations,

Far from the doom planning of World Economic Forum elites of 1971 – 2023.

Witness their towers and powers falling away, like

The tide takes the sandcastles upon the shore.

Peace, Peace, Peace for a thousand years or more.

*(From Hilary Allen's Pendulum – Natural Force + 1 = creation (NF+1=C))

The 'body' is an instrument of the Lord of Life, bio-feedback,

Not the WEFs to control.

Free will is already given.

Let it not be taken by corporate pirates and undercover deals!?

Be gone! You foul and false lords of pestilence and pennies,

Be gone!

4/4/2022 6.29am

The Lords of Love and Light, see all there is to see.

The World Economic Forum, its businesses, affiliates and influence,

Fall away, as if by magic, instantly and effortlessly.

These World Economic Foreskin plans are less than nothing to the Great Spirit of All things.

No matter how much they smile and dress up the stinking cadaver:- the W.E.F carcass is dead.

A bunch of 'smiling arrogance', living excessive indulgent lives, at the expense of The Great Spirit's creativity, through Man/Woman and Child…

At the expense of Peace and Harmony.

The W.E.F false overlay is a prison system, entrapping innocents.

Such a bottleneck of limited, plastic fantastic thinking is garish and clumsy, in comparison to; the Great Fractal of Living Things.

If this is where economy of the richest of rich, leads?

Perhaps, it is time to develop an economy on the understanding of "small is beautiful".

An economy as if People matter.

The W.E.F towers of power are built on sand, of flimsy understanding,

No matter how they attempt to 'sure-up' their foundations and patch holes in their net trap, they are not supported by the Great and Towering Good around and about us.

They have used their intellect to do harm to others, again and again.

A big, No No!

Abuse of intellect and free will is an abomination upon the Great Spirits Creation and Continuum.

10/4/2022 9:08am

If I had to report on progress, I confess that in some respects little has changed...

"Those that live by the sword, die by the sword." A famous old saying...

The swords have become tiny pricks, upon which people leap,

Willingly against some unknown foe?

Indeed, it does seem strange, you know,

To see the people, so many, farmed for money in tiny boxes as with minks, not so long ago?

And the elites and their businesses, cause great destruction and imbalance to satisfy their lust and profits, and then they blame the minions they marketed to, trapped in their financial game? And now The Blame Game?

People stare and act-out living, with little screens that force hypnotic focus into unreal dead end digital worlds?

Great wonder and sadness at the focal bottleneck of modern living.

Psychopathic leadership and support is unsustainable, in its delusion of right from wrong.

One business empire, The World Economic Forum, invests in entrapment and poison programmes, their arms reaching through governments, to The People, like a giant Kraken that crushes ships.

Everything is in the open and yet few people see? Hidden in full view.

So plays, 'the long game', a strangulation of civil liberties while hammering the screaming harp of fear.

The Krakin has replaced the Sheppard in world affairs... If only for a short time.

We await the rising tide of fullness in the hearts and minds as the Sheppard comes from within...

Then all the externalized falsehoods crumble as to dust. A mere object to be stepped over or swept aside by the Lord of Lords... Which will reside, acknowledged once again, in the Heart and Mind and Actions of "Man".

Love is the Law of One.

13/4/2022

The tale of two snakes,

The cobra and the crake. Mononuclear peptides.

Part of the Cov-id injectable recipe, One clots the other bleeds –

Organs affected are Kidneys and Cardio Pulmonary, Pancreas, Liver and Brain.

The Alpha and Omega of modern medicine – snake oil merchants to

Snake venom synthetic injectables!? Is this the World Snake eating its tail?

Providing a clean slate for the new economic reset on debt and unsecured tender?

Decision making of the WEF/FEW? Thanks go to Dr Evil and his young world leader Mini-Mees,

For conscription by prescription to WEF formula for slow cooked death.

Now Vote with your wallet and your feet to set future children and choice free.

May 2022 Monopolies of profitable suffering...

A monopoly in medicine has been created since 1913 and while the toxic eddy has grown,

Healthy humanity has diminished, along with the natural flow..

It is time to flush the toxic eddy of medical monopoly away, to allow an expansion of

Natural and less harmful modalities, to restore balance and thus restore flow.

Today Rockefeller medicine is a toxic bottleneck, like a fish trap, for profits.

While it is true that no thing is, all good or all bad, it is also true, that used in isolation and ignorance, the popularized, globalist chemical management, of every human condition is a Dead End!

Natures Pharmacopeia has no loud, Sell, Sell Sell! Its ways are more gentle and

Promoted by 'word of mouth', Natures Pharmacopeia remains ever effective.

When transcribing the human DNA, scientists put the letters together and they said –

GOD IS ETERNAL. Written in our DNA.

The Infinite and Eternal Garden of Mother Earth has all the nourishment a human body needs, together with the light of the living Sun.

Why would anyone t rust fake propaganda of the airways, from profit machines, that make ever more restrictive –fake laws? Really? Well, in compassion it can be witnessed that, generations of abuse creates its own bottleneck of consciousness and comfort addictions to survive, until Catharsis arrives – Then the storm flushes away false understandings about any separateness.

A new beginning via a breakthrough not breakdown.

I encourage any person to do their own research and resist the profiteers that don't like questioning. Truth can withstand questioning, Lies cannot.

Follow the Foundations – The Money – To see why Cures are not encouraged nor promoted.

Why monsterous Fear is needed to promote elite globalist adgenda. The Racket Formula.

War, Alcohol addiction, Opiate addiction, Gambling addiction, TV addiction, keep up with the Jone's fashion and Technology addiction. All Industry driven.

Addictions are promoted by boredom, fear and pain or discomfort. The tighter they pack the human sardines, the more dependency and debilitation, societal control and profit.

The newest management system involves social credit tracking and chemical management via addiction to vaccines, they hope… The best way to achieve their ends is to create a problem and provide their preferred solution…Just the One. An Entrapment. A Plandemic of profiteers.

Another Ten years of hammering out the disease bombs and the common folks will fall into line nicely or so some big wig desires?

The Holy of Holies has other plans and this little black mark on the Tapestry of Life is providing an 'accent' that shall remain, to highlight an appreciation, a new wisdom yet to come…

Love is the Law. What you Will wilt be Law; Maintain Love underpinning Will.

First Intend No Harm.

Correction, Forgiveness and Compassion; is Loves expression for mistakes and misunderstandings.

Throw-away technology and Throw-away culture can be Thrown-Away, quite safely and easily.

Manage the Tools in order of usefulness, don't allow a 'Tool' to 'manage' You.!

Certain technology will be discarded and new modalities will arrive to fill, renewed focus and more realistic needs, naturally.

Falsehoods will fall away, just a baby lets go of a pacifier, when it's ready…

All the Foundations; Clintons, Gates, Cancer Council, Kidney, Leukaemia and Diabetic Foundations are, upon scrutiny, rackets, complicit in injury and manslaughter. They need to be openly scrutinized under the Nuremberg Code of International Law. All these foundations admit to and submit to zero cures, therefore no individual nor child, should be forced, coerced nor encouraged to take experimental medicine.

No compensation exists for any of the experimental cancer treatments that do more harm than good. Wipe the Smile off that Clown Face. Free Will is Sacrosanct.

June 2022

Informed Intent

Let the Prime Directive and true intent of human form

As a tool of communication, remain true.

Let the intent of healing modalities – First Do No Harm, remain true.

Let the clothes of TRUTH fall from around the bodies of Lies, we all behold.

Be It So. Long Live the Nuremberg Code and

Free will in human form, as basic goodness is fundamental and

Psychopathy is redundant to any sacred 'Union'.

Reflection upon the life of a beloved boy

By the time this work reaches the eyes of others, it will be 12 years since I last held his warm hand in mine.

This work may not be everyone's 'cup of tea', but I was guided to write, I feel by the spirit of my son and other wise compassionate ones.

It is a 'Perspective' piece that intends helpfulness hopefully.

The repetition is deliberate, to mimic the nature of advertising so many are influenced by these days.

While our story is only one perspective, it deserves to be told, despite the fact so called 'Authorities' prefer to keep such witness statements hidden.

Dylan has come to me over the years in spirit, and his message is often the same.. "It's not your fault mum"..."The system is rigged". As with all rackets, 'scrutiny' is its breaking point.

So I speak for those who witness silently, the Rackets of profit and pain, coveted by Foundations again and again...

Perspective has Power and Truth in its Living and Dylan Lived!

Eight Years old and his wisdom was beyond his years and now more than ever,

It is not just the "I" but 'Humanity', that must move beyond Fear to do what is right!

For Biological Life's' sake! Yes Really.

So it is unlikely anyone will find me at a book signing or celebrating celebrity in any way.

I made the effort, it was not easy, to send an SOS to everybody.

A Message now Sent.

In using grief to help others, this book is my version of 'Dashram Pass',

Carving a neural pathway of understanding and vision through the Mountain of bullshit and falsehoods, that the modern world's demands and media puts before our eyes and on our plates.

I pray this perspective pathway; Is of benefit to all our fates.

June 2022

WEF WHO?

This is the Lords House and Kingdom who are you?!

With your corporate blathe set to ensnare and enslave,

Paving only the pathway to Hell?!

This 'template of life' is not for your poisons management and focused theft, of minds controlled!

Business should be left in the market place and not implanted in every home, body or cell!

Some areas of 'Life' should not be the dictate of market shares; i.e.

Good civil governance in 'service provision', family health or education.

Respect is Civil, division is corporate management and control. Remove the corporate pollution and waste, including weapons of mass destruction, with sensible haste.

Develop schools for learning life skills, good will and Respect,

Diverting away from lessons in Warcraft, for

Humanity's mutual benefit. It's called PEACE.

Develop schools of natural healing and wellness, diverting money away from the poisons manufacturers and eugenicists, again

For the benefit of humanity. It's called Wellness before profits.

Develop schools and models in marketing and economics that are balanced, taking funding away from psychopathic economic management, to enlist

Small is beautiful economies that support diverse regions and People generally. Again,

For the mutual respect and benefit of all humanity.

Sacred Agreements

Each Soul has its own agreements and contracts to deliver:- corporate master deceptions should not presume to interfere.

'Love' under 'Will' for Love is the Law, not fear my dears.

Fear Divides – Love Unifies

And if one must break and egg to make cake, what so ever you do, be focused on Love;

As a mother is grateful for every ingredient in their life-sustaining baking.

Sacred focus in everyday doings.

Right thought, right words, right actions.

Discipline. Contemplation.

Let no person without Love in their hearts, touch your food or its preparation.

Do you make your food or does a corporation?

Loves food = vibrant health

Zero love food = poison at worst, low nutrient availability at best.

'Bless' All that you take into your vessels, with Loving intent.

The sexualisation of children

The sexualisation of children in recent times is a damaging and distressing distortion.

Celine Dion it seems has sold her soul for drugs. Now promoting Horror and Transhumanism for babies?!

Directing their sick sexuality towards malleable youth, to enhance

A dead end trend, before they are able to think for themselves, let alone feed themselves?!

An assault and curse upon the human family line?

Celene Dion 2022 clothing advertising represents Extreme Insanity!

This too shall pass.

1.July. 2022

Reclaiming the Rainbow

For those that disagree in the living library, about which book

The librarian has given;

Accept the text as informative to the enquiry made, upon entry.

When finished a further text may be issued.

Never judge a book by its cover, they say, yet content is all about the cover these days?

Or one could equate the imbalance to all Icing but no cake. One is sickly sweet and addictive and the other is satisfying in its filling. So too, human psych is more meat than pastry, more content than cover.. Back to the living library.

There are those that do not accept the body the Great Sprit/Librarian has given…

You can graffiti all over the cover of your book, but such decoration does not change the text within, as it is written.

If one rips the pages away, the reader soul may miss the important message.

Defilement of the physical form, crumple and tears important passages.

The true meaning of HU MAN; is the breeding couple, which is why the sacred union is celebrated as 'marriage'.

The physical joining of Woman (HU) and Man is the Sacred Marriage.

Only the sacred marriage can bear the fruit of children.

Not everyone gets the opportunity to Co Create a Family. But All come from a Sacred Family Tree.

The Rainbow was a saving sign, sent to an ancient Family.

Non breeders are termination/endpoints in the fractal of a family tree.

Be proud of your efforts in alleviating the suffering of others, but

Do not parade and make important, defilement, disease or dysfunctionality, and distraction from 'meaningful reality'. Sexualising a word for 'Joy', 'the rainbow' and now 'children'?

What gross distortion is this? Has 'Universe 21' gone from rat experiment to human?

As if seeing life through the neon-techno-lycra-makeup caked, broken lens.?

Men and Women worshiping broken assholes, sounds like the new normal is a

New-wave 'nappy brigade'!

The only thing at the end of their plastic glitter rainbow is a crock of shit.

Compassionately now, nothing is all good or all bad, but as with GBLTG and cosmetics, less is more. Too much is garish and dysfunctional.

Making Love, implies respect and care, not defilement.

The Sacred Tantra /TAO is a pathway to great understandings, healing and peace, but it is The Sacred Union that is the catalyst for this.

Smiling with your heart. A woman will shine unawares when meeting her true Love. Avoid powerful perfumes to enable natural chemistry, aromatics that aid the cupids true aim.

There are special stages of life. Sexuality is a Sacred Sharing and children should not be part of adult play in sexuality. Image: The damage of attempting to open a rose bud before it's ready to bloom naturally.

Thank the Drama Queens for helping us to see more love and compassion for our fellows. Every kingdom needs funny men/jesters. The experiment titled 'Universe 21' may provide an understanding of the increase in the beautiful boys.

Be kind and pay attention…

Population density and overcrowding has an effect of creating less and less breeders until societal collapse. Too many beautiful boys is a sign of endings, when they get into power, they make themselves and their preferences or habits, more important than broad spectrum civil service provision. Arrogance and over indulgence… was also an influence in The Fall of Rome.

A healthy humanity is served better by smaller communities.

In future times cities will be transit centres and market place. People will take leave from the city for dwelling purposes. Biological beings, preferring biological friendly habitats.

Owning the Rainbow?.. Is as likely as capturing the flow of the stream when your fingers close to a fist.

The Rainbow once a sign of survival, hope and joy, is not owned by any gay group or selfish society.

Free the Rainbow from bondage, unfettered for all to enjoy.

Allow boys and girls to Just be themselves, unlabeled and un-coerced by globalist eugenicist education.

Plotters, politicians, complicit business and authority influencers

Justice would be for them to watch from their self- made FEMA/Lockstep prisons, while

The World reconfigures, happily recognizing different cultures and regions of the world as essential to the Whole.

The Worlds People unite as One, while honouring differences and diversity as true 'Richness'.

This will be prominently celebrated with food and cultural gift exchanges. Enjoyment and wonder through travel and creativity. Hidden treasures revealed.

Humanity will pick the best of technology and economic systems that support life and prevent psychopathy from taking root in societal systems again.

People have a fresh understanding of the meaning of maintaining Love as the foundation of acts of will.

Love is the Law and the basis of all creation.

May Peace. Peace. Peace,

Be always everywhere.

Kung Fu Panda quote: Re-Stated.

"One often meets his destiny on the road he takes to avoid it."

A lesson for humanity – observably true

In many situations…

Decisions have been made that create problems worse than the situations they seek to address.

Zika mosquitos, pasteurization, heat treated fats, contaminated vaccines, war, psycho global economy, chemical agriculture, mandatory cancer treatments, opiate use, changes of government and politicians…to what?

Good reason for consideration of the effects on decisions for Seven (7) generations hence…

Whether in individual lives or societal progression, the pathway of decision, is represented by the statement which is profoundly and observably true, for humanity.

Hippocrates saw true when he stated “First Do No Harm”.

A statement of ‘Care’ that is only honoured by consideration of consequences upon future generations.

Carelessness is the only enemy of Man.

In fast paced times, one may be too concerned with what was and what will be..

This is the time to refocus on ‘Now’;

The only time for action, consideration or wisdom.

Another beautiful quote from the Kung Fu Panda:

“Yesterday is history, tomorrow is a mystery,

Today is the ‘gift’, which is why they call it

The Present.”

Be here Now.

RIP - Dylan .F.S

And Thank you for being. XXX

Blessings to Elaine, Hilary, Eli, Mandy and Bec, Kate and Mel. All of my Beloved Extended Family too, for patience and educated assistance in this message delivery. A special thanks to my old community, men for building services and impromptu fishing trips and the generous women of my community that delivered home cooked meals to the children and myself, after our loss. Blessings to you and yours.

Final recap: Medicine appears to have become another arm of the industrial military complex, using medicine as weapons of mass destruction (WMD). A profitable racket of disease and death.

Billions of children along with my son, received vaccinations contaminated with SV40 from foreign animal proteins mixed with adjuncts of heavy metals and surfactants. SV40 is confirmed as associated causality of blood cancers. My child developed lymphoblastic leukaemia once a rare condition, but now an extremely common disease.

The terminal toxic treatment protocol for this disease damages DNA and PUBMED documentation admits it creates repeated cancers. My son got cancer a second time and the terminal toxic treatment protocol, second round, killed my son but not the cancer cells. The system is rigged and not for wellness, but profitability.

Authorities have "No Evidence" of ever testing any childhood vaccine for Safety or Efficacy and their treatment of disease is making far more disease and death. Profitable mandates have created an unquestionable corporate racket. Modern medicines 'management' of disease is Not Safe and Not Effective, but highly profitable.

First Aid and trauma medicine is the only space where medicine succeeds in ethics and efficacy, most of the time.

Again, the Wolf in Sheep's clothing, vaccines are contaminated with foreign proteins (animal and human) and SV40 along with other toxic adjuncts and they give rise to cancer, as research has shown but not promoted. The toxic treatment protocol for cancers damages the DNA and immune system. When the cancers return, the subsequent treatment protocol kills the person, not the cancer.

Medicine in its 'management' of health and disease is – Not Safe – Not Effective.

The selectiveness of favourable data makes mockery of truth, providing No 'Evidence' of Safety Data or Efficacy ever! Unless you count efficacy regarding population controls and a multi-billion dollar dependency economy?

Medicine should stick to what is go good service to humanity, First Aid. Medicines 'management' of disease has big corporate profits but poor success rates for human beings, and being such educated smart people within that industry, it can only be a deliberate economic ploy. A place where Lies are dressed up as Truth and to question the racket is illegal. The formula used against questioners is to progressively; Ignore, Discredit and Destroy.

Corporate medicine and the private business, The World Health Organisation, peddles disease for profits, showing 'Duty Of Care' to shareholders, Not our children.

The Killing of Care - Doctors that comply without question are party to the problem and the profits. Doctors that question are gas-lit and silenced, their careers ended by deregistration.

The Covid mandates of MRNA technology (also found to contain SV40), caused my mother to Die Suddenly, she had months of 'stroke like' symptoms that did not show up on any brain scans nor blood testing? No autopsy of these victims of experimental MRNA are encouraged in Australia, indicating the lack of science behind the use of this product.

My niece also, was fit, healthy and health conscious, a university mandated the MRNA jab for her to continue her degree, and she was pregnant. She has now been diagnosed with Pericarditis and at age 27 has pace-maker! God Help Humanity's Children, everywhere.

Dr Sucharit – Japan. Calls for the cessation of all MRNA technology in all vaccines on earth, including cancer vaccines. He Denounces the World Health Organisation (WHO) as a private club with intent to introduce MRNA into all vaccines. "The whole danger of the vaccine stems from the ability of the immune system to recognize Non-Self". He states that this technology changes personality as it affects the brain, damages the heart and genome. He also states that Bill Gates and the German taxpayer are the top financiers of the World Health Organisation (WHO) which is forcing vaccinations on populations.

Dr Sucharit says, "All MRNA vaccines are dangerous and only threaten life."

"Changing mankind, all your personalities being changed, your brain is being changed and your heart weakened." "This cannot be allowed to happen even if the WHO says so."

"All MRNA vaccination is damaging the body and must be forbidden."

Senator Malcom Roberts. In one of his 2025 social media posts. **Failure to Warn**: How Federal agencies downplayed the risk of myocarditis and other adverse events following COVID-19 vaccinations. US Senate Permanent Subcommittee Chairman Ron Johnson, Majority Staff Interim Report released in conjunction with the Permanent Subcommittee on investigations. May 21, 2025 Hearing.

The Truth Will Set Us Free.

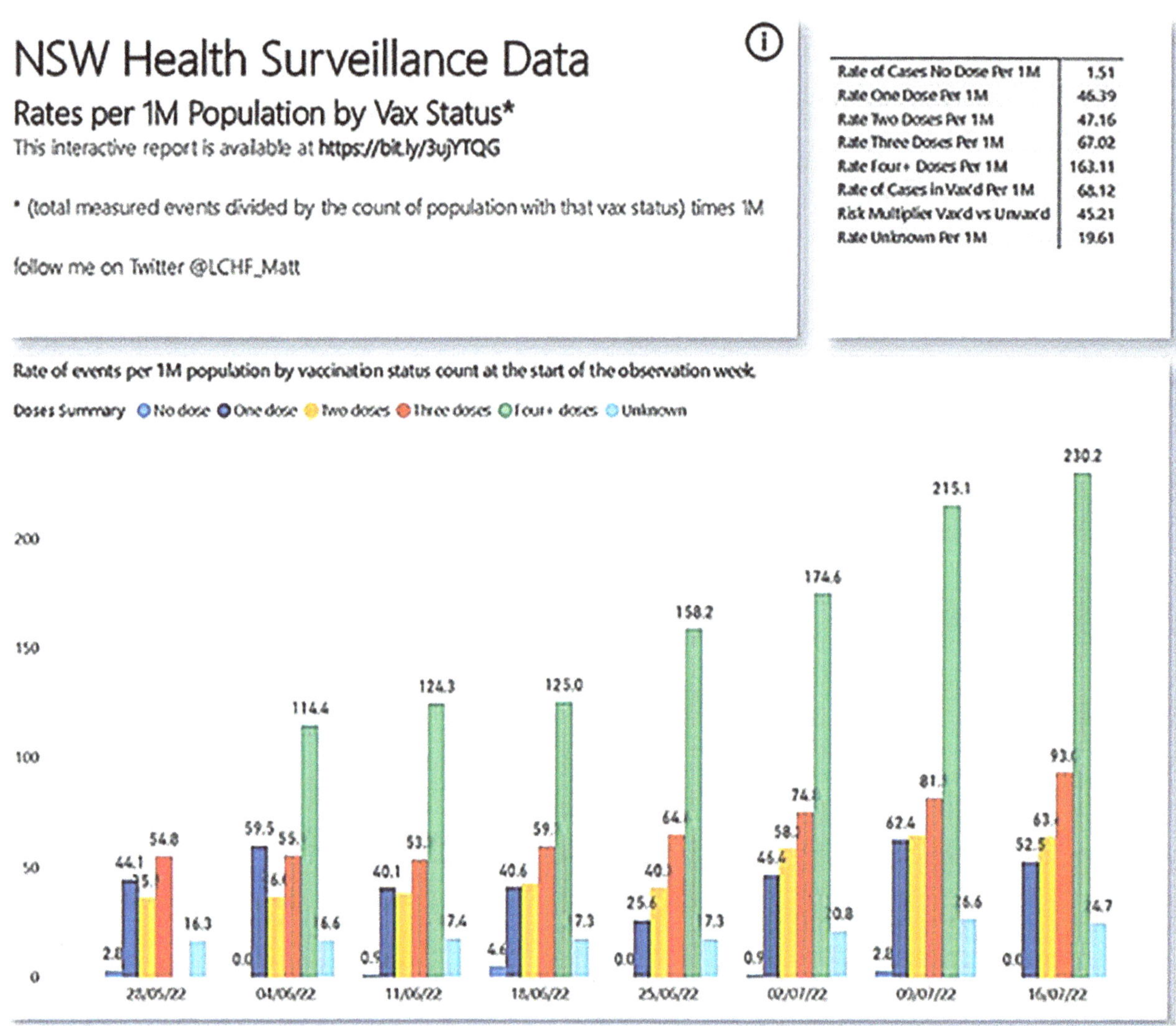

"Like the data sheet of the Pfizer shot, Fauci/Gates/WEF paper on ethics is – "Intentionally Blank".

"Discombobulation Aids the Violation."

"Suppression of facts and discussion is an act of corporate terrorism. Not Science."

CDC Recommended Vaccine Schedule for U.S. Children

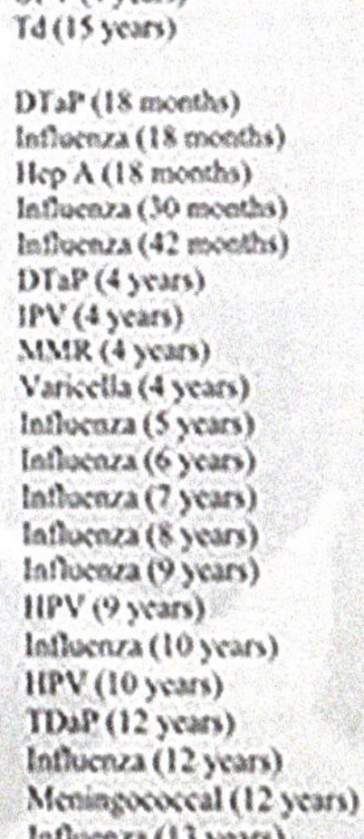

Year		
1962	Polio Smallpox DTP	
1983	DTP (2 months) OPV (2 months) DTP (4 months) OPV (4 months) DTP (6 months)	MMR (15 months) DTP (18 months) OPV (18 months) DTP (4 years) OPV (4 years) Td (15 years)
2019	Influenza (pregancy) TDaP (pregnancy Hep B (birth) Hep B (2 months) Rotavirus (2 months) DTaP (2 months) HiB (2 months) PCV (2 months) IPV (2 months) Rotavirus (4 months) DTaP (4 months) HiB (4 months) PCV (4 months) IPV (4 months) Hep B (6 months) Rotavirus (6 months) DTaP (6 months) HiB (6 months) PCV (6 months) IPV (6 months) Influenza (6 months) Influenza (7 months) HiB (12 months) PCV (12 months) MMR (12 months) Varicella (12 months) Hep A (12 months)	DTaP (18 months) Influenza (18 months) Hep A (18 months) Influenza (30 months) Influenza (42 months) DTaP (4 years) IPV (4 years) MMR (4 years) Varicella (4 years) Influenza (5 years) Influenza (6 years) Influenza (7 years) Influenza (8 years) Influenza (9 years) HPV (9 years) Influenza (10 years) HPV (10 years) TDaP (12 years) Influenza (12 years) Meningococcal (12 years) Influenza (13 years) Influenza (14 years) Influenza (15 years) Influenza (16 years) Meningococcal (16 years) Influenza (17 years) Influenza (18 years)

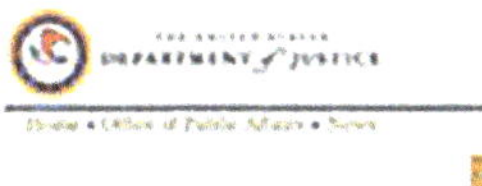

JUSTICE NEWS

Department of Justice

Office of Public Affairs

FOR IMMEDIATE RELEASE Wednesday, September 2, 2009

Justice Department Announces Largest Health Care Fraud Settlement in Its History

Pfizer to Pay $2.3 Billion for Fraudulent Marketing

WASHINGTON – American pharmaceutical giant Pfizer Inc. and its subsidiary Pharmacia & Upjohn Company Inc. (hereinafter together "Pfizer") have agreed to pay $2.3 billion, the largest health care fraud settlement in the history of the Department of Justice, to resolve criminal and civil liability arising from the illegal promotion of certain pharmaceutical products, the Justice Department announced today.

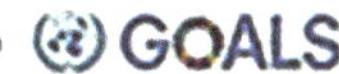

UN agenda 21-2030 GOALS

- One World Government
- One global controlled cashless currency
- One global central bank
- One global military
- The end of national sovereignty
- End ALL private owned property (except some elites)
- The end of the family unit
- Depopulation, control of population growth and density
- Endless mandatory vaccines
- Universal basic income (austerity)
- Microchipped society (for trade, travel, tracking and control)
- Implementation of a world social credit system
- Internet of things, everything hooked to 5G monitoring
- Government raised children
- Government owned and controlled schools (education)
- End private transportation (no more owning cars etc...)
- All businesses owned by government/corporations
- Restriction of nonessential air travel
- Settlement zones (concentration of humans in cities only)
- End of private farms livestock and irrigation
- Restricted land use, end of single family homes
- Ban of natural non synthetic drugs and medicines

WORLD ECONOMIC FORUM

You will own nothing and be happy

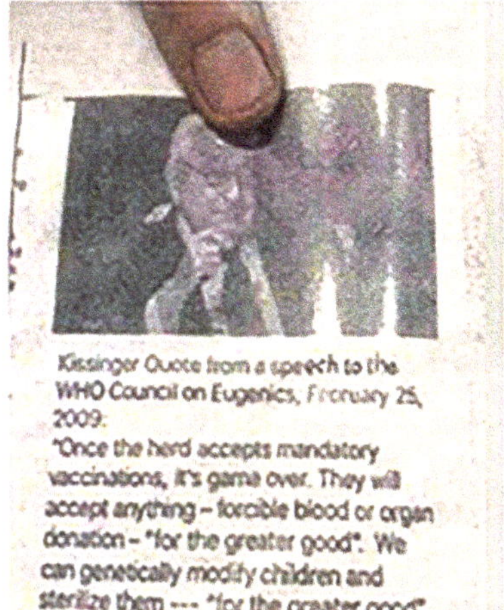

Kissinger Quote from a speech to the WHO Council on Eugenics, February 25, 2009:

"Once the herd accepts mandatory vaccinations, it's game over. They will accept anything – forcible blood or organ donation – "for the greater good". We can genetically modify children and sterilize them --- "for the greater good". Control sheep minds and you control the herd. Vaccine makers stand to make billions. And many of you in this room are investors. It's a big win-win. We thin out the herd and the herd pays us for extermination services."

Forwarded message
From Zeee Media

May we never forget Monkeypox is an Autoimmune Blistering Disease listed on the Pfizer side effects documents they tried to hide for 75 years.

Follow @zeeemedia
Website | Gettr | Instagram | Rumble

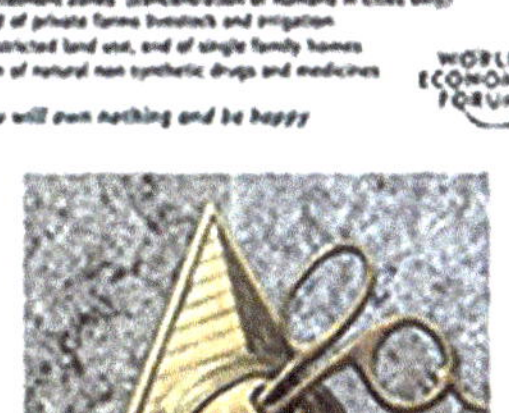

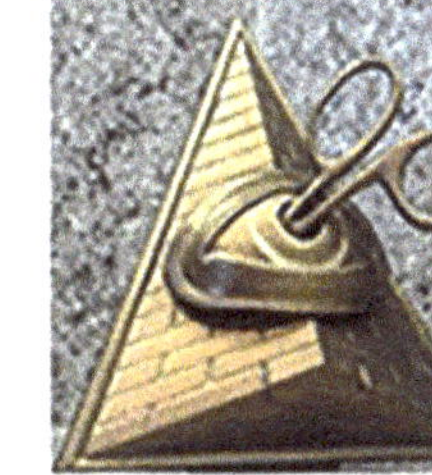

WHO Releases Plan For Global Digital Vaccine Passports Funded By Bill Gates & Rockefeller Foundation

By The European Union Times

The World Health Organization (WHO) has released a proposal backed by two major globalist organizations that serves as a blueprint for governments to implement a worldwide vaccine passport verification system.

The document, called "Digital Documentation of COVID-19 Certificates: Vaccination Status," funded by none other than the Bill & Melinda Gates Foundation and the Rockefeller foundation, describes the technical guidance for governments to roll out the program to usher in a global digital ID – in the name of COVID, of course.

"It's notable how the only groups actively pushing for global vaccine passports are also the main proponents of the so-called Great Reset"

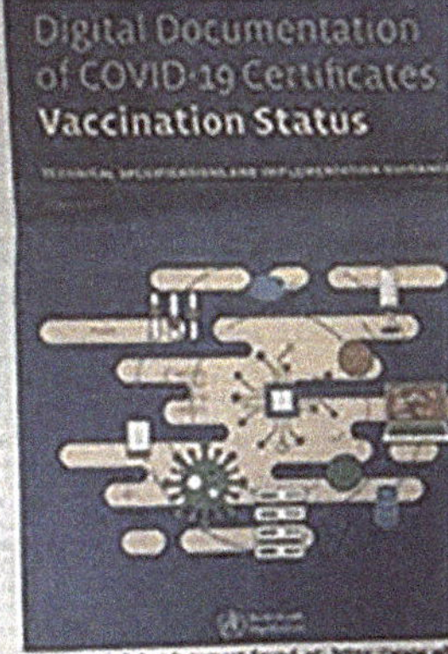

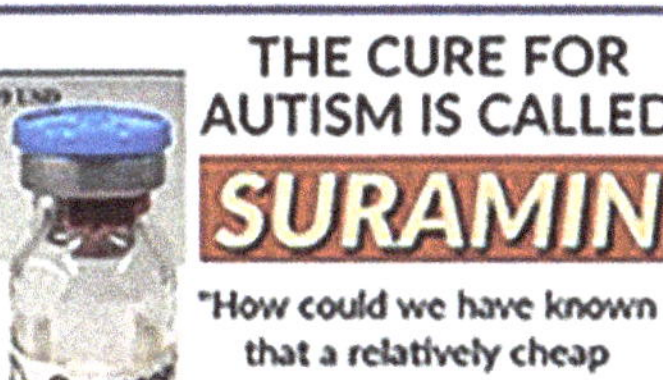

The Investor

Without responsibility nor care he applies his wealth and influence as if he is King of the Lords domain, his vanity attempts to create a false overlay, a template of doom for all living things in this superior realm of Life. His so called 'best intentions' are in deed paving the way towards Hell on Earth.

Bill Gates is not a scientist nor master of truth, but an investor in Trojan horse technologies.

He invests in depopulation and antifertility medications. He invests in blocking out the sun, using toxic substances that corrupt the atmosphere all creatures breath and damages all of life from the mountains to the sea affecting food and water supply. He invests in deforestation, destruction of farming and weakening the genome of Humanity.

He aids war and pestilence, misusing his power through investments in toxic GM products and digital technology, for the benefit of the few and the downfall of the many. The consequences of these investments are of no good. These investments have a disabling effect on all natural systems. It began with the 'con' of convenience and ends with the 'con' 'it's for your own good/safety'.

A man without an original idea, he follows the decree of the globalist technoprat plan for control of every thought, word and action of Man, and makes money from it all.

Like the proverbial wolf in sheep's clothing he smiles his sly smile, while delivering the planned prescription to hell on Earth and the death of human free will. Transhumanism is a dead end, to the living fractal of Man.

Bill Gates and his fellow investors are classic technoprats delivering Trojan horse technology for the illness of all systems except their own digital creations, that the demons work through, to ply the cravings and aversions, the source of suffering and misery for all humans.

Pray for the living Lord of All Things to shine its Love into the hearts and minds of all Humanity, man, woman and child, such that they have eyes to see and ears to hear True. Then the falsehoods will surely crumble away and the new dawn of this consciousness in physicality will embody Peace on Earth and Joy.

Each person born has been given a 'Gift' to bring, let not the narcissist technoprats diabolical plans get in the way, of the Heart of the World. The fractal matrix of GOD is far superior to anything the technoprats can build.

Peace and Blessings to all beings of goodness. Let the plan of Love and Light that the Master Emissaries know and serve, work out, sealing the door where evil dwells.

Dr John Campbell interview with Dr Malhotra - Public health and truth & The Hope Accord.

https://www.youtube.com/live/J64dujeIBdQ

With Dr. Aseem Malhotra, Links to article https://covid19.onedaymd.com/2025/07/

https://www.telegraph.co.uk/news/2025 https://doctoraseem.com/its-time-for-...

"Ancient wisdom teaches us that evil is rooted in ignorance but as Steven Hawking alluded to, the greatest enemy of knowledge is not ignorance, but the illusion of knowledge.

In other words the greatest barrier to the truth is psychological, not intellectual. Two of those major psychological barriers have become most prevalent at an individual, population and institutional level over the past 5 years since the world was turned upside down at the start of the covid pandemic. The first of these which we can all relate to is the emotional phenomenon of fear. Then in a state of fear it impedes one's ability to engage in critical thinking and simultaneously makes us more compliant to authoritarian rule.

For example leaked WhatsApp messages (published on the front page of the Daily Telegraph) revealed as regards to covid the Secretary of State's plan was to " frighten the pants off the public". Such tactics replicated by government bodies around the world amplified by the media grossly exaggerated covid risk in the minds of the public.

For example 30-50% of American's when surveyed believed their risk of being hospitalised with covid was 50%, when the actual risk was much below 1% even during the worst strain. Cutting through all the noise research from the most cited medical researcher in the world (someone I describe as the Stephen Hawking of medicine) Professor John Ioannidis revealed that by the end of 2020 in under 70's the infection fatality rate was 0.05%, in other words 1 in 2000, less than the overall infection fatality rate than the flu at 1 in 1000.

As the director of health literacy at the Max Planc institute in Berlin, Gerd Gigerenzer has previously stated " without understanding the numbers involved the public are vulnerable to exploitation of their hopes and fears by political and commercial interests".

The second psychological barrier to the truth which we are all potentially susceptible to is one of wilful blindness. This is when human beings turn a blind eye to the truth in order to feel safe, avoid conflict, reduce anxiety and to protect prestige and fragile egos. Examples of this on an individual level can be turning a blind eye to the affair of your partner. On an institutional level historical examples include the BBC and Jimmy Saville, Hollywood and Harvey Weinstein, and the Catholic Church and child molestation.

Why do I mention this? Because it is in my view these psychological barriers (which I also temporarily suffered from) that are hindering policy makers, journalists and influential sections of the medical establishment to acknowledge the greatest medical mistake with ongoing catastrophic harm to public health that we will likely witness in our lifetime.

Yes, I'm talking about the covid mRNA vaccine which in reality is more accurately a prophylactic gene therapy. As someone who took two doses and supported its use for high risk and the elderly on Good Morning Britain in February 2021 my revelation came the hard way. On the 26th of July 2021, my father, Dr Kailash Chand Malhotra OBE, retired GP and honorary vice president of the British Medical Association, a very fit and healthy man in comparison to his 73 year old peers suffered a sudden cardiac arrest.

Subsequent post mortem confirmed severe coronary artery disease that had significantly accelerated within a few years of having relatively mild disease. As an expert in coronary artery disease and its progression, this didn't make any sense to me and I even remember angrily blocking someone on twitter who suggested this was because of the covid vaccine. "What a stupid and mad thing to write" I thought.

But a few months later three pieces of evidence made me change my opinion. The first was that an abstract published in the Journal Circulation by Steven Gundry revealed that within 8 weeks of his middle aged patients receiving two doses of the mRNA vaccines their baseline risk jumped from 11% risk of heart attack in 5 years to 25%. This was through measuring well validated inflammatory blood markers of coronary risk.

The second piece of evidence around the same time was a cardiologist whistle blower from a prestigious institution contacted me to tell me that a group of researchers in his department had accidentally discovered through the use of high tech heart imaging modality that there was a signal of coronary inflammation seen in the vaccinated that was not present in the unvaccinated."

Dr. John Campbell @Campbellteaching

By Frank Bergman/Slaynews.com October 1, 2025 12:57pm

Germany Issues Red Alert: mRNA 'Vaccines' Triggered Global Population Implosion - Slay News

Germany's top scientists, doctors, and academics have sounded the alarm, issuing a joint red alert that the experimental Covid mRNA injections are fuelling a global health catastrophe and driving a population implosion.

At a press conference in Berlin, nine leading experts called for an immediate halt to mRNA vaccinations, citing overwhelming evidence of excess mortality, rising disease rates, and collapsing birth rates tied directly to the rollout of the shots.

The panel of experts was supported by more than 200 doctors, scientists, lawyers, and health professionals.

"Today, we are issuing an urgent risk warning and calling for a moratorium on mRNA vaccines, an immediate halt, and an evidence-based reassessment," the group declared.

"The evidence for these demands exists on multiple levels."

"Epidemiologically, there are high correlations between vaccination and booster rates and an increase in excess mortality, disease rates, as well as a decline in birth rates."

A shorter clip of the full press conference was edited, subtitled, and published by Aussie17.com

WATCH: **A Panel of Eminent Experts**

The panel included some of the most credentialed voices in Europe:

Prof. Dr. Gerald Dyker, Professor of Organic Chemistry at Ruhr University Bochum, who has published over 160 papers, warned about the toxic chemical processes in vaccine production and testing.

Dr. Andreas Sönnichsen, Professor of Internal Medicine and Evidence-Based Medicine, called out governments for ignoring real-world data in favour of ideology.

Prof. Dr. Konstantin Beck, a health economist from the University of Lucerne, presented statistics showing that the injections are directly tied to declining fertility rates and excess deaths across Europe.

Dr. Michael Nehls, molecular geneticist, exposed how the spike protein's genetic manipulation disrupts human immunity and may accelerate degenerative diseases.

Prof. Dr. Dr. Christian Schubert, medical psychologist and psychoneuroimmunologist, warned of long-term damage to both body and mind from repeated mRNA exposure.

They were joined by dermatologists, occupational medicine specialists, pharmacists, and frontline doctors who have personally witnessed the harm.

A Globalist Nightmare

The findings mirror growing international data: birth rates have plunged in nearly every highly vaccinated nation, from Germany and Switzerland to Canada and Japan.

As Slay News reported earlier, Canada has just published data revealing that the nation suffered its lowest birth rate in history in 2024, for the second year in a row.

Experts warn this is not a coincidence but a direct result of damage to fertility and immunity caused by the spike protein from mRNA "vaccines."

Yet governments, the World Health Organization (WHO), and pharmaceutical giants remain silent, doubling down on their push for mRNA-based vaccines for everything from the flu to RSV to future pandemics.

Critics argue that this is not simply a public health failure, but a globalist scheme to weaken populations, suppress fertility, and normalize genetic manipulation under the guise of "science."

The Call to Action

The German experts demanded an immediate moratorium on all mRNA injections and a full-scale, independent investigation into "vaccine" harms.

They also warned that without urgent action, humanity faces a looming demographic collapse that could destabilize entire nations within a single generation.

This is not just about Covid, however.

The panel warned that mRNA technology is being quietly expanded into food production, animal vaccines, and even fertility interventions.

The expansions to mRNA injections, such as self-replication technology, are giving biotech corporations and global elites unprecedented control over life itself.

Meanwhile, the birth rate collapse, excess mortality, and explosion of chronic disease are flashing red warning signs.

As the warnings continue to be ignored, the world is headed for a population crisis of historic proportions.

READ MORE - **Top Doctor Sounds Alarm: Covid 'Vaccines' Triggered 'Sudden Unexpected Death Pandemic'** Slaynews.com "

Bombshell Testimony: CDC Data Proves Covid 'Vaccines' Caused 'More Harm Than Benefits'

Frank Bergman October 2, 2025 - 12:57 pm

A top expert has issued explosive testimony warning that CDC data shows Covid mRNA shots caused far more harm to public health than any supposed benefit.

Dr. Toby Rogers, Ph.D., provided the bombshell testimony during a Senate hearing last month.

However, a short clip of a powerful statement from Rogers has recently emerged.

Rogers, a fellow with the Brownstone Institute and independent journalist, explains that the CDC's own research determined that mRNA injections have **"negative efficacy."**

Yet, the CDC and other health officials continued to push the "safe and effective" narrative.

"Tell me how a vaccine with negative efficacy is saving lives," Rogers demanded to cheers and applause.

Bombshell Testimony: CDC Data Proves Covid 'Vaccines' Caused 'More Harm Than Benefits'

Rogers' warning about mRNA injections is now gaining renewed attention, but he had been called to testify about the links between childhood vaccines and autism.

As a researcher, Rogers has spent nearly a decade studying the rise of autism.

He told senators that published evidence shows vaccines and environmental toxins are the most likely culprits behind the epidemic now affecting millions of American children.

Rogers, who began researching autism in 2015 after his then-partner's son was diagnosed, said his review of the CDC references revealed glaring contradictions.

"I went to the CDC's webpage on the causes of autism," Rogers explained.

"As a Ph.D. student, I was trained to focus on primary source documents, so I read all of the references in their footnotes.

"To my surprise, I quickly discovered that the CDC's narrative did not add up."

He also noted the lack of urgency from the federal government, despite autism's cost already reaching "hundreds of billions of dollars."

Rogers changed his doctoral thesis to focus on the Political Economy of Autism and spent four years analysing published research on prevalence, causation, and cost.

His 2019 thesis passed peer review and became one of the most-downloaded dissertations in the history of the University of Sydney.

Vaccine Studies Without Real Controls

Presenting to lawmakers, Rogers said: **"Here are the facts."**

He noted that 22 studies frequently cited by officials claim vaccines don't cause autism.

However, none of those studies included an entirely unvaccinated control group.

"So unfortunately, if you want to understand what's causing the autism epidemic, these studies are of no use," he testified.

By contrast, six published studies that did use unvaccinated control groups found an increased risk of autism among the vaccinated.

Rogers said these studies "have been systematically suppressed and ignored by the mainstream media and the medical establishment."

He also pointed to additional research showing autism spikes following vaccination.

Regression Linked to Acute Toxic Exposure

One study from 2018 revealed that up to 88% of autism cases involve regression.

The issue caused children to lose skills like speech and eye contact after previously developing normally.

"This suggests an acute toxic exposure triggered the development of autism," Rogers said.

"We now have eyewitness testimony from thousands of parents that the acute toxic exposure that preceded the autistic regression was a 'well-baby' vaccine appointment."

He dismissed the argument that autism is primarily genetic.

"Genes don't suddenly create epidemics — the human genome just doesn't change that fast," Rogers noted.

Most studies that combine genetics with toxins such as pesticides and heavy metals, Rogers warned, fail to account for vaccines as a confounding factor, making it "impossible to tease out the true impact."

Vaccines and Other Toxicants Identified

"The best available evidence suggests that anything that causes an immune activation event — an infectious disease, an industrial toxicant, or a vaccine — can cause autism," Rogers explained.

According to his analysis, autism is "most likely caused by vaccines and about a dozen additional toxicants."

He concluded with a blunt warning:

"If we stop exposing children to these hazards in the first place, that would stop the epidemics of chronic illness in children."

"Now we must summon the political will to act."

Slaynews.com

A Pathway Forward

https://www.youtube.com/watch?v=TcbuqQd57rY

Decentralised medicine/ Jack Kruse / Assembly 2023

Jack Kruse is a Neurosurgeon and here he is talking about a historical pathway of centralised medicine that is being used to manipulate, trap and make sick, humanity. He also speaks of the use of blue light as a tool of manipulation. Circadian Biology being affected by technology. Probably the best link you could be aware of today.

His talk includes his experience with Linier accelerator and Blue Light control of human behaviour via screens. Dr Jack Kruse speaks of the origins of the Polio Vaccine, SV40 and cancer. He discusses MRNA shots. How electro radiation makes cancer worse, Fort Deitrich's 'gain-of-function' research, DNA plasmids, SV40 and cancer industry profits. President Regan, the Bob Dole Act and profits from research. He mentions Kevin McKernan, a molecular biologist that confirmed DNA fragments in MRNA shots and Phillip Buckhaults a molecular biologist & cancer geneticist at the University of South Carolina.

Jack Kruse discusses decentralised medicine and how El Salvidor have written into their constitution, a medical freedoms Act, to ensure its Republic remains free of medical tyranny.

A quote from that act, he shared: **"Public Health Freedom Act 2023. The People of El Salvidor do enact as follows; Unless we put Decentralised Medical Freedom into the Constitution, the time will come where licensed institutions in health care will organise into an underground covert authoritarian bureaucracy, it will restrict the art of science and healing to one class of people and deny privileges to others. It will constitute the Bastille of medical science. All such laws are contrary to freedom and liberty. They are despotic and have no place in a Constitutional Republic. The Constitution of the Republic should make special privileges for medical freedom and religious freedoms related to the practice of healing therefore, these laws should be added to our founding documents to protect the Public Health from tyranny form this day forward."**

Dr Kruse also references "The Ethical Sceptic" on twitter/X as noteworthy in content and discussions.

About the Author

Kalubriah is an educated, concerned mother of three and has endured a number of life-changing experiences that led to this writing, about matters that concern us all, much of which is hidden in full view.

Kalubriah now enjoys a quiet rural life. Her background prior to tragedy was Property Law, Taxation Excise, Tourism Management/ Marketing and afterward a Aquaculture Hatchery Technician. Property Law enabled advanced research skills, Taxation, attention to detail and Tourism Marketing provided psychological insight of promotional advertising upon differing populations. After the tragedy, as a Hatchery Technician, growing the smallest creatures in intensive cell culture environments, Kalubriah gained an intimate understanding of the 'fine balance' required, to maintain health and reduce the effects of toxic bio-accumulation, directly observable at micro and macro levels of biological life.

www.ingramcontent.com/pod-product-compliance
Lightning Source LLC
Chambersburg PA
CBHW042337030426
42335CB00030B/3378

* 9 7 8 1 9 6 7 8 2 0 1 7 7 *